S0-AEE-853

CHILD
and
ADOLESCENT DEVELOPMENT:
Clinical Implications

VICTOR C. VAUGHAN III, M.D.

Clinical Professor of Pediatrics, Stanford University
School of Medicine, Stanford, California; Formerly
University Professor and Chief, Department of Pediatrics,
Temple University School of Medicine, and Medical Director,
St. Christopher's Hospital for Children, Philadelphia, Pennsylvania

IRIS F. LITT, M.D.

Professor of Pediatrics and Chief, Division of Adolescent
Medicine, Stanford University School of Medicine,
Stanford, California

1990
W. B. SAUNDERS COMPANY
Harcourt Brace Jovanovich, Inc.

Philadelphia, London, Toronto, Montreal, Sydney, Tokyo

W. B. SAUNDERS COMPANY
Harcourt Brace Jovanovich, Inc.

The Curtis Center
Independence Square West
Philadelphia, PA 19106

Library of Congress Cataloging-in-Publication Data

Vaughan, Victor C., 1919–
    Child and adolescent development : clinical implications / Victor
C. Vaughan III, Iris F. Litt.
    p.   cm.
    Bibliography: p.
    ISBN 0-7216-1394-2
    1. Child development.   2. Adolescence.   I. Litt, Iris F., 1940–
    II. Title.
    [DNLM: 1. Child Development. WS 105 V369c]
RJ131.V39   1990
612'.65--dc19
DNLM/DLC   89-6056
for Library of Congress   CIP

Acquisition Editor: Lisette Bralow

CHILD AND ADOLESCENT DEVELOPMENT: Clinical Implications

ISBN 0-7216-1394-2

Printed in the United States of America.

Last digit is the print number: 9   8   7   6   5   4   3   2   1

To our teachers
to our students
to our children and grandchildren
to each other

*from all of whom we have learned
happy and priceless lessons*

PREFACE

Recent years have seen a prodigious increase in the number of studies of the growth and development of infants, children and adolescents, and in our understanding of the underlying processes and principles. No single volume could contain an adequate review of the observations made, even if that were limited to the most insightful and important among them.

In this volume we have attempted, through sifting what is new as well as what is old in our understanding, to gather together those features of growth and development that have particular significance for the clinical work of health professionals who deal with normal infants, children and adolescents. Emphasis will be given to the interactions between physiologic, neurodevelopmental, cognitive, and psychosocial components of growth and development. We hope that a new description of these interactions for the fetus, infant, child and adolescent may yield a more comprehensive view of the developmental process than is afforded by traditional reviews that have often addressed serially the paths of development in various anatomic or physiologic systems, one system after the other. Here, by contrast, our aim is to enrich for each age or stage the context within which child care professionals may understand and evaluate infants, children, or adolescents, and within which they may give interpretation and advice to children and their parents in various areas of clinical practice. We have been particularly concerned to examine growth and development in their **contemporary sociocultural context,** and have addressed the ways in which aspects of community life in the United States have impact upon the development of children and adolescents.

The chapters to follow will sequentially examine certain models and themes that have provided perspectives within which growth and development have been viewed. These perspectives will be followed by comprehensive descriptions of infants, children, and adolescents at various stages of development, with emphasis upon the interrelationships between the biologic and the environmental and upon those aspects of growth and development that help us best to interpret its features to parents, children, and adolescents. We hope to make the field of growth and development more interesting and to foster growth-promoting attitudes and behavior, both in the clinical arena and within the home and community.

For the material presented here we have drawn selectively from many sources, informal as well as formal. We have learned from our students as well as from our patients. The experience of teaching medical students about human growth and development over a quarter of a century has been invaluable. A substantial portion of our joint effort was initiated while one of us (IFL) was a Fellow at the Center for Advanced Studies in the Behavioral Sciences at Stanford University (1984–1985). We are grateful to the Center for the opportunity to share its archival and human resources.

VICTOR C. VAUGHAN, M.D.
IRIS F. LITT, M.D.

CONTENTS

Chapter 1
  INTRODUCTION 1

Chapter 2
  FETUS AND PREMATURE 131

Chapter 3
  THE NEWBORN INFANT 145

Chapter 4
  THE FIRST YEAR 163

Chapter 5
  THE SECOND YEAR 179

Chapter 6
  THE PRESCHOOL CHILD... 193

Chapter 7
  THE SCHOOL-AGED CHILD... 213

Chapter 8
  EARLY ADOLESCENCE... 229

Chapter 9
  MIDDLE ADOLESCENCE... 293

Chapter 10
  LATE ADOLESCENCE 317

  APPENDIX A 329

  APPENDIX B... 331

BIBLIOGRAPHY... 333

INDEX... 345

Chapter 1

INTRODUCTION

The elements and principles of growth and development constitute a basic science for those professions that deal with the health, education, or welfare of infants, children, or adolescents, and of their parents and families. The term *growth and development* embraces a complex continuum that has many components, ranging in level of organization from the molecular to the social and cultural or the political. *Growth* generally refers to the processes that result in increases in size, whereas *development* refers to increases in complexity of form or function.

The elements of normal growth and development flow in exquisite harmony from conception to maturity. The pattern that evolves is unique, however, for every person, as innate structures and processes are modified by interaction with the environment.

Growth and development can be regarded as a process of gradual differentiation of the child from the parents, beginning with the union of parents at conception, and followed by fetal dependency. Initial physical separation from the mother at birth establishes a parasitic relationship that evolves gradually through various grades and orders of dependency and independency to end with the special relationship that parents have with their adult children.

The elements of growth and development can be organized into various categories within which they share common physiologic or experiential structures or processes. These categories include genetic, embryologic, physical, physiologic, metabolic, nutritional, neurodevelopmental, cognitive, psychosocial, cultural, and political. These are all interrelated. We have varying degrees or levels of understanding of the processes involved; the molecular basis of genetics, for example, is much better understood than the molecular basis of cognition. Accordingly, the classification of the various aspects of growth and development should be regarded as in considerable measure conceptual, rather than as a description of clearly discrete entities. It may be best to regard efforts at classification as presenting models that can help us understand some of the intricacies of the developmental process.

Models

No single description of growth and development in the infant, child, or adolescent is adequate to the complexity of the processes involved. The

1

variety of viewpoints from which these processes may be observed have provided models that attempt to create orderly descriptions and that make assumptions as to the dynamics of the process and as to the relationships between the contributing factors, whether biologically innate or experiential. Some models have permitted the development of scales for the evaluation of the pace of growth and achievement and of the level achieved. Some models serve some aspects of the process better than others, or serve the child or adolescent of one age better than those of other ages.

The *physiologic model* embraces changes in both structure and function. *Physical* growth and development comprises the changes in structure and size that occur after the fertilization of the ovum. It is initiated and at first governed principally by genetic endowment. It is modified by a host of experiences that will ultimately determine to what extent genetic potential is realized. Structural changes are closely related to *physiologic* phenomena that are related in turn to increasing age. Changes in function range from those that occur at the molecular level, such as the activation of enzyme systems in the course of differentiation, to the complex interplay of metabolic and physical changes associated with puberty and adolescence. They are modified by nutrition and by experience (including traumatic experiences that may be physical, infectious, chemical, or radiologic), as well as by emotional, social, and cultural factors.

Physiologic growth and development involves also the homeostatic mechanisms that safeguard the internal environment and regulate the interactions of the individual with the environment. Developmental changes in physiologic activities will determine the time and pattern of many features of development.

The neurodevelopmental model of growth and development comprises elements of the developmental process that underlie behavior at its most basic level, with particular attention to those elements that seem to evolve for the most part as the result of maturation rather than as the consequences primarily of environmental conditions or experiences. Neurodevelopmental aspects include such rudimentary behaviors of the newborn and young infant as visual activity, head control, reaching, grasping, or rolling over, or, in the older child, such behaviors as walking, talking, manipulating toys, or drawing. As the child matures, it becomes more difficult to distinguish between behaviors that depend for their appearance upon maturity alone and those that depend in some measure upon experience.

The *cognitive model* of growth and development is closely related to the neurodevelopmental, and gives consideration to the physiologic and mental structures and processes that permit thought, learning, knowing, and problem-solving. It includes the behaviors that are the outcomes of these activities. *Intelligence* may be thought of as the capacity for complex cognitive function.

Another view of intelligence (Gardner, 1983) holds that it may not be appropriate to speak of a single, global "intelligence," but rather that there may be several more or less discrete intelligences. It is proposed that the organization of the neurophysiologic structures of the brain may support different forms of intelligence in different degrees. Gardner suggests that "a human intellectual competence must entail a set of skills of problem solving—enabling the individual *to resolve genuine problems or difficulties* that he or she encounters and, when appropriate, to create an effective product—and must also entail the potential for *finding or creating problems*—thereby laying the groundwork for the acquisition of new knowledge" (p. 60–61). Gardner presents the evidence that there may be discrete intelligences for linguistic, musical, logical-mathematical, spatial, bodily-kinesthetic, and personal (interpersonal and intrapersonal) intelligences.

Current practice with older children and adolescents assesses cognitive level or achievement through measurement of communicative skills and the ability to handle abstract and symbolic material. The most commonly used descriptor of intelligence, the *intelligence quotient (IQ),* usually samples a variety of skills.

The *developmental task* model of growth and development views the process as a succession of steps taken in mastery of self and of the environment, beginning with the meeting of physiologic needs in infancy, and progressing through such steps as mastery of locomotion or of social or academic skills to the accomplishment of the changes in self-image that are made in adolescence. The need to face developmental tasks continues in adulthood, as lives are changed by marriage, parenthood, and the like.

The *psychosocial model* considers the interactions of the infant, child, or adolescent with the environment, with particular attention to emotional and interpersonal relationships, and to the relationship of these to behavior, personality, and character. The earliest relationships are those with parents; to these are added those with siblings, other family members, and friends. *Cultural* growth and development is an aspect of the psychosocial that follows the way in which infant, child, and adolescent take their places in the community, in accordance with the community's traditions, practices, expectations, and resources. There is an interaction of the *political* structure and life of every community with all aspects of growth and development, with the cultural and political lives of the community determining how children are valued, and what measures will be taken to safeguard their interests and their futures.

An *ethologic model* has enriched the perspective within which human growth and development can be viewed. Ethologists have focused their attention upon the study of overt behavior of animals in their natural settings, with particular attention to patterns of bonding and attachment between the very young and their parents, and in later life to such patterns of behavior as greeting, play, courtship, mating, and defense of territory. The study of such behaviors in animals has suggested some *analogies* with human behavior. The further possibility has been raised that some of these behaviors may represent not just analogies but *homologies,* in the sense that innate physiologic mechanisms defining and directing animal behavior for which there seems to be an analogy in man may be in some measure shared in DNA, as an evolutionary development that represents a biologic link between man and other primates, or with other species.

Themes

Besides the models that provide frameworks for visualization of the developmental process, there are a variety of developmental *themes* that may receive consideration within the various models or independently of them. Such themes include, for example, the roles of temperament and of learning style; the development of autonomy, of self-esteem, of body-image, of gender identity, and of sexuality; the roles of play and of friendships; the role of work in child and adolescent development; the place of aggression and violence in the lives of children; the changing nature of the fears of children, as a reflection of their conceptions of the reality of the world that surrounds them; and the changing views of the child regarding such life events as birth, death, and illness. Children do not advance at the same rate with respect to each of these aspects of development. Themes tend to be embedded in models, to be rather variable in expression or content, and to generate few milestones of age against which to measure the child's achievement.

PHYSICAL AND PHYSIOLOGIC ASPECTS OF GROWTH AND DEVELOPMENT

Genetic, nutritional, traumatic, social, and cultural forces, unique for each child, may produce profoundly different patterns of growth for individual children who fall within the broad limits that designate "normality." The wide variation in patterns of growth often requires that some of the elements of growth be examined in statistical comparison with population standards, rather than in absolute terms.

Assessment of Variability in Growth and Development

When biologic data, such as those that describe growth and development, vary over a range of normal values, the largest number of measurements tend to cluster about an *average* or *mean* value. When such data are plotted on a graph, the result is often a close approximation of the theoretic or gaussian, bell-shaped curve (Fig. 1–1) that describes the ideal distribution of continuously variable values about a population mean. Statistical treatment of such data may generate a number of useful measurements, the most important of which are the *mean* or *average* value and the *standard deviation of the mean.*

The *standard deviation* (SD) measures the degree of dispersion of observed values around the mean value. In an ideal gaussian distribution the values lying between the points 1 SD below and 1 SD above the mean value will include about 68 per cent of all values. The range *mean ± 2 SD* will include about 95 per cent of values distributed about this mean, and the range *mean ± 3 SD* will include about 99.7 per cent of such values.

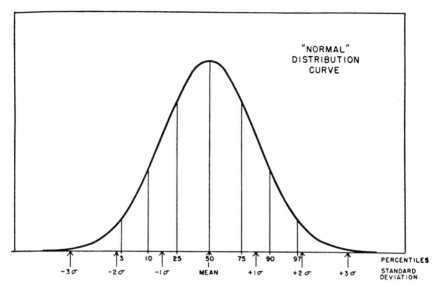

"NORMAL" DISTRIBUTION CURVE

PERCENTILES: 3, 10, 25, 50, 75, 90, 97

STANDARD DEVIATION: -3σ, -2σ, -1σ, MEAN, $+1\sigma$, $+2\sigma$, $+3\sigma$

Figure 1-1. "Normal" (gaussian) distribution curve. This theoretical curve represents a type of distribution characteristic of the range of variability between values for many measurements obtained from groups of children at a given age. The percentiles indicate certain positions within this distribution, as do the standard deviations from the mean.
(From Nelson WE (ed): *Textbook of Pediatrics,* 7th ed. Philadelphia, WB Saunders Company, 1959, p. 18)

In an ideal distribution of random normal values the mean or average value will be the one most commonly found (i.e., the *modal* or *normal* value [*mode* or *norm*]) within the population under study. If, on the other hand, a set of values includes a disproportionately larger number of high values than low, or vice versa, the average value may not be the most representative (modal) for the population being investigated. Asymmetric curves are generated, which are said to be *skewed,* or to show *kurtosis.* Under these circumstances the *median* or central value (see below) may be more representative of the population. When a bimodal curve is found, it may generally be inferred that not one but two populations are being measured, which have some feature differentiating them from each other.

When quantitative data are arranged in order of ascending or descending magnitude, a value, the *median,* can be found, on either side of which lie half of the observations. In the distribution described by the symmetric normal curve, the median, the mean, and the mode fall at the same point. Values may also be designated that divide the data into two groups at the first *quartile* point, below which will lie one quarter of the values, at the second quartile point (the median), and at the third quartile point, below which lie three quarters of the observed values. The *percentile* points in a distribution of ordered data have similar meaning, 1/10th of observations falling below the 10th percentile, 3/10th below the 30th percentile, 1/20th above the 95th percentile, and so on.

Percentile location is commonly used to designate where an individual member of a population stands with respect to the other members. The growth charts in common use for following the course of physical development of children show curves at a number of different positions corresponding to deviations from average values, either above or below the mean. About 10 per cent of normal persons will fall either above the 95th percentile (5 per cent) or below the 5th (5 per cent) for any normally distributed measurement.

When two samples or populations differ with respect to average values for some biologic trait, it is often difficult to evaluate the meaning of this difference unless the distribution or dispersion of values in each sample is known. When the standard deviations of the two samples are known, the *probability* (p) can be calculated that an observed difference between them might have occurred by chance alone, the samples having been drawn from a homogeneous population. When the observed difference is very unlikely to have occurred by chance, it may be inferred that the observed difference is likely to represent a significant differential factor between the two groups.

For example, if two groups of children on different diets were to have different frequencies of occurrence of the common cold, then, with knowledge of the difference between the means, the standard deviations of the means, and the sizes of the groups, one could calculate the likelihood that such a difference in mean frequencies could arise in two samples drawn at random from a population in which there was no relationship between diet and frequency of colds. (The presumption of no relationship is known as the *"null hypothesis."*)

A high level of unlikelihood (p less than 0.05, or less than 0.001, for example) that a given difference would have occurred by chance does not prove that the difference is real rather than an artifact. Nor does the finding of an unexpectedly high likelihood (p greater than 0.95 or 0.99, for example) of agreement prove that no difference exists nor that the populations being compared are the same. When the likelihood that an observed deviation from a mean value or a difference between two means would be expected by chance less than 1 time in 20 comparisons of random data (e.g., an observation is above the 95th percentile or below the 5th percentile, or examination of a difference generates a p less than 0.05), the deviation or difference is often said to be "statistically significant." For many purposes, "$p<0.01$" or "$p<0.001$" will be the preferred criterion and will carry more confidence that a deviation or difference is significant or real. But any choice of a value of p is arbitrary, and if "statistical significance" is defined as p less than 0.05, such "significance" will be found by chance in about 1 in 20 examinations made in a homogeneous population with normally distributed values for some variable.

The above considerations set the basis for use of percentile designations in following the growth and development of children. Examination of their percentile location will help identify children whose substantial distance from the norm (say, above the 95th percentile or below the 5th percentile) suggests that their developmental progress may need careful evaluation before any judgment is made as to whether their deviation from the norm represents a variant normal growth pattern or is the result of an abnormality.

Growth disturbances may be signaled also by changes in growth parameters that occur well within the limits of normal; for example, the movement of a child from a 75th percentile location to a 25th percentile location is likely to reflect a more serious problem than the finding of a child on a single occasion to be below the 10th percentile.

In making such judgments, it is essential that the standards against which a given child will be compared are the appropriate ones. There are genetic, nutritional, and sociocultural differences between populations that will generate different standards for comparison. For some populations, standards must be developed that apply only to *their* normal growth (see below).

Assessment of Physical Growth and Development

Studies of the patterns of physical growth of normal children in the United States, with indications of the variability of height and weight with age, were done a generation ago. These led to the Harvard and Iowa growth charts (Jackson and Kelly, 1945; Stuart and Meredith, 1946), data for which were derived from Caucasian children predominantly of northern European origin, and to the Wetzel grid (Wetzel, 1941), which drew from a wider assortment of sources. Such charts may not reflect the growth patterns of contemporary ethnic, genetic, or socioeconomic groups. There can be no universally adequate standard. There is, for example, evidence that in various parts of the world ethnic differences depend in largest measure upon differences in prevalence of malnutrition and infectious disease, with the expectation that standards will change as these prevalences are altered.

The National Center for Health Statistics (NCHS) has conducted a large survey of children in the United States (Hamill et al., 1979), which has produced the data in Tables 1–1, 1–2A, and 1–2B, and in Figures 1–2A through 1–2D and 1–3A through 1–3D. The children studied represented a cross-section of ethnic (black and Caucasian) and economic groups; accordingly, some genetic, ethnic, and socioeconomic differences are imbedded in the data. The derived charts cannot be regarded as descriptive of any particular group of children but they can serve well as general *reference standards,* since 1) they are reasonably up to date, 2) they reflect the status of generally well-nourished children whose health has been about as good as is likely to be achieved in an industrially developed country, and 3) they appear to indicate conditions close to asymptotic for the trend toward increasing height that has been evident for several centuries. In this last respect their usefulness may be relatively long-standing.

TABLE 1–1. Length, Weight, and Head Circumference by Age, Boys and Girls: Birth to 36 Months*,†

	Boys: Percentiles								Girls: Percentiles						
	5th	*10th*	*25th*	*50th*	*75th*	*90th*	*95th*	Measurement	*5th*	*10th*	*25th*	*50th*	*75th*	*90th*	*95th*
	46.4 (18¼)	47.5 (18¾)	49.0 (19¼)	50.5 (20)	51.8 (20½)	53.5 (21)	54.4 (21½)	Length-mm (in)	45.4 (17¾)	46.5 (18¼)	48.2 (19)	49.9 (19¾)	51.0 (20)	52.0 (20½)	52.9 (20¾)
BIRTH	2.54 (5½)	2.78 (6¼)	3.00 (6½)	3.27 (7¼)	3.64 (8)	3.82 (8½)	4.15 (9¼)	Weight-kg (lb)	2.36 (5¼)	2.58 (5¾)	2.93 (6½)	3.23 (7)	3.52 (7¾)	3.64 (8)	3.81 (8½)
	32.6 (12¾)	33.0 (13)	33.9 (13¼)	34.8 (13¾)	35.6 (14)	36.6 (14½)	37.2 (14¾)	Head C-cm (in)	32.1 (12¾)	32.9 (13)	33.5 (13¼)	34.3 (13½)	34.8 (13¾)	35.5 (14)	35.9 (14¼)
	50.4 (19¾)	51.3 (20¼)	53.0 (20¾)	54.6 (21½)	56.2 (22¼)	57.7 (22¾)	58.6 (23)	Length-cm (in)	49.2 (19¼)	50.2 (19¾)	51.9 (20½)	53.5 (21)	54.9 (21½)	56.1 (22)	56.9 (22½)
1 month	3.16 (7)	3.43 (7½)	3.82 (8½)	4.29 (9½)	4.75 (10½)	5.14 (11¼)	5.38 (11¾)	Weight-kg (lb)	2.97 (6½)	3.22 (7)	3.59 (8)	3.98 (8¾)	4.36 (9½)	4.65 (10¼)	4.92 (10¾)
	34.9 (13¾)	35.4 (14)	36.2 (14¼)	37.2 (14¾)	38.1 (15)	39.0 (15¼)	39.6 (15½)	Head C-cm (in)	34.2 (13½)	34.8 (13¾)	35.6 (14)	36.4 (14¼)	37.1 (14½)	37.8 (15)	38.3 (15)
	56.7 (22¼)	57.7 (22¾)	59.4 (23½)	61.1 (24)	63.0 (24¾)	64.5 (25½)	65.4 (25¾)	Length-cm (in)	55.4 (21¾)	56.2 (22¼)	57.8 (22¾)	59.5 (23½)	61.2 (24)	62.7 (24¾)	63.4 (25)
3 months	4.43 (9¾)	4.78 (10½)	5.32 (11¾)	5.98 (13¼)	6.56 (14½)	7.14 (15¾)	7.37 (16¼)	Weight-kg (lb)	4.18 (9¼)	4.47 (9¾)	4.88 (10¾)	5.40 (12)	5.90 (13)	6.39 (14)	6.74 (14¾)
	38.4 (15)	38.9 (15¼)	39.7 (15¾)	40.6 (16)	41.7 (16½)	42.5 (16¾)	43.1 (17)	Head C-cm (in)	37.3 (14¾)	37.8 (15)	38.7 (15¼)	39.5 (15½)	40.4 (16)	41.2 (16¼)	41.7 (16½)
	63.4 (25)	64.4 (25¼)	66.1 (26)	67.8 (26¾)	69.7 (27½)	71.3 (28)	72.3 (28½)	Length-cm (in)	61.8 (24¼)	62.6 (24¾)	64.2 (25¼)	65.9 (26)	67.8 (26¾)	69.4 (27¼)	70.2 (27¾)
6 months	6.20 (13¾)	6.61 (14½)	7.20 (15¾)	7.85 (17¼)	8.49 (18¾)	9.10 (20)	9.46 (20¾)	Weight-kg (lb)	5.79 (12¾)	6.12 (13½)	6.60 (14½)	7.21 (16)	7.83 (17¼)	8.38 (18½)	8.73 (19¼)
	41.5 (16¼)	42.0 (16½)	42.8 (16¾)	43.8 (17¼)	44.7 (17½)	45.6 (18)	46.2 (18¼)	Head C-cm (in)	40.3 (15¾)	40.9 (16)	41.6 (16½)	42.4 (16¾)	43.3 (17)	44.1 (17¼)	44.6 (17½)
	68.0 (26¾)	69.1 (27¼)	70.6 (27¾)	72.3 (28½)	74.0 (29¼)	75.9 (30)	77.1 (30¼)	Length-cm (in)	66.1 (26)	67.0 (26½)	68.7 (27)	70.4 (27¾)	72.4 (28½)	74.0 (29¼)	75.0 (29½)
9 months	7.52 (16½)	7.95 (17½)	8.56 (18¾)	9.18 (20¼)	9.88 (21¾)	10.49 (23¼)	10.93 (24)	Weight-kg (lb)	7.00 (15½)	7.34 (16¼)	7.89 (17½)	8.56 (18¾)	9.24 (20¼)	9.83 (21¾)	10.17 (22½)
	43.5 (17¼)	44.0 (17¼)	44.8 (17¾)	45.8 (18)	46.6 (18¼)	47.5 (18¾)	48.1 (19)	Head C-cm (in)	42.3 (16¾)	42.8 (16¾)	43.5 (17¼)	44.3 (17½)	45.1 (17¾)	46.0 (18)	46.4 (18¼)

Age	Measurement														
12 months	Length-cm (in)	69.8 (27½)	70.8 (27¾)	72.4 (28½)	74.3 (29¼)	76.3 (30)	78.0 (30¾)	79.1 (31¼)	71.7 (28¼)	72.8 (28¾)	74.3 (29¼)	76.1 (30)	77.7 (30½)	79.8 (31½)	81.2 (32)
	Weight-kg (lb)	7.84 (17¼)	8.19 (18)	8.81 (19¼)	9.53 (21)	10.23 (22½)	10.87 (24)	11.24 (24¾)	8.43 (18½)	8.84 (19½)	9.49 (21)	10.15 (22½)	10.91 (24)	11.54 (25½)	11.99 (26½)
	Head C-cm (in)	43.5 (17¼)	44.1 (17¼)	44.8 (17¾)	45.6 (18)	46.4 (18¼)	47.2 (18½)	47.6 (18¾)	44.8 (17¾)	45.3 (17¾)	46.1 (18¼)	47.0 (18½)	47.9 (18¾)	48.8 (19¼)	49.3 (19½)
18 months	Length-cm (in)	76.0 (30)	77.2 (30½)	78.8 (31)	80.9 (31¾)	83.0 (32¾)	85.0 (33½)	86.1 (34)	77.5 (30½)	78.7 (31)	80.5 (31¾)	82.4 (32½)	84.3 (33¼)	86.6 (34)	88.1 (34¾)
	Weight-kg (lb)	8.92 (19¾)	9.30 (20½)	10.04 (22¼)	10.82 (23¾)	11.55 (25½)	12.30 (27)	12.76 (28¼)	9.59 (21¼)	9.92 (21¾)	10.67 (23½)	11.47 (25¼)	12.31 (27¼)	13.05 (28¾)	13.44 (29½)
	Head C-cm (in)	45.0 (17¾)	45.6 (18)	46.3 (18¼)	47.1 (18½)	47.9 (18¾)	48.6 (19¼)	49.1 (19¼)	46.3 (18¼)	46.7 (18½)	47.4 (18¾)	48.4 (19)	49.3 (19½)	50.1 (19¾)	50.6 (20)
24 months	Length-cm (in)	81.3 (32)	82.5 (32½)	84.2 (33¼)	86.5 (34)	88.7 (35)	90.8 (35¾)	92.0 (36¼)	82.3 (32½)	83.5 (32¾)	85.6 (33¾)	87.6 (34½)	89.9 (35½)	92.2 (36½)	93.8 (37)
	Weight-kg (lb)	9.87 (21¾)	10.26 (22½)	11.10 (24½)	11.90 (26¼)	12.74 (28)	13.57 (30)	14.08 (31)	10.54 (23¼)	10.85 (24)	11.65 (25¾)	12.59 (27¾)	13.44 (29¾)	14.29 (31½)	14.70 (32½)
	Head C-cm (in)	46.1 (18¼)	46.5 (18¼)	47.3 (18½)	48.1 (19)	48.8 (19¼)	49.6 (19½)	50.1 (19¾)	47.3 (18½)	47.7 (18¾)	48.3 (19)	49.2 (19¼)	50.2 (19¾)	51.0 (20)	51.4 (20¼)
30 months	Length-cm (in)	86.0 (33¾)	87.0 (34¼)	88.9 (35)	91.3 (36)	93.7 (37)	95.6 (37¾)	96.9 (38¼)	87.0 (34¼)	88.2 (34¾)	90.1 (35½)	92.3 (36¼)	94.6 (37¼)	97.0 (38¼)	98.7 (38¾)
	Weight-kg (lb)	10.78 (23¾)	11.21 (24¾)	12.11 (26¾)	12.93 (28½)	13.93 (30¾)	14.81 (32¾)	15.35 (33¾)	11.44 (25¼)	11.80 (26)	12.63 (27¾)	13.67 (30¼)	14.51 (32)	15.47 (34)	15.97 (35¼)
	Head C-cm (in)	47.0 (18½)	47.3 (18½)	48.0 (19)	48.8 (19¼)	49.4 (19½)	50.3 (19¾)	50.8 (20)	48.0 (19)	48.4 (19)	49.1 (19¼)	49.9 (19¾)	51.0 (20)	51.7 (20¼)	52.2 (20½)
36 months	Length-cm (in)	90.0 (35½)	91.0 (35¾)	93.1 (36¾)	95.6 (37¾)	98.1 (38½)	100.0 (39¼)	101.5 (40)	91.2 (36)	92.4 (36½)	94.2 (37)	96.5 (38)	98.9 (39)	101.4 (40)	103.1 (40½)
	Weight-kg (lb)	11.60 (25½)	12.07 (26½)	12.99 (28½)	13.93 (30¾)	15.03 (33¼)	15.97 (35¼)	16.54 (36½)	12.26 (27)	12.69 (28)	13.58 (30)	14.69 (32½)	15.59 (34½)	16.66 (36¾)	17.28 (38)
	Head C-cm (in)	47.6 (18¾)	47.9 (18¾)	48.5 (19)	49.3 (19½)	50.0 (19¾)	50.8 (20)	51.4 (20¼)	48.6 (19¼)	49.0 (19¼)	49.7 (19½)	50.5 (20)	51.5 (20¼)	52.3 (20½)	52.8 (20¾)

* From Behrman RE, Vaughan VC III (eds): Nelson Textbook of Pediatrics, 13th ed. Philadelphia, WB Saunders Company, 1987, p 12.

† These data are those of the National Center for Health Statistics (NCHS), Health Resources Administration, DHEW. They were based on studies of The Fels Research Institute, Yellow Springs, Ohio. Metric data have been smoothed by a least-squares cubic spline technique. For details see Hamill PVV, et al: NCHS Growth Charts, 1976. Monthly Vital Statistics Report 25(3):1, 1976. These data and those in Tables 1-2A, 1-2B, 1-4A, and 1-4B were first made available to us with the help of William M. Moore, MD, of Ross Laboratories, who supplied the conversion from metric measurements to approximate inches and pounds. This help is gratefully acknowledged.

TABLE 1-2A. Stature and Weight by Age*,† Boys: 2 to 18 Years (Stature: centimeters and [inches] first entry, Weight: kilograms and [pounds] second entry)

Boys: Percentiles

Age years	5th		10th		25th		50th		75th		90th		95th	
2.0†	82.5 10.49	(32½) (23¼)	83.5 10.96	(32¾) (24¼)	85.3 11.55	(33½) (25½)	86.8 12.34	(34¼) (27¼)	89.2 13.36	(35) (29½)	92.0 14.38	(36¼) (31¾)	94.4 15.50	(37¼) (34¼)
2.5†	85.4 11.27	(33½) (24¾)	86.5 11.77	(34) (26)	88.5 12.55	(34¾) (27¾)	90.4 13.52	(35½) (29¾)	92.9 14.61	(36½) (32¼)	95.6 15.71	(37¾) (34¾)	97.8 16.61	(38½) (36½)
3.0	89.0 12.05	(35) (26½)	90.3 12.58	(35½) (27¾)	92.6 13.12	(36½) (29¾)	94.9 14.62	(37¼) (32¼)	97.5 15.78	(38½) (34¾)	100.1 16.95	(39½) (37¼)	102.0 17.77	(40¼) (39¼)
3.5	92.5 12.84	(36½) (28¼)	93.9 13.41	(37) (29½)	96.4 14.46	(38) (32)	99.1 15.68	(39) (34½)	101.7 16.90	(40) (37¼)	104.3 18.15	(41¼) (40)	106.1 18.98	(41¾) (41¾)
4.0	95.8 13.64	(37¾) (30)	97.3 14.24	(38¼) (31½)	100.0 15.39	(39¼) (34)	102.9 16.69	(40½) (36¾)	105.7 17.99	(41½) (39¾)	108.2 19.32	(42½) (42½)	109.9 20.27	(43¼) (44¾)
4.5	98.9 14.45	(39) (31¾)	100.6 15.10	(39½) (33¼)	103.4 16.30	(40¾) (36)	106.6 17.69	(42) (39)	109.4 19.06	(43) (42)	111.9 20.50	(44) (45¼)	113.5 21.63	(44¾) (47¾)
5.0	102.0 15.27	(40¼) (33¾)	103.7 15.96	(40¾) (35¼)	106.5 17.22	(42) (38)	109.9 18.67	(43¼) (41¼)	112.8 20.14	(44¼) (44½)	115.4 21.70	(45½) (47¾)	117.0 23.09	(46) (51)
5.5	104.9 16.09	(41¼) (35½)	106.7 16.83	(42) (37)	109.6 18.14	(43¼) (40)	113.1 19.67	(44½) (43¼)	116.1 21.25	(45¾) (46¾)	118.7 22.96	(46¾) (50½)	120.3 24.66	(47¼) (54¼)
6.0	107.7 16.93	(42½) (37¼)	109.6 17.72	(43¼) (39)	112.5 19.07	(44¼) (42)	116.1 20.69	(45¾) (45½)	119.2 22.40	(47) (49½)	121.9 24.31	(48) (53½)	123.5 26.34	(48½) (58)
6.5	110.4 17.78	(43½) (39¼)	112.3 18.62	(44¼) (41)	115.3 20.02	(45½) (44¼)	119.0 21.74	(46¾) (48)	122.2 23.62	(48) (52)	124.9 25.76	(49¼) (56¾)	126.6 28.16	(49¾) (62)
7.0	113.0 18.64	(44½) (41)	115.0 19.53	(45¼) (43)	118.0 21.00	(46½) (46¼)	121.7 22.85	(48) (50¼)	125.0 24.94	(49¼) (55)	127.9 27.36	(50¼) (60¼)	129.7 30.12	(51) (66½)
7.5	115.6 19.52	(45½) (43)	117.6 20.45	(46¼) (45)	120.6 22.02	(47½) (48½)	124.4 24.03	(49) (53)	127.8 26.36	(50¼) (58)	130.8 29.11	(51½) (64¼)	132.7 32.73	(52¼) (72¼)
8.0	118.1 20.40	(46½) (45)	120.2 21.39	(47¼) (47¼)	123.2 22.09	(48½) (51)	127.0 25.30	(50) (55¾)	130.5 27.91	(51½) (61½)	133.6 31.06	(52½) (68½)	135.7 34.51	(53½) (76)
8.5	120.5 21.31	(47½) (47)	122.7 22.34	(48½) (49¼)	125.7 24.21	(49½) (53¼)	129.6 26.66	(51) (58¾)	133.2 29.61	(52½) (65¼)	136.5 33.22	(53¾) (73¼)	138.8 36.96	(54¾) (81½)
9.0	122.9 22.25	(48½) (49)	125.2 23.33	(49¼) (51½)	128.2 25.40	(50½) (56)	132.2 28.13	(52) (62)	136.0 31.46	(53½) (69¼)	139.4 35.57	(55) (78½)	141.8 39.58	(55¾) (87¼)
9.5	125.3 23.25	(49¼) (51¼)	127.6 24.38	(50¼) (53¾)	130.8 26.88	(51½) (59¼)	134.8 29.73	(53) (65½)	138.8 33.46	(54¾) (73¾)	142.4 38.11	(56) (84)	144.9 42.35	(57) (93¼)

10.0	127.7 (50¼) 24.33 (53¾)	130.1 (51¼) 25.52 (56¼)	133.4 (52½) 28.07 (62)	137.5 (54¼) 31.44 (69¼)	141.6 (55¾) 35.61 (78½)	145.5 (57¼) 40.80 (90)	148.1 (58¼) 45.27 (99¾)
10.5	130.1 (51¼) 25.51 (56¼)	132.6 (52¼) 26.78 (59)	136.0 (53½) 29.59 (65¼)	140.3 (55¼) 33.30 (73½)	144.6 (57) 37.92 (83½)	148.7 (58½) 43.63 (96¼)	151.5 (59¾) 48.31 (106½)
11.0	132.6 (52¼) 26.80 (59)	135.1 (53¼) 28.17 (62)	138.7 (54½) 31.25 (69)	143.33 (56½) 35.30 (77¾)	147.8 (58¼) 40.38 (89)	152.1 (60) 46.57 (102¾)	154.9 (61) 51.47 (113½)
11.5	135.0 (53¼) 28.24 (62¼)	137.7 (54½) 29.72 (65½)	141.5 (55¾) 33.08 (73)	146.4 (57¾) 37.46 (82½)	151.1 (59½) 43.00 (94¾)	155.6 (61¼) 49.61 (109¼)	158.5 (62½) 54.73 (120¾)
12.0	137.6 (54¼) 29.85 (65¾)	140.3 (55¼) 31.46 (69¼)	144.4 (56¾) 35.09 (77¼)	149.7 (59) 39.78 (87¾)	154.6 (60¾) 45.77 (101)	159.4 (62¾) 52.73 (116¼)	162.3 (64) 58.09 (128)
12.5	140.2 (55¼) 31.64 (69¾)	143.0 (56¼) 33.41 (73¾)	147.4 (58) 37.31 (82¼)	153.0 (60¼) 42.27 (93¼)	158.2 (62¼) 48.70 (107¼)	163.2 (64¼) 55.91 (123¼)	166.1 (65½) 61.52 (135¾)
13.0	142.9 (56¼) 33.64 (74¼)	145.8 (57½) 35.60 (78½)	150.5 (59¼) 39.74 (87½)	156.5 (61½) 44.95 (99)	161.8 (63¾) 51.79 (114¼)	167.0 (65¾) 59.12 (130¼)	169.8 (66¾) 65.02 (143¼)
13.5	145.7 (57¼) 35.85 (79)	148.7 (58½) 38.03 (83¾)	153.6 (60½) 42.40 (93½)	159.9 (63) 47.81 (105½)	165.3 (65) 55.02 (121¼)	170.5 (67¼) 62.35 (137½)	173.4 (68¼) 68.51 (151)
14.0	148.8 (58½) 38.22 (84¼)	151.8 (59¾) 40.64 (89½)	156.9 (61¾) 45.21 (99¾)	63.1 (64¼) 50.77 (112)	168.5 (66¼) 58.31 (128½)	173.8 (68½) 65.57 (144½)	176.7 (69½) 72.13 (159)
14.5	152.0 (59¾) 40.66 (89¾)	155.0 (61) 43.34 (95½)	160.1 (63) 48.08 (106)	166.2 (65½) 53.76 (118½)	171.5 (67½) 61.58 (135¾)	176.6 (69½) 68.76 (151½)	179.5 (70½) 75.66 (166¾)
15.0	155.2 (61) 43.11 (95)	158.2 (62¼) 46.06 (101½)	163.3 (64¼) 50.92 (112¼)	169.0 (66½) 56.71 (125)	174.1 (68½) 64.72 (142¾)	178.9 (70½) 71.91 (158½)	181.9 (71½) 79.12 (174½)
15.5	158.3 (62¼) 45.50 (100¼)	161.2 (63½) 48.69 (107¼)	166.2 (65½) 53.64 (118¼)	171.5 (67½) 59.51 (131¼)	176.3 (69½) 67.64 (149)	180.8 (71¼) 74.98 (165¼)	183.9 (72½) 82.45 (181¾)
16.0	161.1 (63½) 47.74 (105¼)	163.9 (64½) 51.16 (112¾)	168.7 (66½) 56.16 (123¾)	173.5 (68¼) 62.10 (137)	178.1 (70) 70.26 (155)	182.4 (71¾) 77.97 (172)	185.4 (73) 85.62 (188¾)
16.5	163.4 (64¼) 49.76 (109¾)	166.1 (65½) 53.39 (117¾)	170.6 (67¼) 58.38 (128¾)	175.2 (69) 64.39 (142)	179.5 (70¾) 72.46 (159¾)	183.6 (72¼) 80.84 (178¼)	186.6 (73½) 88.59 (195¼)
17.0	164.9 (65) 51.50 (113½)	167.7 (66) 55.28 (121¾)	171.9 (67¾) 60.22 (132¾)	176.2 (69¼) 66.31 (146¼)	180.5 (71) 74.17 (163½)	184.4 (72½) 83.58 (184¼)	187.3 (73¾) 91.31 (201¼)
17.5	165.6 (65¼) 52.89 (116½)	168.5 (66¼) 56.78 (125¼)	172.4 (67¾) 61.61 (135¾)	176.7 (69½) 67.78 (149½)	181.0 (71¼) 75.32 (166)	185.0 (72¾) 86.14 (190)	187.6 (73¾) 93.73 (206¾)
18.0	165.7 (65¼) 53.97 (119)	168.7 (66½) 57.89 (127½)	172.3 (67¾) 62.61 (138)	176.8 (69½) 68.88 (151¾)	181.2 (71¼) 76.0 (167¾)	185.3 (73) 88.41 (195)	187.6 (73¾) 95.76 (211)

* From Behrman RE, Vaughan VC III (eds): *Nelson Textbook of Pediatrics,* 13th ed. Philadelphia, WB Saunders Company, 1987, p 18.

† Data in Tables 1–2A and 1–2B are those of the National Center for Health Statistics, Health Resources Administration, DHEW, collected in its Health Examination Surveys. Metric data have been smoothed by the least-squares cubic spline technique. For details see footnote to Table 1–1.

‡ Stature data for 2.0 to 3.0 years include some recumbent length measurements, which make values slightly higher than if all measurements had been of stature.

TABLE 1–2B. Stature and Weight by Age*,†, Girls: 2 to 18 Years (Stature: centimeters and [inches] first entry, Weight: kilograms and [pounds] second entry)

Girls: Percentiles

Age years	5th		10th		25th		50th		75th		90th		95th	
2.0	81.6 9.95	(32¼) (22)	82.1 10.32	(32¼) (22¾)	84.0 10.96	(33) (24¼)	86.8 11.80	(34¼) (26)	89.3 12.73	(35¼) (28)	92.0 13.58	(36¼) (30)	93.6 14.15	(36¾) (31¼)
2.5	84.6 10.80	(33¼) (23¾)	85.3 11.35	(33½) (25)	87.3 12.11	(34½) (26¾)	90.0 13.03	(35½) (28¾)	92.5 14.23	(36½) (31¼)	95.0 15.16	(37½) (33½)	96.6 15.76	(38) (34¾)
3.0	88.3 11.61	(34¾) (25½)	89.3 12.26	(35¼) (27)	91.4 13.11	(36) (29)	94.1 14.10	(37) (31)	96.6 15.50	(38) (34¼)	99.0 16.54	(39) (36½)	100.6 17.22	(39½) (38)
3.5	91.7 12.37	(36) (27¼)	93.0 13.08	(36½) (28¾)	95.2 14.00	(37½) (30¾)	97.9 15.07	(38½) (33¼)	100.5 16.59	(39½) (36½)	102.8 17.77	(40½) (39¼)	104.5 18.59	(41¼) (41)
4.0	95.0 13.11	(37½) (29)	96.4 13.84	(38) (30½)	98.8 14.80	(39) (32¾)	101.6 15.96	(40) (35¼)	104.3 17.56	(41) (38¾)	106.6 18.93	(42) (41¾)	108.3 19.91	(42¾) (44)
4.5	98.1 13.83	(38½) (30½)	99.7 14.56	(39¼) (32)	102.2 15.55	(40¼) (34¼)	105.0 16.81	(41¼) (37)	107.9 18.48	(42½) (40¾)	110.2 20.06	(43½) (44¼)	112.0 21.24	(44) (46¾)
5.0	101.1 14.55	(39¾) (32)	102.7 15.26	(40½) (33¾)	105.4 16.29	(41½) (36)	108.4 17.66	(42¾) (39)	111.4 19.39	(43¾) (42¾)	113.8 21.23	(44¾) (46¾)	115.6 22.62	(45½) (49¾)
5.5	103.9 15.29	(41) (33¾)	105.6 15.97	(41½) (35¼)	108.4 17.05	(42¾) (37½)	111.6 18.56	(44) (41)	114.8 20.36	(45¼) (45)	117.4 22.48	(46¼) (49½)	119.2 24.11	(47) (53¼)
6.0	106.6 16.05	(42) (35½)	108.4 16.72	(42¾) (36¾)	111.3 17.86	(43¾) (39¼)	114.6 19.52	(45) (43)	118.1 21.44	(46½) (47¼)	120.8 23.89	(47½) (52¾)	122.7 25.75	(48¼) (56¾)
6.5	109.2 16.85	(43) (37¼)	111.0 17.51	(43¾) (38½)	114.1 18.76	(45) (41¼)	117.6 20.61	(46¼) (45½)	121.3 22.68	(47¾) (50)	124.2 25.50	(49) (56¼)	126.1 27.59	(49¾) (60¾)
7.0	111.8 17.71	(44) (39)	113.6 18.39	(44¾) (40½)	116.8 19.78	(46) (43½)	120.6 21.84	(47½) (48¼)	124.4 24.16	(49) (53¼)	127.6 27.39	(50¼) (60½)	129.5 29.68	(51) (65½)
7.5	114.4 18.62	(45) (41)	116.2 19.37	(45¾) (42¾)	119.5 20.95	(47) (46¼)	123.5 23.26	(48½) (51¼)	127.5 25.90	(50¼) (57)	130.9 29.57	(51½) (65¼)	132.9 32.07	(52¼) (70¾)
8.0	116.9 19.62	(46) (43¼)	118.7 20.45	(46¾) (45)	122.2 22.26	(48) (49)	126.4 24.84	(49¾) (54¾)	130.6 27.88	(51½) (61½)	134.2 32.04	(52¾) (70¾)	136.2 34.71	(53¼) (76½)
8.5	119.5 20.68	(47) (45½)	121.3 21.64	(47¾) (47¾)	124.9 23.70	(49¼) (52¼)	129.3 26.58	(51) (58½)	133.6 30.08	(52½) (66¼)	137.4 34.73	(54) (76½)	139.6 37.58	(55) (82¾)
9.0	122.1 21.82	(48) (48)	123.9 22.92	(48¾) (50½)	127.7 25.27	(50¼) (55¾)	132.2 28.46	(52) (62¾)	136.7 32.44	(53¾) (71½)	140.7 37.60	(55½) (83)	142.9 40.64	(56¼) (89½)
9.5	124.8 23.05	(49¼) (50¾)	126.6 24.29	(49¾) (53½)	130.6 26.94	(51½) (59½)	135.2 30.45	(53¼) (67¼)	139.8 34.94	(55) (77)	143.9 40.61	(56¾) (89½)	146.2 43.85	(57½) (96¾)

Age							
10.0	127.5 24.36 (50¼)(53¾)	129.5 25.76 (51)(56¾)	133.6 28.71 (52½)(63¼)	138.3 32.55 (54½)(71¾)	142.9 37.53 (56¼)(82¾)	147.2 43.70 (58)(96¼)	149.5 47.17 (58¾)(104)
10.5	130.4 25.75 (51¼)(56¾)	132.5 27.32 (52¼)(60¼)	136.7 30.57 (53¾)(67½)	141.5 34.72 (55¾)(76½)	146.1 40.17 (57½)(88½)	150.4 46.84 (59¼)(103¼)	152.8 50.57 (60¼)(111½)
11.0	133.5 27.24 (52½)(60)	135.6 28.97 (53½)(63¾)	140.0 32.49 (55)(71¾)	144.8 36.95 (57)(81½)	149.3 42.84 (58¾)(94½)	153.7 49.96 (60½)(110¼)	156.2 54.00 (61½)(119)
11.5	136.6 28.83 (53¾)(63½)	139.0 30.71 (54¾)(67¾)	143.5 34.48 (56½)(76)	148.2 39.23 (58¼)(86½)	152.6 45.48 (60)(100¼)	156.9 53.03 (61¾)(117)	159.5 57.42 (62¾)(126½)
12.0	139.8 30.52 (55)(67¼)	142.3 32.53 (56)(71¼)	147.0 36.52 (57¾)(80½)	151.5 41.53 (59¾)(91½)	155.8 48.07 (61¼)(106)	160.0 55.99 (63)(123½)	162.7 60.81 (64)(134)
12.5	142.7 32.30 (56¼)(71¼)	145.4 34.42 (57¼)(76)	150.1 38.59 (59)(85)	154.6 43.84 (60¾)(96¾)	158.8 50.56 (62½)(111½)	162.9 58.81 (64½)(129¾)	165.6 64.12 (65¼)(141¼)
13.0	145.2 34.14 (57¼)(75¼)	148.0 36.35 (58¼)(80¼)	152.8 40.55 (60¼)(89½)	157.1 46.10 (61¾)(101¾)	161.3 52.91 (63½)(116¾)	165.3 61.45 (65)(135½)	168.1 67.30 (66)(148¼)
13.5	147.2 35.98 (58)(79¼)	150.0 38.26 (59)(84¼)	154.7 42.65 (61)(94)	159.0 48.26 (62½)(106½)	163.2 55.11 (64¼)(121½)	167.3 63.87 (65¾)(140¾)	170.0 70.30 (67)(155)
14.0	148.7 37.76 (58½)(83¼)	151.5 40.11 (59¾)(88½)	155.9 44.54 (61½)(98¼)	160.4 50.28 (63¼)(110¾)	164.6 57.09 (64¾)(125¾)	168.7 66.04 (66½)(145½)	171.3 73.08 (67½)(161)
14.5	149.7 39.45 (59)(87)	152.5 41.83 (60)(92¼)	156.8 46.28 (61¾)(102)	161.2 52.10 (63½)(114¾)	165.6 58.84 (65¼)(129¾)	169.8 67.95 (66¾)(149¾)	172.2 75.59 (67¾)(166¾)
15.0	150.5 40.99 (59¼)(90¼)	153.2 43.38 (60¼)(95¾)	157.2 47.82 (62)(105½)	161.8 53.68 (63¾)(118¼)	166.3 60.32 (65½)(133)	170.5 69.54 (67¼)(153¼)	172.8 77.78 (68)(171½)
15.5	151.1 42.32 (59½)(93¼)	153.6 44.72 (60½)(98½)	157.5 49.10 (62)(108¼)	162.1 54.96 (64)(121¼)	166.7 61.48 (65¾)(135½)	170.9 70.79 (67¼)(156)	173.1 79.59 (68¼)(176½)
16.0	151.6 43.41 (59¾)(95¾)	154.1 45.78 (60¾)(101)	157.8 50.09 (62¼)(110½)	162.4 55.89 (64)(123¼)	166.9 62.29 (65¾)(137¼)	171.1 71.68 (67¼)(158)	173.3 80.99 (68¼)(178½)
16.5	152.2 44.20 (60)(97½)	154.6 46.54 (60¾)(102½)	158.2 50.75 (62¼)(112)	162.7 56.44 (64)(124½)	167.1 62.75 (65¾)(138¼)	171.2 72.18 (67½)(159¼)	173.4 81.93 (68¼)(180½)
17.0	152.7 44.74 (60)(98¾)	155.1 47.04 (61)(103¾)	158.7 51.14 (62½)(112¾)	163.1 56.69 (64¼)(125)	167.3 62.91 (65¾)(138¾)	171.2 72.38 (67½)(159½)	173.5 82.46 (68¼)(181¾)
17.5	153.2 45.08 (60¼)(99½)	155.6 47.33 (61¼)(104¼)	159.1 51.33 (62¾)(113¼)	163.4 56.71 (64¼)(125)	167.5 62.89 (66)(138¾)	171.1 72.37 (67¼)(159½)	173.5 82.62 (68¼)(182¼)
18.0	153.6 45.26 (60½)(99¾)	156.0 47.47 (61½)(104¾)	159.6 51.39 (62¾)(113¼)	163.7 56.62 (64¼)(124¾)	167.6 62.78 (66)(138½)	171.0 72.25 (67¼)(159¼)	173.6 82.47 (68¼)(181¾)

* From Behrman RE, Vaughan VC III (eds): *Nelson Textbook of Pediatrics*, 13th ed. Philadelphia, WB Saunders Company, 1987, p 19.
† See footnotes to Table 1–2A.

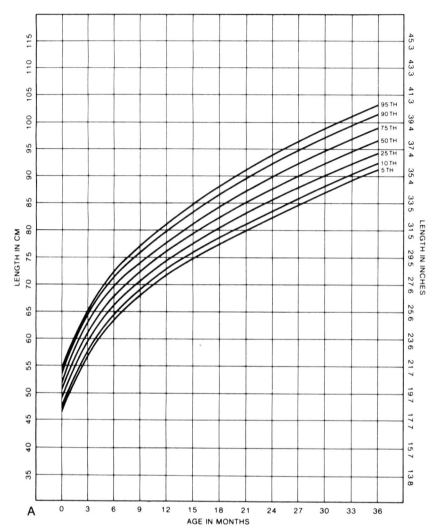

Figure 1–2A. Length by age percentiles for boys ages birth to 36 months.
(From Hamill PVV, Drizd TA, Johnson CL, Reed RB, Roche AF, Moore WM: Physical growth: National Center for Health Statistics percentiles. Am J Clin Nutr 32:610, 1979.)

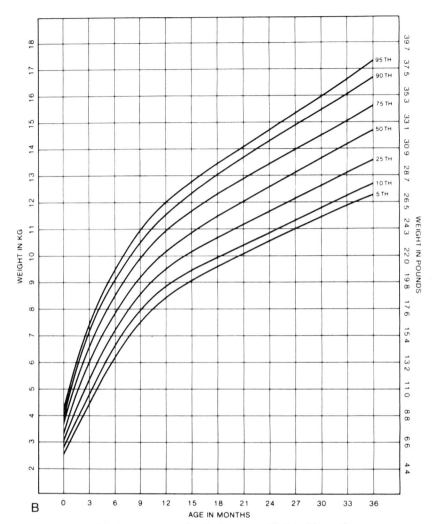

Figure 1–2B. Weight by age percentiles for boys ages birth to 36 months. (From Hamill PVV, Drizd TA, Johnson CL, Reed RB, Roche AF, Moore WM: Physical growth: National Center for Health Statistics percentiles. Am J Clin Nutr 32:612, 1979.)

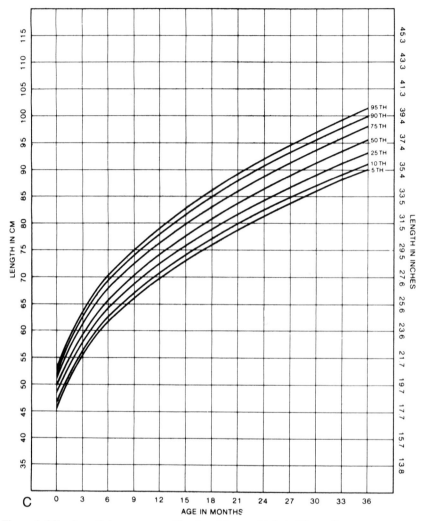

Figure 1–2C. Length by age percentiles for girls ages birth to 36 months. (From Hamill PVV, Drizd TA, Johnson CL, Reed RB, Roche AF, Moore WM: Physical growth: National Center for Health Statistics percentiles. Am J Clin Nutr 32:609, 1979.)

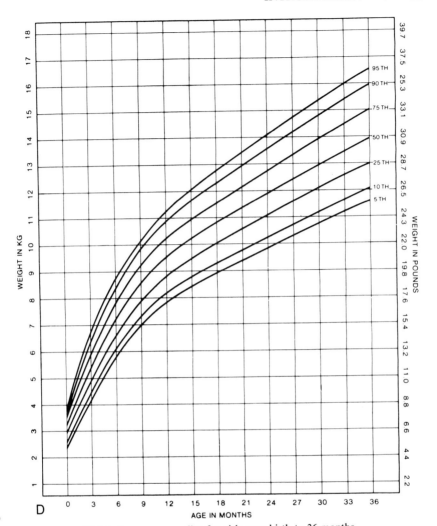

Figure 1–2D. Weight by age percentiles for girls ages birth to 36 months. (From Hamill PVV, Drizd TA, Johnson CL, Reed RB, Roche AF, Moore WM: Physical growth: National Center for Health Statistics percentiles. Am J Clin Nutr 32:611, 1979.)

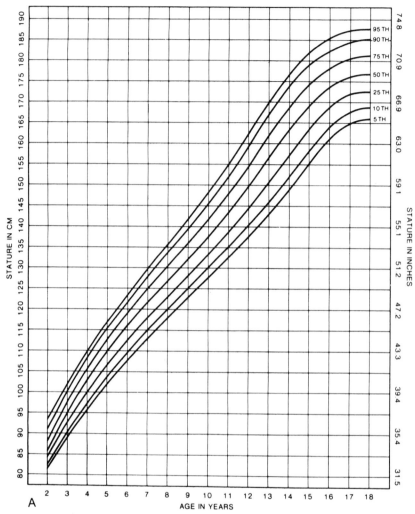

Figure 1–3A. Stature by age percentiles for boys ages 2 to 18 years. (From Hamill PVV, Drizd TA, Johnson CL, Reed RB, Roche AF, Moore WM: Physical growth: National Center for Health Statistics percentiles. Am J Clin Nutr 32:619, 1979.)

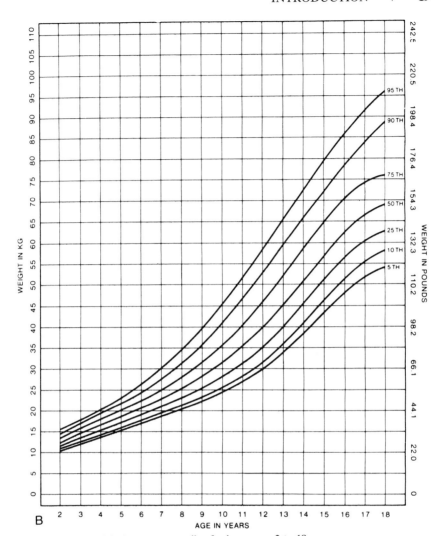

Figure 1–3B. Weight by age percentiles for boys ages 2 to 18 years.
(From Hamill PVV, Drizd TA, Johnson CL, Reed RB, Roche AF, Moore WM: Physical growth: National Center for Health Statistics percentiles. Am J Clin Nutr 32:621, 1979.)

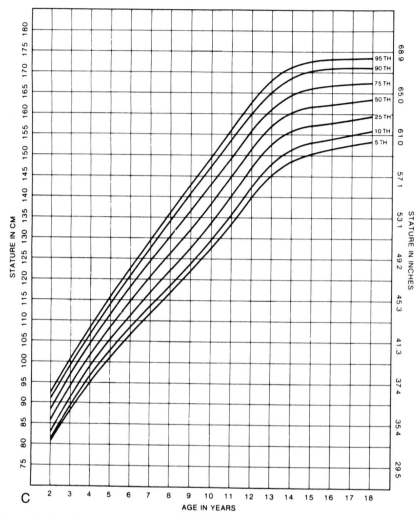

Figure 1–3C. Stature by age percentiles for girls ages 2 to 18 years.
(From Hamill PVV, Drizd TA, Johnson CL, Reed RB, Roche AF, Moore WM: Physical growth: National Center for Health Statistics percentiles. Am J Clin Nutr 32:618, 1979.)

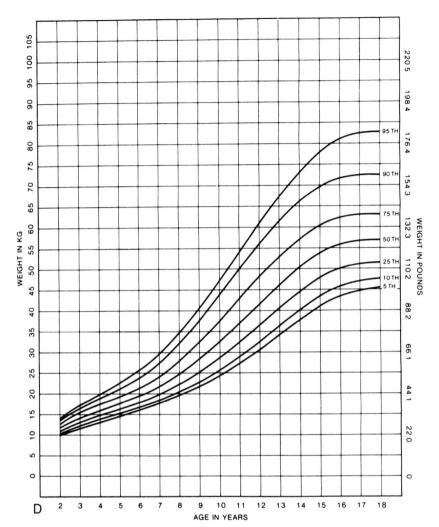

Figure 1–3D. Weight by age percentiles for girls ages 2 to 18 years.
(From Hamill PVV, Drizd TA, Johnson CL, Reed RB, Roche AF, Moore WM: Physical growth: National Center for Health Statistics percentiles. Am J Clin Nutr 32:620, 1979.)

Interrelationships between Parameters of Growth

Tables 1–1, 1–2A, and 1–2B and Figures 1–2A through 1–2D and 1–3A through 1–3D present data regarding the relationship of length (or stature) and weight to age. Formulas giving approximations of the mean data for normal infants and children are given in Table 1–3.

Tables 1–4A and 1–4B and Figures 1–4A through 1–4D and 1–5A and 1–5B present data with respect to the relationships between weight and length (or stature), irrespective of age. Separate data are given for boys and girls.

In conjunction with data relating height to age, the data relating weight to height may be particularly informative. For example, children with low heights for age who have normal weight for height may have experienced nutritional or endocrine causes of growth failure in the past, whereas if both height for age and weight for height are strikingly low, then both past and current nutritional or growth failure may be suspected. By contrast, children with normal height for age who have conspicuously low weight for height are likely to have either relatively acute nutritional or growth problems or variant physiques.

Children whose weights are at less than the 5th or over the 95th percentile for their actual heights should have their growth status evaluated. A physical assessment, along with a review of history of illness, dietary habits, family patterns of growth, and the psychosocial circumstances of the family, will suggest whether more extensive studies are indicated.

Measurements of weight, height, and head circumference will indicate the status of a child with respect to other children of the same age and sex. So long as measurements remain within normal limits, however, only *sequential* measurements will be able to indicate whether the status of any

TABLE 1–3. Formulas for Approximate Average Height and Weight of Normal Infants and Children (After Weech)*

Weight	Kilograms	(Pounds)
(a) at birth	3.25	(7)
(b) 3–12 mo	$\dfrac{age(mo) + 9}{2}$	$(age(mo) + 11)$
(c) 1–6 yr	$age(yr) \times 2 + 8$	$(age(yr) \times 5 + 17)$
(d) 7–12 yr	$\dfrac{age(yr) \times 7 - 5}{2}$	$(age(yr) \times 7 + 5)$

Height	Centimeters	(Inches)
(e) at birth	50	(20)
(f) at 1 yr	75	(30)
(g) 2–12 yr	$age(yr) \times 6 + 77$	$(age(yr) \times 2\frac{1}{2} + 30)$

* From Behrman RE, Vaughan VC III (eds): *Nelson Textbook of Pediatrics,* 13th ed. Philadelphia, WB Saunders Company, 1987, p 11.

given child is likely to represent achievement of his or her innate growth potential.

For example, a child below the 10th percentile in weight for age may be suspected of being undernourished, but 10 per cent of normal children will be below this level. If such children manifest regular growth in height and weight within certain limits, and if sequential measurements follow growth lines that are parallel to the growth lines of the general population, then their growth patterns may be normal in the sense that such children are genetically programmed for such growth. On the other hand, children whose heights and weights are at higher percentiles for their ages (for example, between the 25th and 75th percentiles) may be found to have significantly deviant growth patterns when sequential measurements are evaluated; for example, movement of head circumference from the 25th to the 75th percentile, or of the height or weight from the 75th to the 25th, is likely to reflect a major change in health status.

Appraisal of growth and development in the infant and child depends upon accurate as well as serial measurements in those areas in which changes can be observed. In the infant the most useful of the physical measurements are head circumference, length, and weight (Figs. 1–4A and 1–4C). These may be supplemented by observation of the nutritional state, dentition, and size or patency of the fontanels. In older children measurements of stature and weight may be supplemented by measurements of lengths of body segments (extremities, span, or sitting height).

For adolescents, evaluation and interpretation of growth status requires assessment of sex maturity rating, height velocity, and body fat content in addition to height and weight. Measurements of skinfold thickness and arm or calf circumference may be useful in the estimation of body fat or muscle mass.

The growth velocity curves shown in Figures 1–5A, 1–5B, 1–6A, 1–6B, and 1–7 are derived (Roche and Himes, 1980) from data that relate the normal rates of gain in height, weight, and head circumference to age. They reflect the rapid growth in the first year, the rather steady growth of middle childhood, and the acceleration of growth at and during adolescence. Such charts may help determine the growth status, particularly in adolescence, but will depend upon serial measurements made relatively close together (at 3- to 6-month intervals), and with both accuracy and precision. This need can be met only by more frequent assessments of adolescents by health professionals, especially in early adolescence.

The NCHS data relating height and weight to age were gathered from cross-sectional study of groups of children at various ages, rather than from longitudinal study of individual children. They represent averages of the population at each age. If such data were used to determine *growth velocity,* the findings would obscure important differences between early- and late-maturing adolescents, for whom the curves that relate growth velocity to age would be considerably different. Moreover, there is a tendency for the curve of every adolescent to show at the age of greatest growth velocity a sharper peak than population-derived curves would suggest. In the early-maturing adolescent not only may the peak velocity occur earlier but the peak of the curve may appear to be sharper, whereas

TABLE 1–4A. Weight by Length*†, Boys and Girls Less Than 4 Years

Recumbent Length	Boys: Weight Percentiles, kg and (lb)							Girls: Weight Percentiles, kg and (lb)						
	5th	10th	25th	50th	75th	90th	95th	5th	10th	25th	50th	75th	90th	95th
48–50 cm (19–19¾ in)										3.02 (6¾)	3.29 (7¼)	3.59 (8)		
50–52 cm (19¾–20½ in)										3.25 (7¼)	3.55 (7¾)	3.89 (8½)		
52–54 cm (20½–21¼ in)										3.56 (7¾)	3.89 (8½)	4.26 (9½)		
54–56 cm (21¼–22 in)	3.49 (7¼)	3.65 (8)	3.95 (8¾)	4.34 (9½)	4.76 (10½)	5.13 (11¼)	5.33 (11¾)	3.54 (7¾)	3.64 (8)	3.93 (8¾)	4.29 (9½)	4.70 (10¼)	5.02 (11)	5.21 (11½)
56–58 cm (22–22¾ in)	3.90 (8½)	4.09 (9)	4.43 (9¾)	4.84 (10¾)	5.29 (11¾)	5.69 (12½)	5.88 (13)	3.93 (8¾)	4.05 (9)	4.37 (9¾)	4.76 (10½)	5.20 (11½)	5.55 (12¼)	5.77 (12¾)
58–60 cm (22¾–23½ in)	4.37 (9¾)	4.58 (10)	4.94 (11)	5.38 (11¾)	5.84 (12¾)	6.28 (13¾)	6.47 (14¼)	4.38 (9¾)	4.50 (10)	4.85 (10¾)	5.27 (11½)	5.73 (12¾)	6.12 (13½)	6.36 (14)
60–62 cm (23½–24½ in)	4.88 (10¾)	5.10 (11¼)	5.49 (12)	5.94 (13)	6.42 (14¼)	6.88 (15¼)	7.08 (15½)	4.85 (10¾)	4.99 (11)	5.37 (11¾)	5.82 (12¾)	6.30 (14)	6.70 (14¾)	6.95 (15¼)
62–64 cm (24½–25¼ in)	5.43 (12)	5.65 (12½)	6.05 (13¼)	6.52 (14¼)	7.02 (15½)	7.50 (16½)	7.72 (17)	5.35 (11¾)	5.50 (12)	5.91 (13)	6.39 (14)	6.89 (15¼)	7.30 (16)	7.55 (16¾)
64–66 cm (25¼–26 in)	5.99 (13¼)	6.20 (13¾)	6.62 (14½)	7.11 (15¾)	7.63 (16¾)	8.13 (18)	8.36 (18½)	5.87 (13)	6.03 (13¼)	6.47 (14¼)	6.97 (15¼)	7.48 (16½)	7.90 (17½)	8.15 (18)
66–68 cm (26–26¾ in)	6.55 (14½)	6.76 (15)	7.19 (15¾)	7.70 (17)	8.23 (18¼)	8.75 (19¼)	8.99 (19¾)	6.38 (14)	6.56 (14½)	7.02 (15½)	7.55 (16¾)	8.07 (17¾)	8.50 (18¾)	8.75 (19¼)
68–70 cm (26¾–27½ in)	7.10 (15¾)	7.31 (16)	7.75 (17)	8.27 (18¼)	8.82 (19½)	9.35 (20½)	9.62 (21¼)	6.89 (15¼)	7.08 (15½)	7.56 (16¾)	8.11 (17¾)	8.64 (19)	9.08 (20)	9.33 (20½)
70–72 cm (27½–28¼ in)	7.63 (16¾)	7.84 (17¼)	8.28 (18¼)	8.82 (19½)	9.39 (20¾)	9.93 (22)	10.21 (22½)	7.37 (16¼)	7.58 (16¾)	8.08 (17¾)	8.64 (19)	9.18 (20¼)	9.63 (21¼)	9.88 (21¾)
72–74 cm (28¼–29¼ in)	8.13 (18)	8.33 (18¼)	8.78 (19¼)	9.33 (20½)	9.92 (21¾)	10.48 (23)	10.77 (23¾)	7.82 (17¼)	8.05 (17¾)	8.56 (18¾)	9.14 (20¼)	9.68 (21¼)	10.15 (22½)	10.41 (23)
74–76 cm (29¼–30 in)	8.58 (19)	8.78 (19¼)	9.24 (20¼)	9.81 (21¾)	10.43 (23)	10.99 (24¼)	11.29 (25)	8.24 (18¼)	8.49 (18¾)	9.00 (19¾)	9.59 (21¼)	10.14 (22¼)	10.63 (23½)	10.91 (24)

76–78 cm (30–30¾ in)	9.00 (19¾)	9.21 (20¼)	9.68 (21¼)	10.27 (22¾)	10.91 (24)	11.48 (25¼)	11.78 (26)	8.62 (19)	8.90 (19½)	9.42 (20¾)	10.02 (22)	10.57 (23¼)	11.08 (24½)	11.39 (25)
78–80 cm (30¾–31½ in)	9.40 (20¾)	9.62 (21¼)	10.09 (22¼)	10.70 (23½)	11.36 (25)	11.94 (26¼)	12.25 (27)	8.99 (19¾)	9.29 (20½)	9.81 (21¾)	10.41 (23)	10.97 (24¼)	11.51 (25¼)	11.85 (26)
80–82 cm (31½–32¼ in)	9.77 (21½)	10.01 (22)	10.49 (23¼)	11.12 (24½)	11.80 (26)	12.39 (27¼)	12.69 (28)	9.34 (20½)	9.67 (21¼)	10.19 (22½)	10.80 (23¾)	11.37 (25)	11.93 (26¼)	12.29 (27)
82–84 cm (32¼–33 in)	10.14 (22¼)	10.39 (23)	10.88 (24)	11.53 (25½)	12.23 (27)	12.83 (28¼)	13.13 (29)	9.68 (21¼)	10.04 (22¼)	10.57 (23¼)	11.18 (24¾)	11.75 (26)	12.35 (27¼)	12.72 (28)
84–86 cm (33–33¾ in)	10.49 (23¼)	10.76 (23¾)	11.27 (24¾)	11.93 (26¼)	12.65 (28)	13.26 (29¼)	13.56 (30)	10.03 (22)	10.41 (23)	10.94 (24)	11.56 (25½)	12.15 (26¾)	12.76 (28¼)	13.15 (29)
86–88 cm (33¾–34¾ in)	10.85 (24)	11.14 (24½)	11.67 (25¾)	12.34 (27¼)	13.07 (28¾)	13.69 (30¼)	14.00 (30¾)	10.39 (23)	10.78 (23¾)	11.33 (25)	11.95 (26¼)	12.55 (27¾)	13.19 (29)	13.57 (30)
88–90 cm (34¾–35½ in)	11.22 (24¾)	11.53 (25½)	12.08 (26¾)	12.76 (28¼)	13.50 (29¾)	14.13 (31¼)	14.44 (31¾)	10.76 (23¾)	11.17 (24½)	11.74 (26)	12.36 (27¼)	12.98 (28½)	13.63 (30)	14.01 (31)
90–92 cm (35½–36¼ in)	11.60 (25½)	11.94 (26¼)	12.52 (27½)	13.20 (29)	13.94 (30¾)	14.58 (32¼)	14.90 (32¾)	11.16 (24½)	11.58 (25½)	12.17 (26¾)	12.80 (28¼)	13.45 (29¾)	14.10 (31)	14.45 (31¾)
92–94 cm (36¼–37 in)	12.00 (26½)	12.37 (27¼)	12.97 (28½)	13.65 (30)	14.40 (31¾)	15.05 (33¼)	15.39 (34)	11.59 (25½)	12.02 (26½)	12.63 (27¾)	13.27 (29¼)	13.95 (30¾)	14.61 (32¼)	14.92 (33)
94–96 cm (37–37¾ in)	12.42 (27½)	12.81 (28¼)	13.45 (29¾)	14.14 (31¼)	14.88 (32¾)	15.54 (34¼)	15.90 (35)	12.05 (26½)	12.48 (27½)	13.12 (29)	13.77 (30¼)	14.48 (32)	15.14 (33½)	15.42 (34)
96–98 cm (37¾–38½ in)	12.88 (28½)	13.28 (29¼)	13.96 (30¾)	14.66 (32¼)	15.39 (34)	16.06 (35½)	16.43 (36¼)	12.55 (27¾)	12.98 (28½)	13.64 (30)	14.31 (31½)	15.04 (33¼)	15.71 (34¾)	15.99 (35¼)
98–100 cm (38½–39¼ in)	13.37 (29½)	13.78 (30½)	14.50 (32)	15.21 (33½)	15.94 (35¼)	16.62 (36¾)	17.00 (37½)	13.10 (29)	13.51 (29¾)	14.19 (31¼)	14.87 (32¾)	15.63 (34½)	16.32 (36)	16.64 (36¾)
100–102 cm (39¼–49¼ in)	13.90 (30¾)	14.30 (31½)	15.06 (33¼)	15.81 (34¾)	16.54 (36½)	17.22 (38)	17.60 (38¾)	13.68 (30¼)	14.08 (31)	14.77 (32½)	15.46 (34)	16.25 (35¾)	16.96 (37½)	17.39 (38¼)
102–104 cm (40¼–41 in)	14.48 (32)	14.85 (32¾)	15.65 (34½)	16.45 (36¼)	17.18 (37¾)	17.87 (39½)	18.24 (40¼)							

* From Behrman RE, Vaughan VC III (eds): *Nelson Textbook of Pediatrics,* 13th ed. Philadelphia, WB Saunders Company, 1987, p 14.

† Data in Tables 1–4A and 1–4B are those of the National Center for Health Statistics (NCHS), Health Resources Administration, DHEW. Data of Table 1–4A are based on studies of The Fels Research Institute, Yellow Springs, Ohio; those of Table 1–4B are based on the Health Examination Surveys of the NCHS. For details see footnote to Table 1–1.

TABLE 1–4B. Weight by Stature*,†, Boys and Girls: Prepubescent

	Boys: Weight Percentiles, kg and (lb)							Girls: Weight Percentiles, kg and (lb)						
Stature	*5th*	*10th*	*25th*	*50th*	*75th*	*90th*	*95th*	*5th*	*10th*	*25th*	*50th*	*75th*	*90th*	*95th*
90–92 cm (35½–36¼ in)	11.70 (25¾)	11.97 (26½)	12.59 (27¾)	13.41 (29½)	14.35 (31¾)	15.25 (33½)	15.72 (34¾)	11.45 (25¼)	11.67 (25¾)	12.28 (27)	13.14 (29)	14.11 (31)	14.98 (33)	15.74 (34¾)
92–94 cm (36¼–37 in)	12.07 (26½)	12.36 (27¼)	13.03 (28¾)	13.89 (30½)	14.84 (32¾)	15.87 (35)	16.41 (36¼)	11.86 (26¼)	12.10 (26¾)	12.74 (28)	13.63 (30)	14.63 (32¼)	15.57 (34¼)	16.42 (36¼)
94–96 cm (37–37¾ in)	12.46 (27½)	12.77 (28¼)	13.49 (29¾)	14.38 (31¾)	15.34 (33¾)	16.45 (36¼)	17.06 (37½)	12.26 (27)	12.53 (27½)	13.21 (29)	14.12 (31¼)	15.14 (33½)	16.13 (35½)	17.05 (37½)
96–98 cm (37¾–38½ in)	12.87 (28¼)	13.21 (29)	13.98 (30¾)	14.89 (32¾)	15.87 (35)	17.01 (37½)	17.69 (39)	12.66 (28)	12.97 (28½)	13.70 (30¼)	14.62 (32¼)	15.66 (34½)	16.69 (36¾)	17.65 (39)
98–100 cm (38½–39¼ in)	13.31 (29¼)	13.67 (30¼)	14.48 (32)	15.43 (34)	16.41 (36¼)	17.56 (38¾)	18.29 (40¼)	13.06 (28¾)	13.42 (29½)	14.19 (31¼)	15.13 (33¼)	16.19 (35¾)	17.24 (38)	18.23 (40¼)
100–102 cm (39¼–40¼ in)	13.77 (30¼)	14.15 (31¼)	15.00 (33)	15.98 (35¼)	16.98 (37½)	18.11 (40)	18.89 (41¾)	13.48 (29¾)	13.88 (30½)	14.69 (32½)	15.65 (34½)	16.73 (37)	17.80 (39¼)	18.80 (41½)
102–104 cm (40¼–41 in)	14.25 (31½)	14.65 (32¼)	15.54 (34¼)	16.65 (36½)	17.57 (38¾)	18.67 (41¼)	19.50 (43)	13.91 (30¾)	14.36 (31¾)	15.21 (33½)	16.20 (35¾)	17.28 (38)	18.38 (40½)	19.38 (42¾)
104–106 cm (41–41¾ in)	14.76 (32½)	15.18 (33½)	16.10 (35½)	17.13 (37¾)	18.18 (40)	19.25 (42½)	20.12 (44¼)	14.36 (31¾)	14.85 (32¾)	15.75 (34¾)	16.75 (37)	17.86 (39¼)	18.98 (41¾)	19.98 (44)
106–108 cm (41¾–42½ in)	15.30 (33¾)	15.73 (34¾)	16.68 (36¾)	17.74 (39)	18.82 (41½)	19.86 (43¾)	20.76 (45¾)	14.84 (32¾)	15.37 (34)	16.30 (36)	17.33 (38¼)	18.46 (40¾)	19.62 (43¼)	20.61 (45½)
108–110 cm (42½–43¼ in)	15.85 (35)	16.31 (36)	17.28 (38)	18.37 (40½)	19.49 (43)	20.51 (45¼)	21.45 (47¼)	15.35 (33¾)	15.91 (35)	16.87 (37¼)	17.94 (39½)	19.09 (42)	20.30 (44¾)	21.29 (47)
110–112 cm (43¼–44 in)	16.43 (36¼)	16.91 (37¼)	17.90 (39½)	19.02 (42)	20.18 (44½)	21.22 (46¾)	22.18 (49)	15.90 (35)	16.48 (36¼)	17.47 (38½)	18.56 (41)	19.76 (43½)	21.03 (46¼)	22.03 (48½)
112–114 cm (44–45 in)	17.04 (37½)	17.53 (38¾)	18.54 (40¾)	19.70 (43½)	20.91 (46)	21.98 (48½)	22.98 (50¾)	16.48 (36¼)	17.09 (37¾)	18.08 (39¾)	19.22 (42¼)	20.47 (45¼)	21.81 (48)	22.84 (50¼)
114–116 cm (45–45¾ in)	17.66 (39)	18.18 (40)	19.20 (42¼)	20.39 (45)	21.66 (47¾)	22.82 (50¼)	23.85 (52½)	17.11 (37¾)	17.72 (39)	18.72 (41¼)	19.91 (44)	21.23 (46¾)	22.67 (50)	23.73 (52¼)

116–118 cm (45¾–46½ in)	18.32 (40½)	18.85 (41½)	19.89 (43¾)	21.11 (46½)	22.45 (49½)	23.73 (52¼)	24.80 (54¾)	17.77 (39¼)	18.40 (40½)	19.40 (42¾)	20.64 (45½)	22.04 (48½)	23.60 (52)	24.71 (54½)
118–120 cm (46½–47¼ in)	18.99 (41¾)	19.55 (43)	20.60 (45½)	21.85 (48¼)	23.28 (51¼)	24.73 (54½)	25.83 (57)	18.48 (40¾)	19.11 (42¼)	20.11 (44¼)	21.42 (47¼)	22.92 (50½)	24.62 (54¼)	25.81 (57)
120–122 cm (47¼–48 in)	19.70 (43½)	20.28 (44¾)	21.34 (47)	22.63 (50)	24.15 (53¼)	25.80 (57)	26.96 (59½)	19.22 (42¼)	19.85 (43¾)	20.87 (46)	22.25 (49)	23.88 (52¾)	25.73 (56¾)	27.03 (59½)
122–124 cm (48–48¾ in)	20.43 (45)	21.03 (46¼)	22.11 (48¾)	23.45 (51¾)	25.07 (55¼)	26.96 (59½)	28.18 (62¼)	19.99 (44)	20.64 (45½)	21.68 (47¾)	23.13 (51)	24.91 (55)	26.95 (59½)	28.37 (62½)
124–126 cm (48¾–49½ in)	21.20 (46¾)	21.82 (48)	22.92 (50½)	24.32 (53½)	26.05 (57½)	28.18 (62¼)	29.50 (65)	20.80 (45¾)	21.47 (47¼)	22.54 (49¾)	24.09 (53)	26.05 (57½)	28.27 (62¼)	29.87 (65¾)
126–128 cm (49½–50½ in)	21.99 (48½)	22.64 (50)	23.77 (52½)	25.24 (55¾)	27.10 (59¾)	29.48 (65)	30.92 (68¼)	21.65 (47¾)	22.34 (49¼)	23.47 (51¾)	25.11 (55¼)	27.28 (60¼)	29.71 (65½)	31.51 (69½)
128–130 cm (50½–51¾ in)	22.82 (50¼)	23.50 (51¾)	24.67 (54½)	26.22 (57¾)	28.21 (62¼)	30.86 (68)	32.44 (71½)	22.53 (49¾)	23.25 (51¼)	24.46 (54)	26.22 (57¾)	28.63 (63)	31.28 (69)	33.33 (73½)
130–132 cm (51¼–52 in)	23.69 (52¼)	24.59 (53¾)	25.62 (56½)	27.26 (60)	29.41 (64¾)	32.31 (71¼)	34.07 (75)	23.44 (51¾)	24.22 (53½)	25.52 (56¼)	27.40 (60½)	30.09 (66¼)	32.99 (72¾)	35.33 (78)
132–134 cm (52–52¾ in)	24.59 (54¼)	25.32 (55¾)	26.62 (58¾)	28.38 (62½)	30.68 (67¾)	33.82 (74½)	35.81 (79)	24.38 (53¾)	25.22 (55½)	26.66 (58¾)	28.68 (63¼)	31.68 (69¾)	34.84 (76¾)	37.53 (82¾)
134–136 cm (52¾–53½ in)	25.53 (56¼)	26.30 (58)	27.68 (61)	29.58 (65¼)	32.05 (70¾)	35.40 (78)	37.67 (83)	25.35 (56)	26.28 (58)	27.88 (61½)	30.06 (66¼)	33.41 (73¾)	36.84 (81¼)	39.93 (88)
136–138 cm (53½–54¼ in)	26.51 (58½)	27.32 (60¼)	28.80 (63½)	30.86 (68)	33.51 (74)	37.05 (81¾)	39.65 (87½)	26.34 (58)	27.39 (60½)	29.19 (64¼)	31.54 (69½)	35.29 (77¾)	39.01 (86)	42.54 (93¾)
138–140 cm (54½–55 in)	27.53 (60¾)	28.38 (62½)	29.99 (66)	32.23 (71)	35.08 (77¼)	38.77 (85½)	41.74 (92)							
140–142 cm (55–56 in)	28.59 (63)	29.48 (65)	31.25 (69)	33.70 (74¼)	36.75 (81)	40.55 (89½)	43.97 (97)							
142–144 cm (56–56¾ in)	29.70 (65½)	30.64 (67½)	32.58 (71¾)	35.27 (77¾)	38.54 (85)	42.39 (93½)	46.32 (102)							
144–146 cm (56¾–57½ in)	30.86 (68)	31.85 (70¼)	34.00 (75)	36.95 (81½)	40.45 (89¼)	44.29 (97¾)	48.80 (107½)							

* From Behrman RE, Vaughan VC III (eds): *Nelson Textbook of Pediatrics,* 13th ed. Philadelphia, WB Saunders Company, 1987, p 15.
† See footnote to Table 1–4A.

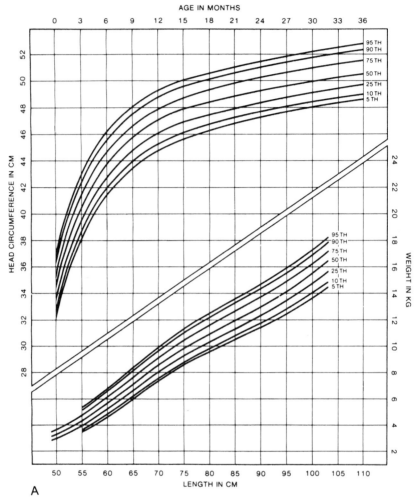

A

Figure 1–4A. *Top,* Head circumference by age percentiles for boys ages birth to 36 months. *Bottom,* Weight by length percentiles for boys ages birth to 36 months.
(From Hamill PVV, Drizd TA, Johnson CL, Reed RB, Roche AF, Moore WM: Physical growth: National Center for Health Statistics percentiles. Am J Clin Nutr 32:614, 1979.)

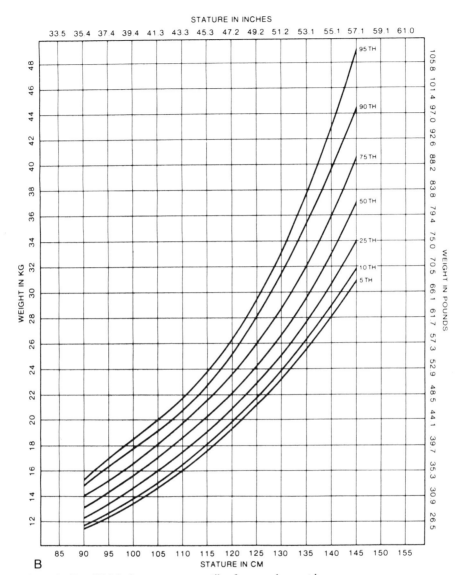

Figure 1–4B. Weight by stature percentiles for prepubescent boys. (From Hamill PVV, Drizd TA, Johnson CL, Reed RB, Roche AF, Moore WM: Physical growth: National Center for Health Statistics percentiles. Am J Clin Nutr 32:626, 1979.)

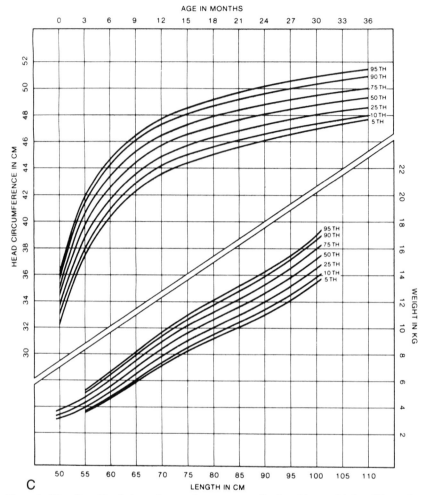

Figure 1–4C. *Top,* Head circumference by age percentiles for girls ages birth to 36 months. *Bottom,* Weight by length percentiles for girls ages birth to 36 months.
(From Hamill PVV, Drizd TA, Johnson CL, Reed RB, Roche AF, Moore WM: Physical growth: National Center for Health Statistics percentiles. Am J Clin Nutr 32:613, 1979.)

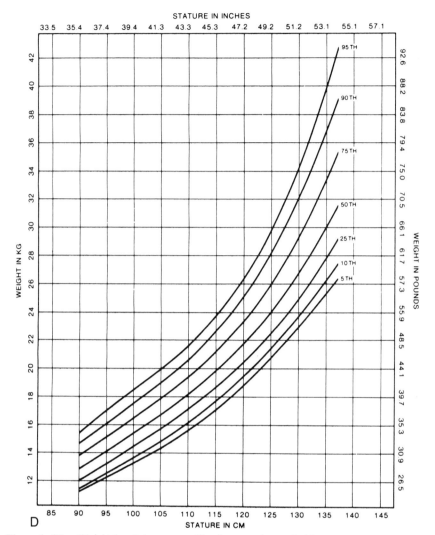

Figure 1–4D. Weight by stature percentiles for prepubescent girls. (From Hamill PVV, Drizd TA, Johnson CL, Reed RB, Roche AF, Moore WM: Physical growth: National Center for Health Statistics percentiles. Am J Clin Nutr 32:625, 1979.)

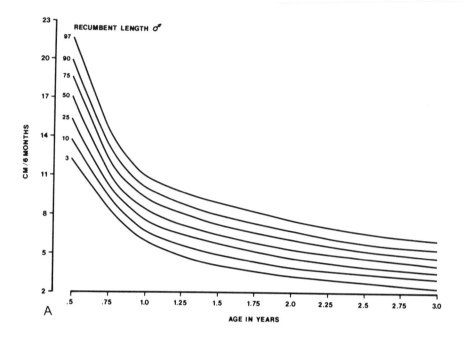

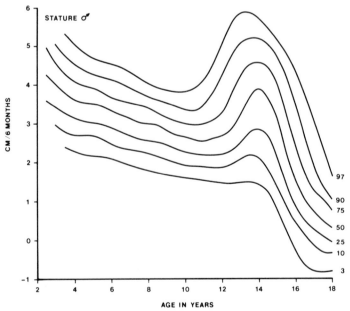

Figure 1–5A. *Top,* Percentiles for 6-month increments in recumbent length from birth to 3 years in boys. *Bottom,* Percentiles for 6-month increments in stature from 2 to 18 years in boys.
(From Roche AF, Himes JH: Incremental growth charts. Am J Clin Nutr 33:2046, 2047, 1980.)

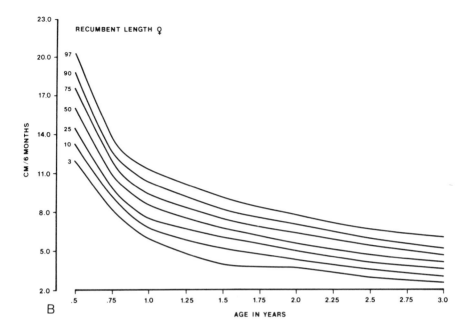

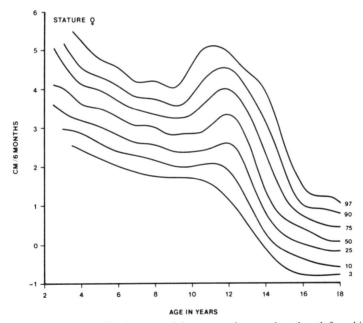

Figure 1–5B. *Top,* Percentiles for 6-month increments in recumbent length from birth to 3 years in girls. *Bottom,* Percentiles for 6-month increments in stature from 2 to 18 years in girls.
(From Roche AF, Himes JH: Incremental growth charts. Am J Clin Nutr 33:2047, 2048, 1980.)

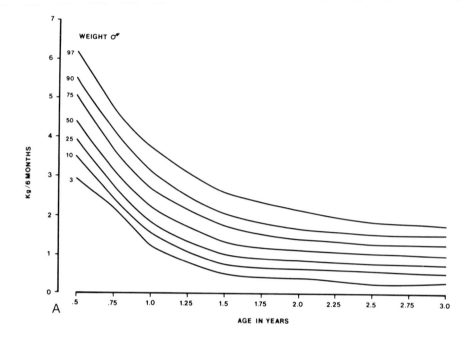

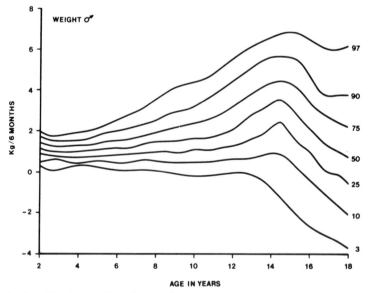

Figure 1–6A. *Top,* Percentiles of 6-month increments in weight from birth to 3 years in boys. *Bottom,* Percentiles of 6-month increments in weight from 2 to 18 years in boys. (From Roche AF, Himes JH: Incremental growth charts. Am J Clin Nutr 33:2043, 2044, 1980.)

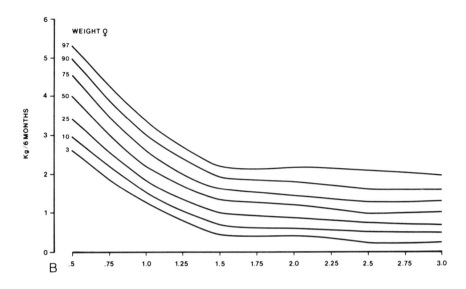

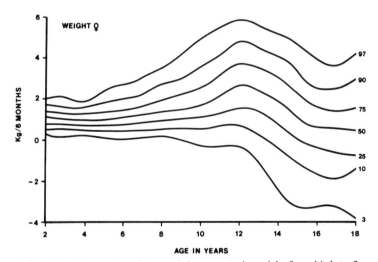

Figure 1–6B. *Top,* Percentiles of 6-month increments in weight from birth to 3 years in girls. *Bottom,* Percentiles of 6-month increments in weight from 2 to 18 years in girls. (From Roche AF, Himes JH: Incremental growth charts. Am J Clin Nutr 33:2044, 2045, 1980.)

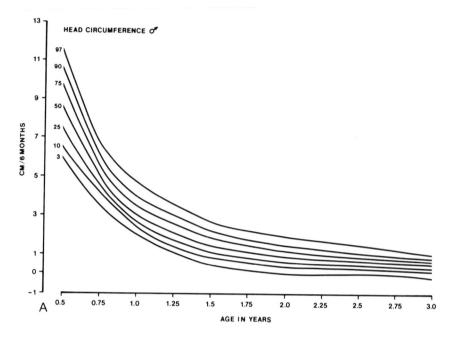

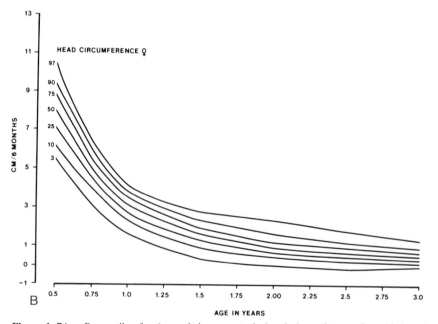

Figure 1–7A. Percentiles for 6-month increments in head circumference from birth to 3 years in boys. **B.** Percentiles for 6-month increments in head circumference from birth to 3 years in girls.
(From Roche AF, Himes JH: Incremental growth charts. Am J Clin Nutr 33:2049, 1980.)

in the late-maturing adolescent the peak may be lower and the total period of growth longer. It is unlikely that any adolescent will follow precisely the standard curve. The data of Roche and Himes were derived from longitudinal studies, but do not differentiate between early and late maturers. Tanner and Davies (1985) present data that do make this distinction.

The growth curves of each healthy child at his or her appropriate percentile point in the normal distribution are sufficiently smooth so that any substantial perturbation of a growth line is likely to reflect physical illness, nutritional disturbance, or psychosocial difficulties. The early recognition of such disturbances may depend heavily upon the care with which regular and accurate measurements are made.

It will be useful in assessing children's height to take into account family patterns. Tanner et al. (1970) have developed for children between the ages of 2 and 9 years standards for height appropriately adjusted for parental height. Wingerd et al. (1973) and Roche et al. (1975) also have indicated how an appraisal of the preadolescent child's height can take parental height into account.

Techniques of Physical Measurement

Since slight variations in technique may result in significant errors in the placement of children according to percentile rank, accurate measurement is essential to the reliable interpretation of growth data. Lohman et al. (1988) have described in detail the appropriate techniques for physical measurements.

Height

Recumbent length can be more accurately measured than standing height in children under the age of 5 years, after which measurement of standing height is generally more convenient. Recumbent length is measured as the child lies on a firm table that has a measuring stick at least 125 cm (50 in) long fastened along one edge. The soles of the feet are held firmly against a fixed upright placed at the zero mark. A movable upright bar that crosses the table above the head is brought firmly against the vertex. If recumbent length is used after 5 years of age, the value obtained may be increased by as much as 1 cm over that for standing height. The difference is greater for younger children, and cannot be relied upon at any age when precision is required.

Standing height is measured as the child stands erect, with heels, buttocks, upper part of the back, and occiput against a vertical upright. The heels should be close together, and the arms should hang naturally at the child's sides. The external auditory meatus and the lower border of the orbit should be in a plane parallel with the floor. A wooden headpiece having two faces at right angles may be placed firmly on the head against a 2-m (6-ft) measuring scale attached to the vertical surface against which the child is positioned.

During adolescence serial measurements of height should be plotted on a *height velocity* chart, in order that the acceleration of growth that should mark the pubertal growth spurt may be documented. The interpretation of findings should take into account the sex maturity rating of the patient in order to determine whether the velocity curve is consistent with that expected for the developmental stage. Standards have been prepared by Tanner and Davies (1985).

Body Composition

Measurements of skinfold thickness (SFT) provide a rough estimate of body fatness. Measurements at several sites may be helpful, since the distribution of fat may vary among individuals, and the measurements at multiple sites will increase the validity of an assessment. The side of the body chosen for measurement of SFT has varied among studies. Measurements of limb circumference may differ between the right and left sides, depending upon the handedness of the subject. The differences are generally inconsequential, but within any study the choice of side should be stated and consistent (Martorell et al., 1988).

Subscapular SFT is measured below the angle of the scapula. Triceps SFT is measured over the posterior surface of the triceps by calipers placed at a point halfway between the acromion and the olecranon as the arm hangs vertically in a relaxed fashion at the child's side. See Figure 8–7. Values obtained may be converted to estimates of body fat using tables such as those of Smith et al. (1978). See Table 8–5.

When evaluation of the body fat content is needed in the diagnosis or evaluation of obesity, the body mass index (BMI or Quetelet index) seems likely to give the most useful current indicator of obesity, inasmuch as the index is correlated closely with the likelihood of ill effects of increasing obesity upon health status. The BMI is calculated from height and weight in accordance with the formula:

$$BMI = weight (kg)/(height [m])^2$$

Values of BMI define obesity of various degrees: mild (BMI 25–29.9), moderate (BMI 30–40), or severe (BMI greater than 40).

Measurements of triceps SFT and arm circumference together can be used to derive estimates of body muscle mass, and have been used in nutritional assessments (Frisancho, 1981). Muscle mass is calculated from the relationship betwen mid-arm circumference (MCA) and an estimate of mid-arm muscle circumference (MAMC).

For example, for older children and adolescents MAMC is approximately equal to

$$MAMC (cm) - (SFT [cm] \times 3.14)$$

Measurements of MAC and MAMC, with adjustment for the probable contribution of bone, allow estimates of the cross-sectional areas of the arm that are devoted to fat or to muscle, and the relationship between these areas can generate estimates of total body fat of muscle.

Other measurements may provide estimates of body composition for research purposes; these include measurements of 24-hour excretion of creatinine or isotopic measurement of total body potassium as indices of lean body mass, measurement of body density by immersion and weighing in water as an index of body fat, or the use of radioisotopes in the assessment of other tissues or tissue components.

Sex Maturity Rating

Inspection of the stage of development of the patient's secondary sex characteristics is generally adequate to establish his or her sex maturity rating (SMR [Tanner stage]). Comparison is made with standards for those secondary sex characteristics that develop in predictable sequence in normal adolescents. Examination includes breasts and pubic hair in girls, and testes, penis, and pubic hair in boys. The criteria for determining SMR, and figures that show the corresponding physical findings, are given later (Figs. 8–12 to 8–14). Staging of testicular size is aided by use of an orchiometer.

Head Circumference

This measurement is particularly valuable in infants; it need not be taken routinely after 3 years of age. A tape measure is applied firmly over the glabella and supraorbital ridges anteriorly and that part of the occiput that gives the maximal circumference. Difficulties will sometimes arise when the head has an unusual or abnormal shape, as in hydrocephalus or with transient molding after vaginal delivery. Under these circumstances serial measurements of the changing size of the head may best be made by positioning the tape over whatever points on the forehead and occiput give *maximal* circumference. If cloth tapes are used, they may stretch with aging and will need to be checked frequently against wooden or metal standards.

Chest Circumference

Measurement is made in midrespiration at the level of the xiphoid cartilage or substernal notch, in a plane at right angles to the vertebral column. Measurement is made with the patient recumbent up to the age of 5 years, and standing thereafter.

Abdominal Circumference

This measurement is taken to 3 years only and will be of value principally in recognizing and following the course of chronic intestinal disturbances. Measurement is made in the plane of the umbilicus when the infant is recumbent.

Other Measurements

Studies of specific growth problems or dysplasias will often require other measurements, such as arm span or relationship of sitting height to length or standing height, pelvic breadth (in adolescence), and the like (see later in this chapter).

Variability in Body Proportions

Figure 1–8 depicts the general changes that take place in body proportions between fetal and adult life. The growth of the brain and head dominates fetal life and the early years; the head comprises one quarter of body length in the newborn infant versus about one eighth in the adult. The midpoint of the body is at the umbilicus in the newborn infant, whereas it will be at the symphysis pubis in the adult. The brain and cranial cavity approach adult sizes much more rapidly than the face or the length of the legs. With the onset of puberty, on the other hand, the early acceleration of skeletal growth is more emphatic in the extremities than in the central skeleton.

The relative preponderance of early growth at the head end of the body (with corresponding early elaboration of cerebral function and later development of the trunk and extremities), has been termed the *cephalocaudad progression*. Besides these changes, there are *individual* differences that express innate growth potential and environmental influences. These variations in body forms of normal persons may be termed *differences in physique*.

Somatotype connotes the development of a particular physique: ectomorphic, mesomorphic, or endomorphic. The ectomorph is characterized by relative linearity, light bone structure, and small mass in respect to body length. The endomorph is characterized by relatively stocky build, with large amounts of soft tissue. The physique of the mesomorph is in between, and is often relatively muscular. Functional features of growth (e.g., late occurrence of menarche in ectomorphs), including some psychologic attributes (e.g., relatively high social popularity of mesomorphs), may reflect somatotype.

Somatotype may be evident in early childhood or become clear only with the termination of the growth period. Somatotype does not seem closely related to the ultimate height or weight achieved, but the endo-

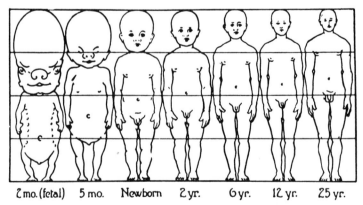

2 mo.(fetal)　5 mo.　Newborn　2 yr.　6 yr.　12 yr.　25 yr.

Figure 1–8. Changes in body proportions from second fetal month to adulthood. (From Robbins WJ, Brody S, Hogan AG, Jackson CM, Greene CW: *Growth*. New Haven, CT, Yale University Press, 1928.)

morph appears to mature earlier than the ectomorph. As a result of this early maturation the endomorphic child may have a tendency to be taller than the ectomorphic one in late childhood, with the differences being reduced as the ectomorph completes growth.

Other variations in body proportions depend on different rates of growth of body parts. Alterations in proportionate sizes of trunk, extremities, and head are characteristic of certain growth disturbances and may give insight into the underlying pathophysiologic processes (e.g., in patients with achondroplasia or other skeletal dysplasias, such as Marfan syndrome). Helpful measurements include sitting and standing heights, arm span, body weight, and head circumference. Normally, sitting height represents about 70 per cent of length in the newborn infant, 57 per cent at 3 years, and about 52 per cent at the time of menarche (SMR [Tanner stage] 3) in girls and at about SMR 4 in boys. There is then a slight increase of 1 to 2 percentage points, as the trunk has some growth after the limbs have ceased growing. Ethnic differences may be conspicuous in these measurements (e.g., between blacks and Caucasians, or among the pygmies, Masai, or Hottentots).

Figure 1–9 illustrates the proportionate rates of growth for several body

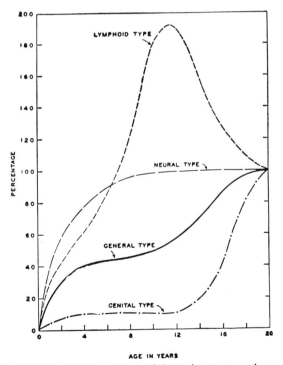

Figure 1–9. Main types of postnatal growth of the various parts and organs of the body. (After Scammon: The measurement of the body in childhood. In Harris et al: *The Measurement of Man*. Minneapolis, University of Minnesota Press, 1930.)
(From Behrman RE, Vaughan VC III (eds): *Nelson Textbook of Pediatrics*, 13th ed. Philadelphia, WB Saunders Company, 1987, p 28.)

systems: the distinctive variations in pattern are often closely correlated with function. The patterns shown have been designated as general, lymphoid, neural, and genital. There may be variations within patterns: whereas the ovary and testis follow the designated genital pattern, the uterus and adrenals are relatively large at birth, and show involution in the early weeks of life.

As Figure 1–9 indicates, the absolute amount of lymphoid tissue in the school-aged child may exceed that in the normal adult, with involution occurring at puberty. The weight of the thymus is labile in childhood, decreasing rapidly during illness. It tends to follow the general pattern of growth during the first 5 years of life, with involution at adolescence. The

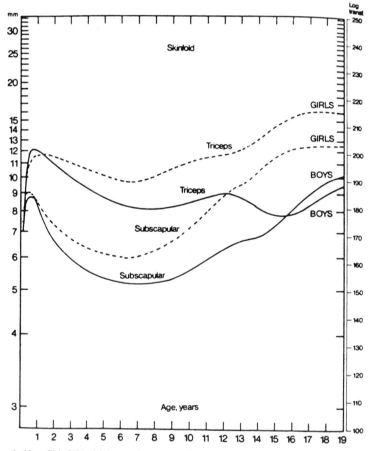

Figure 1–10. Skinfold thickness by age and sex, as measured by Harpenden skinfold calipers over triceps and under scapula. Scale is in mm on the left and logarithmic transformation units on the right side. The lines shown are the 50th percentiles for British children.

From Tanner JM (1978), p. 18. The data generating these curves are those of Tanner and Whitehouse (1975).

spleen appears to follow the lymphoid pattern, and the liver the general pattern. Skeletal muscle follows the general pattern, with a pubertal growth spurt in males, but may be slow to achieve its ultimate mass. Cardiac muscle is initially proportionately large in relation to body size and after the neonatal period follows the general growth curve.

The proportionate mass of subcutaneous tissue is greatest (about 25 per cent of body mass) at about 9 months; it decreases steadily to about 6 years, when the increase begins that presages the "fat spurt" of preadolescence, at which time sex differences in body composition become more apparent (Fig. 1–10). The usefulness of SFT as a measure of fat content diminishes somewhat during adolescence. The ratio of total body water to body weight may be a more accurate measurement of body fat, correlating at about 0.62 with SFT. In office practice, however, measurements of triceps and subscapular SFT will generally suffice, and can be compared with standards such as those prepared by Tanner and Whitehouse (1976).

Evaluation of Osseous Maturation

A general index of growth status is given by the bone age, as determined from roentgenograms. Bone age is based on 1) the number and size of epiphyseal centers; 2) the size, shape, density, and sharpness of outline of the ends of bones; and 3) the distance separating the epiphyseal center and the zone of provisional calcification or the degree of fusion between these two elements. Examination of the hand and wrist is useful at all ages; useful information can also be derived from the leg (knee), especially in early infancy.

Ossification of the fetal skeleton begins at about the fifth month and makes increasing demands upon the maternal supply of bone-forming substances. Ossification appears first in the clavicles and membranous bones of the skull, and follows rapidly in long bones and spine. The distal femoral and proximal tibial epiphyses are usually ossified in the normal full-term infant; failure of their ossification in the full-term newborn infant will suggest the possibility of hypothyroidism. The fusion of the humeral capitellum with the shaft is said to mark the end of the period of most rapid growth in girls and to predict menarche within a year, as does appearance of sesamoid bones of the thumbs and closure of the epiphysis of the iliac crest.

Tables 1–5 and 1–6 show expected times of appearance and fusion of various ossification centers, with their normal variation. Since girls are more advanced than boys in skeletal development at all ages, separate standards are necessary. Variability is less for girls than for boys, especially in later childhood. In boys the standard deviation of bone age around chronologic age is about 2 months in the first year of life; it increases to 4 months during the second year, to 6 months during the third year, and to 10 months by the seventh year. Thereafter, for the rest of the growth period, the standard deviation is about 12 to 15 months. Larger standard deviations during adolescence reflect the different rates of pu-

TABLE 1–5. Time of Appearance in Roentgenograms of Centers of Ossification in Infancy and Childhood[*][†]

Bones and Epiphyseal Centers	Boys—Age at Appearance Mean ± Std. Deviation ‡	Girls—Age at Appearance Mean ± Std. Deviation ‡
Humerus, head	3 wk	3 wk
Carpal bones		
Capitate	2 mo ± 2 mo	2 mo ± 2 mo
Hamate	3 mo ± 2 mo	2 mo ± 2 mo
(Triangular) §	(30 mo ± 16 mo)	(21 mo ± 14 mo)
(Lunate) §	(42 mo ± 19 mo)	(34 mo ± 13 mo)
(Trapezium) §	(67 mo ± 19 mo)	(47 mo ± 14 mo)
(Trapezoid) §	(69 mo ± 15 mo)	(49 mo ± 12 mo)
(Scaphoid) §	(66 mo ± 15 mo)	(51 mo ± 12 mo)
(Pisiform) §	(no standards available)	(no standards available)
Metacarpal bones		
II	18 mo ± 5 mo	12 mo ± 3 mo
III	20 mo ± 5 mo	13 mo ± 3 mo
IV	23 mo ± 6 mo	15 mo ± 4 mo
V	26 mo ± 7 mo	16 mo ± 5 mo
I	32 mo ± 9 mo	18 mo ± 5 mo

Fingers (epiphyses)		
Proximal phalanx, 3rd finger	16 mo ± 4 mo	10 mo ± 3 mo
Proximal phalanx, 2nd finger	16 mo ± 4 mo	11 mo ± 3 mo
Proximal phalanx, 4th finger	17 mo ± 5 mo	11 mo ± 3 mo
Distal phalanx, 1st finger	19 mo ± 7 mo	12 mo ± 4 mo
Proximal phalanx, 5th finger	21 mo ± 5 mo	14 mo ± 4 mo
Middle phalanx, 3rd finger	24 mo ± 6 mo	15 mo ± 5 mo
Middle phalanx, 4th finger	24 mo ± 6 mo	15 mo ± 5 mo
Middle phalanx, 2nd finger	26 mo ± 6 mo	16 mo ± 5 mo
Distal phalanx, 3rd finger	28 mo ± 6 mo	18 mo ± 4 mo
Distal phalanx, 4th finger	28 mo ± 6 mo	18 mo ± 5 mo
Proximal phalanx, 1st finger	32 mo ± 7 mo	20 mo ± 5 mo
Distal phalanx, 5th finger	37 mo ± 9 mo	23 mo ± 6 mo
Distal phalanx, 2nd finger	37 mo ± 8 mo	23 mo ± 6 mo
Middle phalanx, 5th finger	39 mo ± 10 mo	22 mo ± 7 mo
Sesamoid (adductor pollicis)	152 mo ± 18 mo	121 mo ± 13 mo

Hip and knee		
Femur, distal	Usually present at birth	Usually present at birth
Tibia, proximal	Usually present at birth	Usually present at birth
Femur, head	4 mo ± 2 mo	4 mo ± 2 mo
Patella	46 mo ± 11 mo	29 mo ± 7 mo

Foot and ankle ‖

* From Behrman RE, Vaughan VC III (eds): *Nelson Textbook of Pediatrics*, 13th ed. Philadelphia, WB Saunders Company, 1987, p 29.

† The norms in Tables 1–5 and 1–6 present a composite of published data from the Fels Research Institute, Yellow Springs, Ohio (Pyle SI, Sontag L. Am J Roentgenol Vol 49, 1943), and unpublished data from the Brush Foundation, Case Western Reserve University, Cleveland, Ohio, and the Harvard School of Public Health, Boston, Massachusetts. Compiled by Lieb, Buehl, and Pyle.

‡ To nearest month.

§ Except for the capitate and hamate bones, the variability of carpal centers is too great to make them very useful clinically.

‖ Standards for the foot are available, but normal variation is wide, including some familial variants, so that this area is of little clinical use.

TABLE 1–6. Modal Age at Onset and Completion of Fusion in Skeletal Areas in Adolescence[*,†]

Boys—Modal Age Between	Area	Girls—Modal Age Between
	Elbow	
13.0–13.5 yr	Onset in humerus	11.0–11.5 yr
15.0–15.5	Complete in ulna	12.5–13.0
	Foot and ankle	
14.0–14.5	Onset in great toe	12.5–13.0
15.5–16	Complete in tibia, fibula	14.0–14.5
	Hand and wrist	
15.0–15.5	Onset in distal phalanges	13.0–13.5
17.5–18.0	Complete in radius	16.0–16.5
	Knee	
15.0–15.5	Onset in tibial tuberosity	13.5–14.0
17.5–18.0	Complete in fibula	16.0–16.5
	Hip and pelvis	
15.5–16.0	Onset in greater trochanter	14.0–14.5
after 18.0	Complete in symphysis	17.5–18.0
	Shoulder and clavicle	
15.5–16.0	Onset in greater tubercle of humerus	14.0–14.5
after 18.0	Complete in clavicle	17.5–18.0

[*] From Behrman RE, Vaughan VC III (eds): *Nelson Textbook of Pediatrics*, 13th ed. Philadelphia, WB Saunders Company, 1987, p 30.
[†] See footnote to Table 1–5.

bertal maturation, with bone age corresponding more closely to SMR than to chronologic age (see also Fig. 9–2).

Recent technologic advances have made it possible more accurately to assess bone density. Previously thought to peak during the fourth or fifth decade of life, it is now apparent that the peak of bone density occurs between late adolescence and the early twenties. The period of maximal accretion of bone mass appears to be during the pubertal growth spurt (Gilsanz et al., 1988). The factors responsible for the phenomenon are multiple and continue to be investigated. Studies have focused almost exclusively on adults and little is yet known about the developmental issues. Calcium and fluoride intake, general nutritional status, levels of growth hormone, somatomedin-C, estradiol, androgens, and genetic factors all appear to affect bone density, whereas, in contrast with earlier studies, aerobic exercise does not. Studies of young adolescent females with anorexia nervosa have shown that two-thirds have severe osteoporosis (Bachrach et al., 1989).

Evaluation of Dental Development

Calcification of teeth begins in about the seventh month of fetal life, and involves deciduous teeth until shortly before term, when calcification begins in the permanent teeth that will be the first to erupt.

Table 1–7 lists the times of eruption of the deciduous and permanent teeth. Delay in eruption of deciduous teeth occurs in hypothyroidism and in other nutritional and growth disturbances, but the normal variability in eruption prevents such delay from being useful as an indicator of growth disorder. In some families the children have conspicuously early or late dentition without other signs of retardation or acceleration of growth.

The first permanent teeth to erupt are the 6-year molars; they may be mistaken for deciduous teeth. The first permanent molars stabilize the dental arch and have a great deal to do with the ultimate shape of the jaw and the orderly arrangement of teeth. Caries or other defects in them should receive prompt attention; extraction of these teeth should be avoided.

Nutritional disorders (protein-calorie malnutrition or rickets) or certain medications (such as tetracyclines) or prolonged illness in infancy may interfere with calcification of deciduous and permanent teeth. Such disturbances, if temporary, may leave defects in the enamel ranging from a line of small pits across the tooth to a broader band of hypoplasia. It is possible at times to date a nutritional disturbance in accordance with the location of these pits or bands.

The formation of healthy tooth structure is fostered by a diet adequate in protein, calcium, phosphate, and vitamins, especially C and D, and depends further upon an adequate supply of thyroid hormone. Resistance to dental caries is increased when the diet contains optimal amounts of fluoride.

TABLE 1-7. Chronology of Human Dentition*†

PRIMARY OR DECIDUOUS TEETH

	Calcification		Eruption		Shedding	
	Begins at	Complete at	Maxillary	Mandibular	Maxillary	Mandibular
Central incisors	5th fetal mo	18–24 mo	6–8 mo	5–7 mo	7–8 yr	6–7 yr
Lateral incisors	5th fetal mo	18–24 mo	8–11 mo	7–10 mo	8–9 yr	7–8 yr
Cuspids (canines)	6th fetal mo	30–36 mo	16–20 mo	16–20 mo	11–12 yr	9–11 yr
First molars	5th fetal mo	24–30 mo	10–16 mo	10–16 mo	10–11 yr	10–12 yr
Second molars	6th fetal mo	36 mo	20–30 mo	20–30 mo	10–12 yr	11–13 yr

Secondary or Permanent Teeth

	Calcification		Eruption	
	Begins at	Complete at	Maxillary	Mandibular
Central incisors	3–4 mo	9–10 yr	7–8 yr	6–7 yr
Lateral incisors	Max., 10–12 mo; Mand., 3–4 mo	10–11 yr	8–9 yr	7–8 yr
Cuspids (canines)	4–5 mo	12–15 yr	11–12 yr	9–11 yr
First premolars (bicuspids)	18–21 mo	12–13 yr	10–11 yr	10–12 yr
Second premolars (bicuspids)	24–30 mo	12–14 yr	10–12 yr	11–13 yr
First molars	Birth	9–10 yr	6–7 yr	6–7 yr
Second molars	30–36 mo	14–16 yr	12–13 yr	12–13 yr
Third molars	Max., 7–9 yr; Mand., 8–10 yr	18–25 yr	17–22 yr	17–22 yr

* From Behrman RE, Vaughan VC III (eds): *Nelson Textbook of Pediatrics,* 13th ed. Philadelphia, WB Saunders Company, 1987, p 30.
† Adapted from chart prepared by PK Losch, Harvard School of Dental Medicine, who provided the data for this chart.

Other Physical and Physiologic Aspects of Growth and Development

Growth in the Respiratory Tract

The status of the sinuses in the newborn infant is described on page 146. The sphenoidal sinuses appear by about the age of 3 years, and the frontal sinuses between 3 and 7 years of age. Figure 1–11 shows the changes in respiratory rate with age, with 10th and 90th percentile lines, and shows how the rates differ for boys and girls, with the distinctive changes at adolescence.

Growth in the Cardiovascular System

The heart is relatively large at birth, and there is a pubertal growth spurt in heart size that parallels that of the body in general. As a result, there may need to be different standards for radiologic interpretation of cardiac diameter in adolescents. Figure 1–12 shows how the pulse rate varies with age, and Figure 1–13 the changes in blood pressure with age and growth status. It is seen that the systolic pressure for boys continues to advance with age after that of girls has begun to reach an asymptote, likely reflecting the earlier completion of maturation. The levels of serum urate increase and those of high-density lipoprotein cholesterol decrease with advancing age in male adolescents.

Metabolism and Nutrition

The metabolic and nutritional needs of fetus, infant, child, and adolescent are based upon the requirements for growth, for activity, and (after birth) for the maintenance of body temperature. Energy requirements are generally measured in kilocalories (kcal), a calorie being the amount of heat needed at standard atmospheric pressure to raise the temperature of 1 g of water 1 degree Celsius. The kilocalorie has replaced the widely used "nutritional" calorie (Cal or 1000 kcal) in modern scientific references.

Caloric needs increase with growth in size but bear relatively constant relationship to the area of the body surface, which provides the principal route for the radiant and convective loss of heat and is as closely correlated with the body's mass of metabolically active tissue as any other simple measurement. Measurements of body surface that correspond to

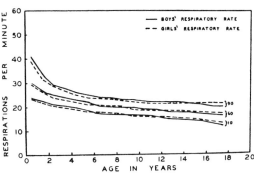

Figure 1–11. Respiratory rates in infants and children. (From Behrman RE, Vaughan VC III (eds): *Nelson Textbook of Pediatrics,* 13th ed. Philadelphia, WB Saunders Company, 1987, p 31.)

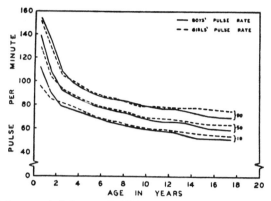

Figure 1–12. Pulse rates in infants and children.
(From Behrman RE, Vaughan VC III (eds): *Nelson Textbook of Pediatrics,* 13th ed. Philadelphia, WB Saunders Company, 1987, p 31.)

given heights and weights are available, and estimates can be obtained from nomograms. Cruder estimates from weight alone can be made for children whose physique is normal; such estimates are given by the simple formulas in Table 1–8.

Basal energy requirement is that needed for the maintenance of body heat in the fasting and resting state in an approximately neutral thermal environment. The apportionment of calories among basal needs, activity, growth, and other needs is indicated in Figure 1–14. Caloric need in proportion to body weight is highest in the smallest infants, in whom the ratio of surface area to weight is highest. When referred to body surface, however, basal caloric needs appear to be somewhat lower in premature infants than in full-term ones. They increase during the first year of life from about 30 kcal/m^2/hr to about 50 by the second year, with a subsequent fall to adult levels of 35 to 40 kcal/m^2/hr. The rate of fall is slowed or may be reversed during prepubertal or adolescent years by the need for additional energy to support the increase in growth rate that occurs at this time, when, at the peak of the height velocity curve, males may need 3000 kcal/day and females 2500 kcal/day. This increased need for calories is matched by increased need for other nutritional factors, including iron for

TABLE 1–8. Approximation of Surface Area (m^2) to Weight (kg)[*,†]

Weight Range	Approximate Surface Area
1 to 5 kg	m^2 = (0.05 × kg) + 0.05
6 to 10 kg	m^2 = (0.04 × kg) + 0.10
11 to 20 kg	m^2 = (0.03 × kg) + 0.20
21 to 40 kg	m^2 = (0.02 × kg) + 0.40

[*] From Behrman RE, Vaughan VC III (eds): *Nelson Textbook of Pediatrics,* 13th ed. Philadelphia, WB Saunders Company, 1987, p 31.
[†] The figures 5, 10, 20, and 40 are given in italics to indicate a simple mnemonic. The formula m^2 = (0.02 × kg) + 40 is reasonably accurate from 21 to 70 kg.

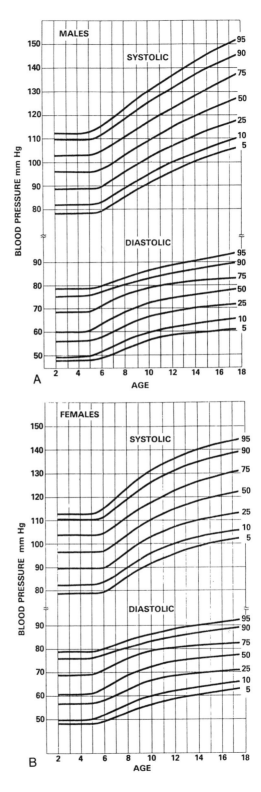

Figure 1–13A. Percentiles of blood pressure in seated males. **B.** Percentiles of blood pressure in seated females.
(From Report of the Task Force on Blood Pressure Control in Children, National Heart, Lung and Blood Institute. Pediatrics (suppl) 59:803, 1987. Copyright American Academy of Pediatrics.)

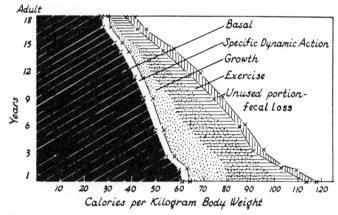

Figure 1–14. Total daily expenditure of calories with approximate distribution among individual factors in relation to age and weight. (Calorie = large calorie = 1 kcal = 1 cal.) (From Behrman RE, Vaughan VC III (eds): *Nelson Textbook of Pediatrics,* 13th ed. Philadelphia, WB Saunders Company, 1987, p 115.)

both sexes (for muscular development in males and to replace menstrual blood loss in postmenarchal females).

Many body functions and needs are intimately related to the level of expenditure of energy. Among these are the requirements for water to replace obligate insensible loss through humidification of inspired air and for control of body temperature through insensible loss through the skin. The daily requirement of water to replace insensible loss amounts to about 40 mL for each 100 kcal produced in energy.

Additional losses of water occur through sweating and the production of urine. The amount of water needed for production of urine will depend

TABLE 1–9. Water Requirements*

URINE SPECIFIC GRAVITY	INFANT—3 KG 300 CALORIES[†] INTAKE			ADULT—70 KG 3000 CALORIES[†] INTAKE		
	Water Intake			Water Intake		
	mL	$mL/100$ $kcal$	$mL/$ kg	mL	$mL/100$ $kcal$	$mL/$ kg
1.005	650	217	220	6300	210	90
1.015	339	113	116	3180	106	45
1.020	300	100	100	2790	93	40
1.030	264	88	91	2430	81	35

* From Behrman RE, Vaughan VC III (eds): *Nelson Textbook of Pediatrics,* 13th ed. Philadelphia, WB Saunders Company, 1987, p 115.
† In this sense Calorie = large calorie = 1 kcal = 1 Cal (see text).

TABLE 1−10. Range of Average Water Requirements of Children at Different Ages Under Ordinary Conditions*

AGE	AVERAGE BODY WEIGHT (KG)	TOTAL WATER IN 24 HOURS (ML)	WATER PER KG BODY WT IN 24 HOURS (ML)
3 days	3.0	250–300	80–100
10 days	3.2	400–500	125–150
3 mo	5.4	750–850	140–160
6 mo	7.3	950–1100	130–155
9 mo	8.6	1100–1250	125–145
1 yr	9.5	1150–1300	120–135
2 yr	11.8	1350–1500	115–125
4 yr	16.2	1600–1800	100–110
6 yr	20.0	1800–2000	90–100
10 yr	28.7	2000–2500	70–85
14 yr	45.0	2200–2700	50–60
18 yr	54.0	2200–2700	40–50

* From Behrman RE, Vaughan VC III (eds): *Nelson Textbook of Pediatrics,* 13th ed. Philadelphia, WB Saunders Company, 1987, p 115.

upon the nature of the diet, and especially upon the dietary content of protein and salt.

Water requirement depends also upon body temperature, many metabolic processes being accelerated by elevations of temperature, the acceleration being approximately 10 per cent for each degree Celsius of elevation. Tables 1–9 and 1–10 show how these considerations are reflected in caloric and water requirements at various ages and under various conditions.

Nutritional disturbances may be acute or chronic. *Acute* disturbances involve water and electrolytes, and may develop over periods of hours or days in response to diarrhea or vomiting, or to other abnormal losses of water, as in sweat (e.g., cystic fibrosis) or with renal disease (e.g., diabetes insipidus). *Chronic* derangements develop over longer periods (days, months, or years), depending upon the degree of deficiency in diet or the substances involved. Both the energy and the structural elements embodied in carbohydrates, fats, proteins, vitamins, minerals, and trace elements are required for growth. These needs are met when a balanced diet of sufficient caloric content is made available to the fetus through the mother or to the infant or child through an appropriate nutritional regimen. Adolescent growth is particularly susceptible to impairment by dietary fads or by behaviors that deprive the youngster of essential calories or other nutritional substances (see pp. 277–281).

Immunologic Development

Development of the immune system begins early in fetal life, but it is normally substantially inactive until birth. During fetal life transplacental transfer of maternal immunoglobulin G (IgG) to the fetus is aided by an active transport mechanism, with the result that the newborn infant has a higher level of IgG than does the mother. These IgG antibodies confer passive immunity upon the newborn infant against many viral and some bacterial infections.

Very little or no maternal IgM, IgA, or IgE reaches the fetus. The fetal system can, however, be stimulated to activity by food proteins or other substances that cross the placenta, or by infection of the placenta or of the fetus by organisms originating in maternal blood. When the fetus is actively infected, the antibody response typically involves first the production of IgM antibodies; accordingly, a significant titer of IgM antibody in cord blood is evidence of intrauterine infection.

When umbilical cord blood has a significant titer of IgE, the likelihood is increased that the infant may develop food allergies. These IgE antibodies are presumptively of fetal origin, their production having been stimulated by the transfer across the placenta of food proteins.

Immunoglobulins G, M, A, and E are produced actively by the infant, beginning with the neonatal period. The infant's high titer of maternal IgG falls as endogenous production of IgG rises. The infant's serum level of total IgG (waning maternal plus new endogenous) falls to a low point at about 3 months, after which all Ig levels rise toward adult levels, with the adult range being generally approached by about 2 years (Table 1–11). There is a secondary peak in IgE level in adolescence; its significance is unknown.

Both humoral and cellular immunity increase in the infant as a result of exposure to exogenous antigens. Aside from the protection received from maternal IgG, however, the infant is relatively unprotected against infection. Protection against some viral illnesses is effective so long as the mother has had the illness or been immunized against it, and conveys antibody against it to the fetus.

The neonate is more susceptible at this age than later to bacterial infection by relatively normal flora (e.g., staphylococci or *Escherichia coli*) or by pathogens that have relatively low virulence in later life (e.g., group B streptococci or *Listeria*). Infection of the newborn infant is, moreover, often highly invasive, with septicemia and meningitis relatively common. This enhanced invasiveness may be as true for normal flora and organisms of low virulence as for more aggressive organisms such as *Streptococcus pyogenes* or *Haemophilus influenzae*. Invasiveness may be encouraged not only by relatively poor humoral and cellular immune protection but by sluggish responses of other normal defense mechanisms, such as leukocytosis, leukotaxis, phagocytosis, and the like.

For some relatively common and often recurrent bacterial infections, such as those due to *S. pyogenes* and *S. pneumoniae,* the invasiveness of early infancy is followed by a rather slow change with age in the nature of the body's response. For these organisms each infection confers a degree of immunity against the specific serotype involved. At the same time, a more general increase in resistance to the organism develops, which in the case of streptococcal or pneumococcal infection is responsible for increasing localization and local intensification of the infectious process. For example, pneumococcal pneumonia in infancy takes the form of bronchopneumonia, a relatively diffuse process; in the adult, lobar pneumonia is more typical, and consists of a more sharply contained infection.

TABLE 1–11. Levels of Immunoglobulins[*][†]

	IgG (mg/dL)	IgM (mg/dL)	IgA (mg/dL)	IgE (IU/mL)
Serum				
Newborn	1031 ± 200[‡]	11 ± 5	2 ± 3	$0-7.5$
6 mo	427 ± 186	43 ± 17	28 ± 18	—
12 mo	661 ± 219	54 ± 23	37 ± 18	—
24 mo	762 ± 209	58 ± 23	50 ± 24	137 ± 147
8 yr	923 ± 256	65 ± 25	124 ± 45	251 ± 167
16 yr	946 ± 124	59 ± 20	148 ± 63	330 ± 212
Adult	1158 ± 305	99 ± 27	200 ± 61	200[§]
Secretions				
Colostrum	10	61	1234	—
Stimulated parotid saliva	0.036	0.043	3.9	—
Unstimulated whole saliva	4.86	0.55	30.4	—
Jejunal fluid	34	70	—	—
Seminal fluid	510	90	116	—
Cerebrospinal fluid				
Normal	3 ± 1	0	0.4 ± 0.5	—
Purulent infection	9	4	4	—
Viral infection	4	0.5	1	—

* From Behrman RE, Vaughan VC III (eds): *Nelson Textbook of Pediatrics*, 13th ed. Philadelphia, WB Saunders Company, 1987, p 456.
† Adapted from Clin Immunobiol 3:13, 1976.
‡ Mean ± 1 standard deviation.
§ Values up to 800 IU/mL are normal.

These changes are particularly well documented in the case of infections due to *S. pyogenes,* and have given rise to the concept of *streptococcosis.* In early infancy (under the age of about 6 months), streptococcosis is often a relatively indolent infection, with low-grade fever and rhinorrhea and little other indication of illness. Young children may come more often to medical attention because of higher fever, sore throat, and vomiting, and are prone to have occasional pyogenic or invasive complications (otitis media, suppurative cervical adenitis, septicemia, or meningitis). In older children and adults, streptococcosis is more likely to be sharply confined to the tonsils or pharynx, with local exudate, and with nonsuppurative cervical adenitis. In older children, a distinctive feature of streptococcosis is the frequency of nonsuppurative complications remote from the site of infection (acute glomerulonephritis, rheumatic fever, etc.). The occurrence of these complications may depend upon host factors besides the state of the immune system or humoral or cellular response to previous streptococcal infection. Genetic factors may play a role.

Other changes with age in the body's response to infection have been less well studied. What we see with differences in age may depend upon many factors, including immunologic, epidemiologic, demographic, sociocultural, and climatic influences. In any case, the integrity of the normal immune system depends upon opportunities for normal exposure to antigens, as foods or other substances (vaccines, for example), or as constituents of pathogenic organisms. It depends as well upon nutritional status, and upon age as a correlate of level of development. Adolescents, for example, have heightened reactivity to some infections (e.g., measles and poliomyelitis) that may be better tolerated by younger children, and they may be at particular risk for reactivation of childhood tuberculosis during pubertal growth. The reasons are not known.

Immunization attempts to create resistance to infection by systematic exposure to the antigens of infectious agents, in the form of attenuated live organisms, killed organisms, or their antigenic products. Recommendations for immunization schedules, revised from time to time, are issued by the American Academy of Pediatrics (*Red Book,* 1988) and by the Centers for Disease Control (CDC). Revisions are made in response to new knowledge of the natural history of each infection, the relationship of immunity to primary immunization or to booster injections, and the occurrence of the infection in the community.

For some infectious organisms (e.g., BCG [Calmette-Guérin bacillus], poliovirus, pertussis, or tetanus) immunization is effective at birth or soon thereafter. For others, against which the infant has received maternal IgG, the procedure must be deferred until maternal antibody has been exhausted and the immunizing agent can reach the infant's antibody-producing cells in sufficient quantity. For measles, this need for delay extends to the end of the first year for many infants. For this reason, immunization against measles is normally deferred until 15 months of age, when it is achieved with a vaccine that immunizes also against mumps and rubella.

Current recommendations for immunization of infants, children, and adolescents are given in Table 8–23.

Developmental Aspects of Drug Metabolism

The reaction of the growing human to drugs varies with age, beginning in fetal life, when some drugs will be teratogenic at certain periods of differentiation of the embryo, or may otherwise adversely affect fetal growth and development. Reactions of the fetus to maternal smoking may involve both carbon monoxide and nicotine, as well as other products of combustion to which the fetus is exposed. (The carbon monoxide may be primarily responsible for the growth retardation that occurs in the offspring of mothers who smoke.) Late in pregnancy the fetus may become addicted to opiates, to cocaine, to phenobarbital, or to alcohol, with behavioral changes in the neonatal period as a result of drug withdrawal.

Changes in metabolic activity with age may significantly alter the response to drugs, and require adjustments of dosage. This is particularly evident with respect to administration of drugs to newborn infants, in whom variability in rates of metabolism of drugs may reflect the rapidity with which the infant acquires normal activity in metabolic pathways that are at birth not yet or only incompletely activated. Normal activities of glucuronidase, phenylalanine transaminase, and other enzymes may be achieved only after days, weeks, or months, sometimes with clinical consequences. In older infants and children, some drugs may impair growth (e.g., stimulants given for attention deficit disorder or learning disabilities [methylphenidate or dextroamphetamines], or corticosteroids).

Changes in body composition during puberty, such as those involving the relative proportions of body fat or water, may affect the patterns of drug distribution in the body, with clinical consequences. The increased levels of sex steroids may alter the activities of enzymes that metabolize drugs. In male adolescents, for example, rising levels of androgens increase the binding capacity of the cytochrome P-450 system. Hein et al. (1985) have found the rate of elimination of theophylline to be more closely related to stage of pubertal maturation than to age. Exposure of the female adolescent to exogenous hormones may similarly affect metabolism of other drugs, both prescribed and illicit.

Genetic variability also may determine the rate of metabolism or the pharmacologic effect of some substances. Acetylation, methylation, demethylation, sulfation, and other processes may be involved. For example, the rapidity of acetylation and excretion of such drugs as isoniazid, hydralazine, and some sulfonamides is genetically set by autosomal recessive genes. Persons who are fast acetylators may need larger doses of drugs and respond poorly to them, whereas slow acetylators are at higher risk of toxic effects associated with elevated levels.

Other developmental aspects of pharmacology that are not well understood include the paradoxic reactions of some children to some drugs; excitement as a response to phenobarbital and abatement of hyperkinesis with amphetamine are examples. Moreover, children appear to have increased sensitivity or reactivity to the effects of some drugs that produce reactions also in adults; children with deficiencies of glucose-6-phosphate dehydrogenase, for example, generally have more severe reactions from ingestion of the offending drugs than do susceptible adults.

NEURODEVELOPMENTAL GROWTH AND DEVELOPMENT

A neurodevelopmental view of growth and development focuses upon elements of behavior that can be regarded as expressive of *maturation,* and that are rooted in those changes in neurobiologic function that evolve with age. This point of view was given major early emphasis by Arnold Gesell and Catherine Amatruda (Knobloch and Pasamanick, 1974), and has been elaborated upon and enriched by the work of many others. Gesell's systematic observations of the responses of infants and young children to the presentation of simple stimuli and tasks led to the description of a variety of behavioral responses that are characteristic of children within specified age ranges. The performances of infants and children at these tasks determined their developmental levels. Gesell and Amatruda standardized a procedure for developmental assessment that produced a *developmental quotient* analogous to the intelligence quotient earlier devised by Binet.

Gesell and Amatruda categorized behavior into four areas: gross and fine motor, adaptive, personal/social, and language. The developmental continuum was presented as a series of steps from one level of function to the next, with ages designated at which one would ordinarily expect each level to be reached. The scale developed by Gesell and Amatruda has been revised and modified by Knobloch and Pasamanick (1974), and items in the scale have been adopted by others. Similar studies led to the development of the Bayley Scales of Infant Development (Bayley, 1969), the Cattell Infant Scale (Cattell, 1960), and others.

The above tests for assessment of infants and young children employ observations of the spontaneous behavior of the infant or child, including gross and fine motor behavior, and the responses when he or she is presented with large and small objects (a rattle or a block, or a raisin, for example) or given opportunities to scribble or to draw. Social responses and interactions are observed, including the use of language.

The examinations are best given by persons with experience in the interpretation of various responses, but knowledge of some of the features and points in such scales can be of help in the informal examination of infants and children in many clinical settings. The arrangements and materials needed are relatively simple (Figs. 1–15 and 1–16). Some useful items for informal assessment are given in Tables 1–12 and 1–13. Details of the manners in which infants and children of various ages should be expected to respond to particular items are given later.

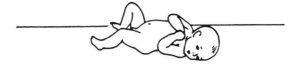

4- and 16-week zones

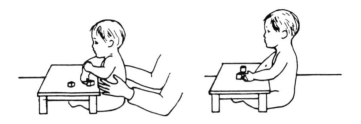

16- and 28-week zones   40-week to 15-month zones

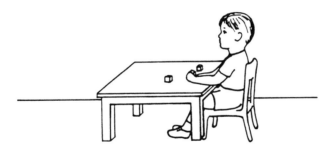

18 months and older

Figure 1–15. Examination arrangements adapted to advanced grades of postural maturity: supine, supported sitting, free sitting, and chair sitting. (Adaptations can be made if special examining equipment is not available.)
(From Knobloch H, Stevens F, Malone AF: *Manual of Developmental Diagnosis.* Hagerstown, Harper & Row, 1980. [Now published by Developmental Evaluation Materials, Inc., P.O. Box 272391, Houston, Texas 77277].)

The neurodevelopmental view is most useful in assessment of the infant and young child, in whom age-specific criteria of neurodevelopmental level evolve rapidly and with considerable temporal precision. On the other hand, the development of many anatomic and physiologic features of the central nervous system is not complete until adolescence or beyond. Various aspects of behavior, cognition, and mentation depend upon this further maturation.

TABLE 1-12. Emerging Patterns of Behavior During the First Year of Life*,†

Neonatal Period (First 4 Weeks)

Prone:	Lies in flexed attitude; turns head from side to side; head sags on ventral suspension
Supine:	Generally flexed and a little stiff
Visual:	May fixate face or light in line of vision; "doll's-eye" movement of eyes on turning of the body
Reflex:	Moro response active; stepping and placing reflexes; grasp reflex active
Social:	Visual preference for human face

At 4 Weeks

Prone:	Legs more extended; holds chin up; turns head; head lifted momentarily to plane of body on ventral suspension
Supine:	Tonic neck posture predominates; supple and relaxed; head lags on pull to sitting position
Visual:	Watches person; follows moving object
Social:	Body movements in cadence with voice of other in social contact; beginning to smile

At 8 Weeks

Prone:	Raises head slightly farther; head sustained in plane of body on ventral suspension
Supine:	Tonic neck posture predominates; head lags on pull to sitting position
Visual:	Follows moving object 180 degrees
Social:	Smiles on social contact; listens to voice and coos

At 12 Weeks

Prone:	Lifts head and chest, arms extended; head above plane of body on ventral suspension
Supine:	Tonic neck posture predominates; reaches toward and misses objects; waves at toy
Sitting:	Head lag partially compensated on pull to sitting position; early head control with bobbing motion; back rounded
Reflex:	Typical Moro response has not persisted; makes defense movements or selective withdrawal reactions
Social:	Sustained social contact; listens to music; says "aah, ngah"

At 16 Weeks

Prone:	Lifts head and chest, head in approximately vertical axis; legs extended
Supine:	Symmetrical posture predominates, hands in midline; reaches and grasps objects and brings them to mouth
Sitting:	No head lag on pull to sitting position; head steady, held forward; enjoys sitting with full truncal support
Standing:	When held erect, pushes with feet
Adaptive:	Sees pellet, but makes no move to it
Social:	Laughs out loud; may show displeasure if social contact is broken; excited at sight of food

At 28 Weeks

Prone: Rolls over; may pivot
Supine: Lifts head; rolls over; squirming movements
Sitting: Sits briefly, with support of pelvis; leans forward on hands; back rounded
Standing: May support most of weight; bounces actively
Adaptive: Reaches out for and grasps large object; *transfers* objects from hand to hand; grasp uses radial palm; rakes at pellet
Language: Polysyllabic vowel sounds formed
Social: Prefers mother; babbles; enjoys mirror; responds to changes in emotional content of social contact

At 40 Weeks

Sitting: Sits up alone and indefinitely without support, back straight
Standing: Pulls to standing position
Motor: Creeps or crawls
Adaptive: Grasps objects with *thumb and forefinger*; pokes at things with forefinger; picks up pellet with assisted pincer movement; uncovers hidden toy; attempts to retrieve dropped object; releases object grasped by other person
Language: Repetitive consonant sounds (mama, dada)
Social: Responds to sound of name; plays peek-a-boo or pat-a-cake; waves bye-bye

At 52 Weeks (1 Year)

Motor: Walks with one hand held; "cruises" or walks holding on to furniture
Adaptive: Picks up pellet with unassisted pincer movement of forefinger and thumb; releases object to other person on request or gesture
Language: A few words besides mama, dada
Social: Plays simple ball game; makes postural adjustment to dressing

---

* From Behrman RE, Vaughan VC III (eds): *Nelson Textbook of Pediatrics*, 13th ed. Philadelphia, WB Saunders Company, 1987, p 33.

† Data are derived from those of Gesell, Shirley, Provence, Wolf, Bayley, and others.

Attention is called to the fact that the Revised Gesell and Amatruda Schedules (Knobloch et al., 1980) set earlier ages for the expected appearance of some of the above behaviors. In particular:

"Creeps or crawls" (40 wk) is now assigned to 28 wk ("crawls or creep-crawls")

"Walks alone" (15 mo) is now assigned to 52 wk ("rises independently, takes several steps").

61

TABLE 1–13. Emerging Patterns of Behavior From 1 to 5 Years of Age*,†

15 Months

Motor:	Walks alone; crawls up stairs
Adaptive:	Makes tower of 2 cubes; makes a line with crayon; inserts pellet in bottle
Language:	Jargon; follows simple commands; may name a familiar object (ball)
Social:	Indicates some desires or needs by pointing; hugs parents

18 Months

Motor:	Runs stiffly; sits on small chair; walks up stairs with one hand held; explores drawers and waste baskets
Adaptive:	Piles 3 cubes; imitates scribbling; imitates vertical stroke; dumps pellet from bottle
Language:	10 words (average); names pictures; identifies one or more parts of body
Social:	Feeds self; seeks help when in trouble; may complain when wet or soiled; kisses parent with pucker

24 Months

Motor:	Runs well; walks up and down stairs, one step at a time; opens doors; climbs on furniture
Adaptive:	Tower of 6 cubes; circular scribbling; imitates horizontal stroke; folds paper once imitatively
Language:	Puts 3 words together (subject, verb, object)
Social:	Handles spoon well; often tells immediate experiences; helps to undress; listens to stories with pictures

30 Months

Motor:	Jumps
Adaptive:	Tower of 8 cubes; makes vertical and horizontal strokes, but generally will not join them to make a cross; imitates circular stroke, forming closed figure
Language:	Refers to self by pronoun "I"; knows full name
Social:	Helps put things away; pretends in play

62

36 Months

Motor: Goes up stairs alternating feet; rides tricycle; stands momentarily on one foot
Adaptive: Tower of 9 cubes; imitates construction of "bridge" of 3 cubes; copies a circle; imitates a cross
Language: Knows age and sex; counts 3 objects correctly; repeats 3 numbers or a sentence of 6 syllables
Social: Plays simple games (in "parallel" with other children); helps in dressing (unbuttons clothing and puts on shoes); washes hands

48 Months

Motor: Hops on one foot; throws ball overhand; uses scissors to cut out pictures; climbs well
Adaptive: Copies bridge from model; imitates construction of "gate" of 5 cubes; copies cross and square; draws a man with 2 to 4 parts besides head; names longer of 2 lines
Language: Counts 4 pennies accurately; tells a story
Social: Plays with several children with beginning of social interaction and role-playing; goes to toilet alone

60 Months

Motor: Skips
Adaptive: Draws triangle from copy; names heavier of 2 weights
Language: Names 4 colors; repeats sentence of 10 syllables; counts 10 pennies correctly
Social: Dresses and undresses; asks questions about meaning of words; domestic role-playing

* From Behrman RE, Vaughan VC III (eds): *Nelson Textbook of Pediatrics*, 13th ed. Philadelphia, WB Saunders Company, 1987, p 34.

† Data are derived from those of Gesell, Shirley, Provence, Wolf, Bailey, and others. After 5 years the Stanford-Binet, Wechsler-Bellevue, and other scales offer the most precise estimates of developmental level. In order to have their greatest value, they should be administered only by an experienced and qualified person.

It should be noted that the Revised Gesell and Amatruda Schedules make the following changes in age of expected appearance of behaviors listed in Table 1–13 (see footnote to Table 1–12):

"Makes a tower of 3 cubes" (18 mo) is now assigned to 15 mo (with 4 cubes at 18 mo)
"Makes a tower of 6 cubes" (24 mo) is now assigned to 21 mo (with 7 cubes at 24 mo)
"Makes a tower of 9 cubes" (36 mo) is now assigned to 30 mo (with 10 cubes at 36 mo)
"Walks up stairs, one hand held" (18 mo) is now assigned to 15 mo
"Jumps" (30 mo) is now assigned to 24 mo
"Goes up stairs alternating feet" (36 mo) is now assigned to 30 mo

For further discussion of the Revised Schedules, the reader is referred to Knobloch et al. (1980), where particular attention should be given to the Preface (pp. ix–xi). Formal testing will appropriately use the Revised Schedules.

63

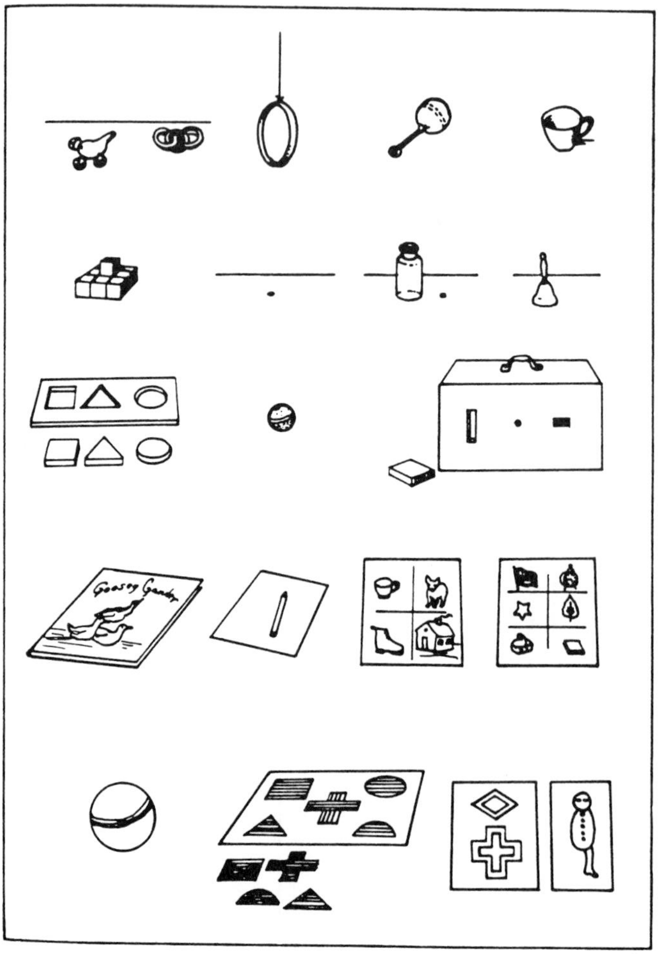

Figure 1–16. Examination materials: catbells and tricolored rings, dangling ring, rattle, cup, cubes, pellet, pellet and bottle, bell, formboard and 3 blocks, small ball, performance box with square block, picture book, paper and crayon, picture cards, large ball, color forms, double diamond and cross, incomplete man. (Additional materials for formal examination are used with the 1980 revision of the Gesell Scale [see Knobloch H, et al., 1980, Figs. B-1 and B-2, pp. 262–263].)
(From Knobloch H, Stevens F, Malone AF: *Manual of Developmental Diagnosis.* Hagerstown, Harper & Row, 1980. [Now published by Developmental Evaluation Materials, Inc., P.O. Box 272391, Houston, Texas 77277].)

COGNITION AND DEVELOPMENT

Nearly a century of increasingly sophisticated study of the ways in which infants and children come to think, to know, and to solve problems has come to fruition in the theories of Piaget, Kohlberg, Skinner, and others. These investigators have differed in their foci of attention, and in the inferences drawn as to the nature of the process. The dominant force in recent years has been the work of Piaget. Because the works of Piaget,

Kohlberg, Skinner, and Bandura seem currently to offer the most relevance to the understanding of children and to child-rearing, they are reviewed in some detail.

Learning lies at the root of cognition. There are a number of theories as to how learning takes place, with some disagreement as to the roles or importance of inner *drives* or *needs* (such as hunger, thirst, or freudian *libido*) or environmental stimuli (skinnerian *consequences* of behavior or banduran *models*). The postulated physiologic mechanisms vary.

Piaget

Piaget (see Flavell, 1963; and Rosen, 1985) devoted a long career to exploring the ways in which infants and children form their impressions of reality; of the relationships between objects, space, and time; and of the operations that can be executed within that reality. Piaget has postulated that the order in which children acquire their notions of reality tends to follow a regular sequence, and that each step is a necessary forerunner to the next, beginning with reflex structures in the newborn infant that become organized into cognitive structures.

Piaget defined four principal periods of development of cognition:

1. The *sensorimotor* period (birth to 2 years)
2. The *preoperational* period (2 to 7 years)
3. The period of *concrete operations* (7 to 11 years)
4. The period of *formal operations* (entered between 11 and 15 years [see pp. 254–257]).

These periods are described below and summarized in Table 8–12.

Piaget used the word "operations" to mean the mental manipulation of objects (*concrete* operations) or of ideas in the absence of objects (*formal* operations); in either case, the mental activity might or might not be accompanied by or lead to motor actions related to the objects or the ideas.

The attachment of ages to the above periods is approximate. Piaget was less interested in finding a detailed time scale for the development of cognitive skills than in finding clues to the process; accordingly, in spite of the richness of Piaget's experimental data, his observations have not led to any evaluative instrument for the determination of a developmental level comparable to that given by the Gesell and Amatruda or Bayley scales. Užgiris and Hunt (1975), however, have made use of Piaget's work in developing an ordinal scale of psychologic development in infancy.

Piaget has described the process at the root of learning as involving *schemes* or *schemata* as basic units. Schemes are visualized as the techniques of adjustment that enable the organism to adapt to the environment; they may be mental or motor or both, and reflect the internal structure and organization of activities in response to environmental stimulation. Schemes may be simple (reflex) or complicated (a series of actions achieving a certain end). They are accompanied by emotional tones as integral elements.

Piaget proposed that the evolution of schemes comes about through the processes of *assimilation* and *accommodation*. Assimilation is the incorporation of a stimulus into whatever set of schemes already exists, with more or less recognition of those elements of the stimulus that correspond to elements of the schemes already established. The assimilation of the new stimulus is accompanied or followed by *accommodation*, a reshaping of the original set of schemes to take into account the new information received. Assimilation and accommodation together give rise to *adaptation*.

Sensory-Motor Intelligence

Piaget identified six stages within the period of sensory-motor intelligence.

Stage 1 is a period of *reflex activity* (birth to 1 month), during which the infant consolidates homeostatic functions such as breathing, crying, and sucking.

Stage 2 (1 to 4 months) sees the first acquired adaptations and the *primary circular reaction*. This stage involves changes in the form of neonatal reflexes as the result of experience. The primary circular reaction is the tendency of the infant to engage in repetitive activity, as if to practice new skills or to reexperience new sensations, such as to grasp and let go of a fold of clothing repeatedly. Stage 2 finds an imitation sequence active: baby behaves, adult imitates, baby imitates adult. Looking, sucking, and grasping become coordinated at about 4 months, with lots of smiling.

Stage 3 (4 to 8 months) involves growing interest in the consequences of acts, and in procedures for making interesting sights last. This stage is marked by the growing differentiation of self from the outside world and by the *secondary circular reactions*, which are learned maneuvers by which the infant brings about some change in the outer world, rather than in the inner. An example would be the deliberate reaching for a bell in order to make a sound, or to look at what is grasped and release it. Like the primary circular reactions, the secondary circular reactions are repetitive.

In Stage 4 (8 to 12 months) Piaget discerns the beginnings of clear intelligence, with the *coordination of secondary schemes*. The infant begins to be able to push obstacles away, to get an object by pulling on a string, or to put a whistle into a parent's mouth to have it blown. By now the infant is able to show his or her belief in the existence and increasingly in the permanence of objects or persons that are out of sight.

Stage 5 (12 to 18 months) is marked by the *tertiary circular reaction* and the discovery of new means of producing familiar results by active experimentation. The primary circular reactions seem designed to preserve events through repetition, the secondary to achieve anticipated results in familiar ways, and the tertiary to find new ways to achieve these ends or new arenas for such activity. There is, moreover, an active quest for the novel, with such experimentation as putting objects into or on top of other objects in different ways, with effects each time different from the original one.

Stage 6 (18 months to 2 years) is marked by the *invention of new means to desired ends* through mental combinations that lead to problem solving in more complex ways. An example would be the preplanned use of a stick to retrieve a toy that is out of reach.

Preoperational Thought

In piagetian theory an *operation* corresponds to a manipulation of an object or set of objects in some relationship to each other, such as number, color, size, or some other feature. The period designated as *pre-*

operational thought (about 2 to 7 years) is marked by increasing sophistication in the use of language, and by growing appreciation of the consequences of manipulations, most dramatically in the way in which the features of the objects are "conserved" in manipulation.

Piaget's most famous demonstrations of the principle of conservation include the pouring of water from a wide into a narrow vessel or the manipulation of a lump of clay. The child of 4 years, for example, will judge that the amount of water has been increased because it rises higher in the narrow vessel. The same child will perceive that the clay is skinnier and lighter if it is rolled out into a long snake. The notions of conservation of volume, weight, and mass develop during this period, and may be unfinished even at its end. The child seems during this period to be dealing with a before-the-eye reality requiring interpretations that the child must learn to master.

The development of language during the preoperational period tends to evolve from an egocentric toward a more social use. The young child often is heard to comment in a monologue upon his or her actions as these are carried out. The older child during this period can use language more effectively as a social tool.

Period of Concrete Operations

The period of concrete operations (about 7 to 11 years) finds the child ready to deal with objects as perceived or imagined, but not yet ready to manipulate concepts not attached to objects. For example, arithmetic manipulations of imagined apples can be carried out on paper, but the child is not ready for a course in abstract logic. By the age of 9 or 10 years the child has learned that the weight of a lump of clay has been conserved in manipulations of shape; by 11 or 12 years the conservation of volume in such deformations is mastered as well.

Period of Formal Operations

The period of formal operations (entered at about 11 to 15 years) is marked by the acquisition of the ability to deal not only with the actual or an imagined reality, but with the potential or hypothetical as well. There is residual egocentrism at the beginning of this period, but at the end of the period all the structures of adult thought are in place. What is learned later will be assimilated into the structures underlying intellectual activity as these now exist.

The adolescent's discovery of logic may lie at the root of much of the optimism and idealism and rebellion that characterize adolescent thought, as if to say that there are ways in which the world can be made a better place, that they are known, and that they can be brought to pass.

No brief treatment of the work of Piaget can do justice to the richness of his studies or to the ingeniousness of the experiments he and his coworkers have designed to investigate the ways in which children see the world and learn to interpret what they see. He has made systematic observations of childrens' views of space, geometry, and the laws of chance, and of their notions of quantity, logic, number, distance, velocity, and time. He has examined the evolution of moral (value) judgments in such areas as the playing of games and the interpretation of relative rights and wrongs. We make reference to some of these studies in the descriptions of the behavior of children that follow. We also (in the discussion of adolescence, p. 256) consider the reservations expressed by Flavell (1985) and others that challenge the piagetian emphasis upon discrete stages of cognitive development.

Kohlberg, Gilligan, Coles

Like Piaget, Kohlberg (1964) has given particular attention to the development of moral judgment in children and adolescents. He has described three levels of moral judgment, with two stages at each level. The levels are: 1) preconventional; 2) conventional; and 3) postconventional, principled, or autonomous.

At the *preconventional* level, Stage 1 finds moral judgments dependent upon an obedience to parental authority and upon an orientation toward reward and punishment. Stage 2 introduces a notion of fairness or *quid pro quo.*

At the *conventional level,* Stage 3 emphasizes helping others and the gaining of approval for proper actions, with Stage 4 finding proper actions responsive to notions of law and order or obedience to the community's authority.

At the *postconventional level,* Stage 5 involves notions of social contract, with legalistic and utilitarian features to which society has given its support, and Stage 6 reaches universal principles of ethics, human rights, and social justice. The ages at which children and adolescents reach these stages of moral development are variable. Stages 5 and 6 belong for the most part to the period of formal operations, as these develop in adolescence (see also pp. 256–257).

Besides level of cognitive development, Kohlberg identifies three other factors that contribute to the form that moral development takes: one is the child's *motivation* or *need,* which, like cognitive function, is dependent in part upon genetic and personal factors; the other two, entirely environmental, are the child's *opportunity to learn social roles,* and the *forms of justice* that the child encounters in the social institutions with which he or she becomes familiar. Kohlberg regards the order of development of stages as invariant across cultures, but the proportion of persons at each stage may differ from one society to another.

Kohlberg believed that women reach stages 5 and 6 less often than men. Gilligan (1982) has suggested that this observation may reflect different perceptions by women of their social roles rather than a less than full realization of moral development. Gilligan believes that women experience or visualize the arena in which moral judgments are made as involving primarily interpersonal relationships rather than systems of rules designed to protect the individual or to ensure social justice in the abstract.

In a series of observations of children in a variety of stressful life situations, Coles (1986) has emphasized that the moral life of children may not so much follow a prescribed developmental sequence as be derived from their unique life experiences. He believes that the type of moral and ethical person who is the resultant of these experiences depends heavily upon the models to which the child is exposed, in parents and others. It has been suggested also that cultural determinants may shape and set limits to moral development as Kohlberg has described it. In a traditional third-world country, for example, the needs of the community may be entirely adequately served by the inculcation or adoption of standards that go no further than Kohlberg's conventional level (stage 4), which emphasizes adoption of the community's standards without appeal to any higher principle, there being within that culture no more compelling standard.

Skinner

Learning theory has a prominent place in our understanding of the ways in which the cognition and behavior of children are formed. The work of Pavlov gave initial direction to examination of the ways in which stimulus and response (S-R) are related to each other. The pavlovian work on the *conditioned reflex* has been supplemented by the work of Skinner (1963) and of others identified with *behavioral* schools of psychology.

The thrust of much behaviorism has been not toward identifying or speculating about inner mechanisms responsible for learning but rather toward learning from behavior itself in controlled environments what the relationship is between stimulus and response.

Pavlov showed that under conditions of need or motivation (e.g., hunger), when an animal who is presented with a natural stimulus (food) and gives the normal response (salivation) receives at the same time another unrelated stimulus (the sound of a bell), the response (salivation) could be transferred in time to the second stimulus alone. There is no doubt that such conditioned learning occurs in man. The work of Skinner, on the other hand, makes it probable that most learning in man is the result not of classical conditioning, but of what Skinner has termed *operant* or *instrumental* conditioning.

Skinner holds that behavior is determined more by its *consequences* than by other considerations. Behavior may be generated by inner needs and tensions, but the learned behavior through which the infant begins to exert control over the environment is regarded as generated by the response of the environment to behavior that may be initially relatively random. The same may be said for learned behavior at any age: behavior is responsive to its consequences—that is, to the ways in which it is rewarded or punished or ignored.

If a pattern of behavior is reliably followed (reinforced) by pleasant circumstances such as reduction of need, or by intrinsically satisfying stimuli, then that pattern of behavior will tend to occur with increasing probability. If, on the other hand, behavior is followed (punished) by unpleasant circumstances, then it will be exhibited with decreasing probability. This relationship exists for both "desirable" and "undesirable" behaviors, whether these judgments are made in personal, parental, or societal perspective.

The *reinforcement* of behavior may be termed *positive* or *negative* in accordance with whether it consists of: 1) a pleasant or rewarding experience (positive); or 2) the termination of some uncomfortable, unpleasant, or aversive situation (negative).

In contrast to negative reinforcement, *punishment* implies the creation of an unpleasant situation upon the exhibition of behavior.

Behavior that produces neither positive nor negative reinforcement, nor punishment, tends not to recur. The disappearance of established or repetitive patterns of behavior with lack of reinforcement is termed *extinction* of such behavior.

Techniques of *behavior modification* and *behavior shaping* have been based upon the above principles, and have broad implications for child rearing, especially for socialization and discipline, and for therapeutic interventions. Behavior shaping involves identifying the behavior ultimately desired and then rewarding actions that move toward or are partially successful in achieving that behavior or that show a willingness to move toward it. As behavior approaches in quality the desired goal, rewards are ultimately given only for behavior that represents goal conditions. Once the desired behavior has been achieved, it can be maintained through *occasional* further positive reinforcement; occasional or random reinforcement may, in fact, become more effective than if reinforcement were to occur with every manifestation of the behavior.

There is a need to set limits to the behavior of children from time to time through restraint or other measures that might be construed as punishment, but there is ample evidence that positive reinforcement is a more effective way than punishment to elicit desirable behavior from children (see also Discipline, pp. 187, 203–208).

Bandura

Another dimension has been added to learning theory by the work of Bandura (1977) and others who have emphasized the importance of social variables in the acquisition of knowledge and the regulation of behavior. Of particular importance is the role that *models* play in learning, and in socialization and acculturation.

Even in the first months of life children are able to imitate the behavior of those about them. As they grow older, they are able to draw lessons and inferences not only from experiencing the consequences of their own behavior, but also from observing that certain forms of behavior have predictable consequences for others.

Some social learning theorists hold that learning can take place *incidentally* or *vicariously,* simply through observation and storage in memory of environmental data that have no immediate personal relevance or reward, but that can be called upon later to guide behavior in an appropriate way when the motivation for that behavior comes into existence. What has been produced is *one-trial learning*. If the initial performance is perfect, it will have been produced without ever having been reinforced; if imperfect, it may be perfected through shaping.

The importance of models to the child can scarcely be overemphasized. There is no doubt that what children see about them in reality, in the behavior of their parents and others, and what they experience through mass media, such as television, newspapers, and literature, may profoundly affect their systems of values and their notions of what is expected of them. It is important that the value systems proposed for children by their parents and other significant persons be congruent with what the children actually see in the behavior that such persons model for them.

Evaluation of Cognitive Function

The evaluation of cognitive function and intellectual ability becomes more complex as the infant and child grow older, both as to the structure, content, and purposes of the tests used and the variety of experiences that the child brings to the testing situation. Both the kinds of tests and their frequency of administration have increased greatly in recent years, in response to a nationwide concern with the quality of education in the schools and the manifest failure of some schools to prepare some students with the academic skills necessary to become effective adults.

Tests of cognitive function are used for any of several purposes. At the most basic level they are used to assess the inherent *ability* or *capacity* of the child for cognitive function. An application of this assessment is their use as *screening tests,* to see whether children have achieved the appropriate developmental levels for entry into school (or preschool, or kindergarten, or first grade). A related use is as *achievement tests,* to see whether the levels of academic performance have met certain standards. *Performance testing* carries the assessment a step further, in trying to determine whether the child with adequate equipment and educational achievement can translate what has been learned into actual practice. The impediments to adequate performance may include physical impairments or emotional disabilities.

Educators and others also use *criterion* or *mastery* testing to determine whether subjects have met predetermined levels of achievement or function, frequently in order to determine whether entry into a next higher level of instruction or an opportunity for further formal education is appropriate.

The relationships between these purposes of tests are indicated as follows:

Screening tests ask: "Is the child ready to learn?"
Ability testing asks: "At what level can the child learn?"
Achievement tests ask: "What has the child learned?"
Criterion testing asks: "Has the child mastered the specific assignment or reached the specified goal?"

Performance tests ask: "Can the child use effectively what he or she has learned?"

The first goal of cognitive testing, the discovery of "native ability," has for many decades had at a conceptual core the notion of "intelligence quotient" (IQ). The IQ is calculated as the ratio (multiplied by 100) of the subject's level of cognitive function or *mental age* (MA), expressed as the age of normal child for whom that level is average, to the subject's *chronologic age* (CA).

$$IQ = [MA/CA] \times 100$$

At each age the average performance at that age generates an IQ of 100, with 1 SD of the mean of the scores corresponding to 15 points of IQ.

Table 1–14 shows how IQ scores would be distributed *theoretically* in a *normal* population and how they might be interpreted. The labels and inferences drawn from such IQ measurements, are presently used by the health professions and agencies that deal with mentally retarded persons in order to assess needs and coordinate services.

Mentally retarded persons are reported to make up from 1 to 5 per cent of the population, a frequency that varies with the population studied and the criteria used to assign that label. Clinically retarded individuals do not simply represent the lower end of the distribution curve for normal persons; rather, they represent both the lower end of the normal distribution *and* a different, larger, and abnormal population whose low IQs are the result of developmental abnormalities, trauma, residua of infectious disease, or socioeconomic or sociocultural deprivation. Their IQs serve to identify them as having special needs.

Of those who have the diagnosis of mental retardation, about 90 per cent have IQs in the borderline or mildly retarded range; about 5 per cent of them have severe or profound disability.

The idea has been rather pervasive that properly designed measurements of IQ could confidently identify the positions at which children fell on a spectrum of abilities ranging from retarded to genius, that the IQ was a relatively stable index of such native potential, and that it reliably predicted future function. In recent years, however, confidence in the conclusions to be drawn from the IQ as conventionally measured has been

TABLE 1–14. Theoretical Distribution of IQ Scores in a Normal Population

IQ RANGE	INTERPRETATION (%)	EXPECTED LEVEL OF FUNCTION
Over 144	Very superior (0.3)	Creative
130–144	Superior (2.25)	Superior (professional)
115–129	Above average (13.5)	Competent (college)
85–114	Normal (68)	Average (high school)
70–84	Borderline (13.5)	Independent living
55–69	Mildly retarded (2.25)	Supervised self-care
<55	Moderate, severe, or profound retardation (0.3)	Need for constant supervision and care

greatly diminished by concern that the tests used to measure it are often biased by the culture and by the previous experiences of the subjects. The predictive value of tests of cognitive function has proved to be limited.

In particular, the developmental quotient (DQ), which expresses the predominantly neurodevelopmental abilities of the infant, does not until the age of about 3 years begin to be substantially predictive of later IQ for children whose abilities are within the normal range. This finding may reflect the tendency of the later tests to incorporate test items the responses to which may in the individual child depend in considerable measure upon his or her experience within the home and community.

From a technical standpoint, in the testing of older preschool and school-aged children increasing reliance has been placed upon multiple-choice tests, which are presumably "objective" in their scoring procedures as well as able to be administered efficiently to large groups and to be scored rapidly by machines. Objections to such tests have included that success depends more often upon simple recognition of the right answers than upon a capacity to analyze a problem and to solve it with creative cognitive activity. Moreover, when they are used to assess large numbers of students, their reliability as instruments for prediction of the future capabilities of individual students is biased by the test-taking experiences of the subjects, as well as by possibly divergent socioeconomic backgrounds and prior educational and emotional experiences of the subjects tested.

Data have suggested that there may be substantial genetic differences in IQ among various normal populations or groups. These differences have been attributed to a variety of causes. Jensen (1980), for example, has attributed the difference in average IQ between black and Caucasian Americans predominantly to genetic factors. Others have thought that the observed differences more likely reflect the fact that most of the tests that give IQs demonstrate cultural bias, particularly in the items that depend upon verbal ability. A variety of attempts have been made to devise "culture-free" intelligence tests, but there is no general agreement that any such test exists.

Other environmental explanations offered for the observed differences include socioeconomic disadvantage, racial prejudice, low expectations, inferior schools, and inferior teaching. The history of black education in the United States gives some support to each of these arguments. The idea that generally lower expectations of the black minority may contribute significantly to the observed differences is particularly interesting in the light of the demonstration that in the normal classroom, when a teacher is given reason to expect superior performance of certain students, those students are particularly likely to do well in spite of the fact that they have been selected at random from the student body (Rosenthal and Jacobson, 1968).

The argument has been advanced recently that differences such as those between black and Caucasian children in the United States may be the pervasive result of the status of the black community as a "caste" within the dominant society. Such status, which implies permanent assignment to a disadvantaged group within the community, is regarded as conferring not merely social, economic, or political disadvantage, nor merely lower expectations on the part of the dominant group, but among the black children themselves lowered self-expectations that become self-fulfilling prophecies. This view holds that the observed differences in measured IQ reflect primarily the defects found in the social structure of the community.

Support for the view that observed differences in IQ between dominant and minority groups reflect the structure of the community rather than the genetic endowment of the minority is found in the observation that the scores of black children in the United States on the conventional tests are improving from one generation to the next. Moreover, it has been observed that when immigrants who have had low caste status in their country of origin immigrate to the United States, if they are accepted into the social structure without significant social or political handicap, the performances of their children resemble those of the dominant group in the community from which they came, rather than any lower performance that may have characterized their function in the country of origin. This has proved to be true, for example, for the Burakumi of Japan, who are given the status of Japanese here rather than the lower caste status accorded in Japan; here they perform on tests of IQ like other immigrant Japanese, rather than giving the depressed performances that have in Japan been a characteristic of their group (DeVos, 1988).

Other persuasive evidence for the predominantly or overwhelmingly environmental origin of group or racial differences in distribution of IQs has been summarized by Hetherington and Parke (1975).

Tests Used in the Evaluation of Cognitive Function

Goldman et al. (1983) have given comprehensive descriptions of many of the tests in common use for infants and children. Features of such tests are summarized here.

REVISED GESELL DEVELOPMENTAL AND NEUROLOGIC EXAMINATION

In its original form this was the first major developmental scale, now recently revised by Knobloch and Pasamanick (1974). It is suitable for testing of infants and children from the ages of 1 to 60 months. It examines behavior in five areas: gross motor, fine motor, adaptive, language, and personal-social. It yields a *developmental quotient* (DQ) analogous to but not equivalent to the IQ.

An abbreviated form of the Gesell examination, the *Revised Developmental Screening Inventory* (RDSI), has been developed by Knobloch et al. (1980) as a *screening test* for infants from 12 to 60 months of age. It produces a DQ, and assigns the infants to Normal (DQ greater than 85), Questionable (DQ 76 to 85), or Abnormal (DQ less than 76) categories. Infants whose performances are questionable or abnormal will need further evaluation.

Knobloch proposes that administration of the RDSI be preceded or supplemented by completion of a questionnaire by parents *(Revised Parent Developmental Questionnaire [RPDQ])*.

BAYLEY SCALES OF INFANT DEVELOPMENT

The Bayley scales (Bayley, 1969) are designed for infants from 2 to 30 months of age. They include a Mental Scale (163 items), a Motor Scale (81 items), and an Infant Behavior Record (30 behaviors). Standard scores are calculated for the Mental and Motor Scales, with 100 the normal mean score for age and a standard deviation of 16. Other ratings are arrived at for the Infant Behavior Inventory.

DENVER DEVELOPMENTAL SCREENING TEST

The Denver Developmental Screening Test (DDST; Frankenburg et al., 1973, 1981) is a screening test suitable for children from 2 months to 5.5 years of age. It does not produce a developmental age, a DQ, or an IQ, but rather produces ratings of Normal, Questionable, or Abnormal, the latter two indicating a need for further assessment.

A Prescreening Developmental Questionnaire (PDQ) related to the DDST consists of questions formulated from items in the DDST. Ten age-appropriate questions are presented to the parent, with "yes" answers to 9 or 10 indicating no problem, to 8 or less indicating the need for retesting, and to 6 or less on two tests indicating the need for full evaluation.

STANFORD-BINET INTELLIGENCE SCALE

This time-honored scale, now in its fourth revision (1988), is designed for the age range from 2 years to adult. The concepts of mental age and IQ were originally developed around this instrument. The items for the younger ages are presented in a gamelike format. The items for older children and adults have considerable dependence on verbal function.

WECHSLER INTELLIGENCE SCALE FOR CHILDREN—REVISED

The Wechsler Intelligence Scale for Children—Revised (WISC-R; Wechsler, 1974) is designed for children from 6 to 16 years of age. It consists of subtests yielding Verbal and Performance scores or quotients (VIQs or PIQs); these are combined to create a Full Scale Intelligence Quotient (FSIQ). Substantial discrepancies between verbal and performance scores may have implications for clinical diagnosis.

The Wechsler Preschool and Primary Scale of Intelligence (WPPSI) (Wechsler 1976) extends the WISC-R, in effect; it is adapted to the age range from 4 to 6.5 years, with similar Verbal, Performance, and Full Scale IQs being derived.

McCARTHY SCALES OF CHILDREN'S ABILITIES

The McCarthy Scales of Children's Abilities (MSCA; McCarthy, 1972) are designed for the age range from 2.5 to 8.5 years. The MSCA consists of 18 subtests, which address Verbal, Performance, Quantitative, Memory, Motor, and General cognitive functions. A General Cognitive Index (GCI) is derived from the Verbal, Performance, and Quantitative scores, with a mean normal at each age of 100 and a standard deviation of 16. The Memory scale assesses short-term memory with items drawn from the Verbal, Performance, and Quantitative scales. The Motor scale assesses fine and gross coordination in a variety of tasks.

KAUFMAN ASSESSMENT BATTERY FOR CHILDREN

The Kaufman Assessment Battery for Children (K-ABC; Kaufman and Kaufman, 1983) embodies a Sequential Processing Scale and a Simultaneous Processing Scale that measure intelligence as mental processing or problem-solving skills, and a third Achievement section that draws upon knowledge and skills that should normally be acquired from the cultural and school environments. A Global Scale is derived from the Sequential and Simultaneous Processing Scales, a Mental Processing composite, and the Achievement score. It is hoped that the separation of items of "intelligence" from those of "acquired knowledge" will permit the test to function as culture free on the one hand, and as an assessor of the environmental element in performance on the other.

PEABODY PICTURE VOCABULARY TEST

The Peabody Picture Vocabulary Test (PPVT; Dunn, 1965) is designed as a measure of hearing or receptive vocabulary, not of general intelligence. It may help to determine future success in school. The results can be expressed as an IQ, but the test is narrow and any broad inferences as to IQ are inappropriate. Its advantages are the ease of administration and a relatively easy adaptability to language or speech impairments or motor disability.

RAVEN PROGRESSIVE MATRICES TEST

The Raven matrices (Raven, 1960) are a widely used nonverbal test, relatively culture free, suitable for an age range from 5.5 years to adult. The test consists of figures to be chosen in accordance with a deducible principle generated by other figures. It may be particularly effective in assessing visual perceptual functioning. The test is easy to administer, and generates an estimate of IQ.

ACHIEVEMENT TESTS

Many achievement tests are available. These are usually administered by teachers or by educational psychologists in the schools. Among them are Metropolitan Readiness Tests, Metropolitan Achievement Tests, the Peabody Individual Achievement Test, Diagnostic Reading Scales, the Stanford Achievement Test, the Wide Range Achievement Test (WRAT), and the Woodcock-Johnson Psycho-Educational Battery (Part II—Tests of Achievement). These are described, with critiques, by Goldman et al. (1983).

Among the above tests, the Stanford-Binet, the Wechsler, the McCarthy, and the Kaufman are generally administered by persons with special training in psychometrics. The same is true of the Gesell and Bayley scales when these are used for formal assessment of developmental level; on the other hand, informal assessment of the infant or child can make effective use of elements of these tests (pp. 58–64). The DDST, the PPVT and the Raven matrices are relatively easy to use; they produce informal, but often useful assessments.

PSYCHOSOCIAL DEVELOPMENT

The process through which the infant, child, and adolescent take their places in their families, communities, and cultures has been a concern of every society. The record of this concern is as old as history itself. The spectrum of views as to how this process should be guided has ranged from a view of the infant as endowed with original sin from which he or she must be delivered by appropriate child-rearing practices to a view of the child as born innocent and needing for the most part only useful models by which to grow and develop. Disciplinary measures (in the original sense [teaching] of the word] have ranged from severe (or even savage, with the incorporation of pain or even death as punishment) to lenient, emphasizing loving guidance and positive reinforcement.

An analogy can be drawn between the physical and the behavioral dimensions of growth and development. For example: each begins with a genetic substrate; each is modified by experience; and each may be regarded as susceptible to abnormalities caused by deficiencies or excesses of essential input.

Calories may be regarded as the most basic life-sustaining input laying the basis for physical growth. By analogy, we may look upon *stimulation* as an equivalent basic need for behavioral development. Calories are not enough for growth, however; protein is required for the formation of new tissues. The analogue of protein may be *positive reinforcement,* which is essential for the evolution of behavior (healthy or otherwise). On the other hand, while protein permits the growth of new tissues, it is not enough to assure that the growth will be of high quality; without vitamins its quality will be defective. The analogue of vitamins for the achievement of high quality in behavioral growth and development may be *loving relationships.*

Behavioral growth and development may be impaired by deficiencies or excesses of stimulation, by excesses of rewards or punishment, or by traumatic life events, such as interpersonal relationships of stressful or hurtful nature, failure to be loved or to learn to love, or the loss of loved ones.

Freud

Our modern understanding of the process of emotional growth and development and acculturation may be said to have begun about a century ago with the work of Sigmund Freud, who may have been the first to give us a view of human development that insists that we take into account the inner experience of the infant and child.

The word *psyche* is now generally used to refer to the human capacity for thought, judgment, and emotion, and is regarded as having both conscious and unconscious aspects.

In an age marked by scientific discovery and by interest in the nature of energy and of material structures, Freud proposed a structure for the psyche that reflected an analogy between an engine of mind and the engines of physical science. The basic energy of the psyche he termed *libido,* and he postulated psychic structures through which this psychic energy was expressed, and for which they competed from time to time.

Of the three psychic structures postulated by Freud, the most basic and primitive is the *id,* within which reside instincts and tendencies for self-preservation. The id is regarded as unconscious, but able to motivate behavior through the *pleasure principle*. Among the important aspects of the id Freud included sexuality, or sexual motivation.

The second basic structure postulated by Freud was the *ego,* in which resides the conscious sense of self, the part of the psyche that experiences and tests reality. The sense of who one is and of what one's goals are, and the maintenance of this identity, reside in the ego. The ego is the repository of conscious strivings and of conscious defense mechanisms.

The third psychic structure postulated was the *superego,* wherein resides the conscience. The superego is made up of elements derived from both the id and the ego, and exerts control over the impulses of the id and the decision-making of the ego. The superego is considered to function largely in the unconscious area of the psyche.

It was through the work of the freudian school that the psychic mechanisms of defense were first identified and defined, the most central of which was *repression,* the tendency to push into the unconscious those experiences or feelings (memories, emotions, or desires) that are imbued with too much anxiety, shame, guilt, or conflict to be acknowledged and dealt with in the conscious life. Repression is a feature of normal as well as of psychopathologic defenses. It occurs, according to theory, at the expense of libido. When this energy devoted to repression can be rechanneled into useful activity, it is said to represent *sublimation* of the repressed instinctual drive.

Other mechanisms of defense include *reaction formation* (the substitution of a conscious attitude opposite to the repressed [unconscious] one), *isolation* (the separation of a fantasy or memory from its emotional component), *regression* (the retreat to an earlier stage of development [becoming more dependent during illness, for example]), *denial* (treating an unbearable situation as if it did not exist), and *projection* (imputing or attributing to others one's own unbearable or repressed thoughts or characteristics).

Regression, denial, and projection, as normal mechanisms of defence, are particularly common among children. Their persistence in the face of a reality with which the child would normally be expected to cope, or their chronic or persistent overuse, may indicate a need for psychologic evaluation and possibly for intervention.

Freud came to his views of the psyche partly through the technique of *psychoanalysis,* elements of which included free association, the interpretation of dreams, and interpretation of the phenomena of resistance and transference. Through these, elements of the unconscious could be exposed and brought to consciousness. As psychoanalytic theory evolved, it defined various stages in the development of the psyche, with particular attention to psychosexual aspects of the libido.

Freud believed that the psychosexual function of the id was operative even in early infancy in response to the pleasure principle, with the sensory zone in which that function was active being primarily the oral area. On the other hand, even in infancy the operation of the pleasure principle may be explicitly sexual, as in the infant who masturbates. Psychoanalytic theory holds that infantile sexuality has important implications for the basic nature of the relationships that grow between family members in infancy and childhood, as well as in adolescence and adult life (see pp. 94–104).

As psychoanalytic theory evolved, the first stage of psychosexual development was viewed as characterized primarily by the need of the dependent infant for nourishment and for a supportive relationship with a primary caretaker, usually the mother. This stage became known as the *oral* stage.

The oral stage was superseded in the second year and later by a stage characterized chiefly by the need of the child to become responsible for control of his or her own bodily functions, with the submission of primitive impulses to the regulatory influences of the family and the culture. This stage is called the *anal* or *anal-sadistic* period because of presumed heavy investment of libido in the eliminatory functions.

The next stage of development dealt with the demands of the growing sexual and gender identities of the child, and for the first time separated boys and girls. It was proposed that this stage (the *phallic*) was marked by penis envy in girls and by castration anxiety in boys, as they became aware of their anatomic differences. The stage was further marked by the child's fantasy that he or she might marry the parent of the opposite sex, supplanting the parent of the same sex. This fantasy appears to grow normally out of the child's growing sense of what might be his or her future role as boy or girl "grown up." The *oedipal complex* represents this need to choose between the parents as models, with rejection of the one in favor of the other.

Psychoanalytic theory held for some time that the next stage (the *latency* period), characteristic of the school-aged child, saw a suppression of libidinal investment in the psychosexual while the educational life became predominant. It is now clear that there is substantial psychosexual activity during the latency period.

The final *genital* period of psychosexual development came with adolescence, in response to physiologic changes, and as a step in the continuum of development set in motion at birth.

This scant description of a psychoanalytic model for child and adolescent development cannot do justice to the complexities of psychoanalytic theory, nor to the rich literature recording how the psychoanalytic approach has illuminated our understanding of the infant, child, and adolescent. On the other hand, the early psychoanalytic model was in considerable measure elaborated out of work with adult patients presenting clinical problems, and drew much of its inference as to infancy and childhood from retrospective analyses of these problems. When psychoanalytic insights began to be examined in the contexts of normal development, at the hands of Erikson, Spitz, and others, the classical freudian views of development began to be, and have now in considerable measure been, supplemented, restructured, or supplanted by models generally given the name *psychosocial*. Psychoanalytic insights remain useful to the clinician, but they may have little day-to-day applicability in routine clinical assessment of children or adolescents.

Erikson

The psychosocial model that has captured major recent attention has been that of Erikson (1985), who has proposed eight stages in psychosocial development, each characterized by certain goals to be met and by certain consequences if they are not met. These stages are depicted in Table 1–15, as presented by Noam (1982). It will be seen that they correspond more or less closely to the early freudian stages described above, but that they go beyond them in detail, particularly for the adolescent and adult.

Erikson's first stage emphasized the infant's need in the first year or so for the development of a basic sense of *trust* through having basic oral and sensory needs adequately met, the evidence for which was to be found in the ease of feeding, the depth of sleep, and perhaps the normal functions of other organ systems. For the infant whose basic needs are not met, there develops a basic *mistrust* of life and of new experiences that may lay the basis for narcissism or psychosis.

The second stage emphasized the development in the second and third years of *autonomy*, particularly as this is manifested in muscular (including anal) and impulse controls. Failure of the setting to provide the opportunities for this autonomy or of the growing child to achieve it are seen as leading to feelings of *doubt* and *shame*.

For the normal child the preschool years are marked by the child's increasing exercise of his or her own *initiative*, not only in activities but also in thought. Some of this initiative is invested in plans for the future, including choice of models between parents, and gives rise to fantasies that may be anxiety-provoking and create *guilt* as the countervailing force to initiative.

With entry into school, the initiative of the earlier stage becomes harnessed to the tasks of learning and of preparation for an actual career, with the development of a sense of *industry* or of *duty and accomplishment*. In this endeavor the child runs the risk of *failure*.

The remaining four eriksonian stages belong to adolescence and adult life. With the onset of puberty comes a need to redefine one's self and one's goals in the context of earlier successful or unsuccessful achievement of initiative and accomplishment and sense of duty. With success at this redefinition comes a sense of *identity;* with failure comes *role diffusion.* The struggle for identity takes many forms, including

TABLE 1–15. Eriksonian Stages of Psychosocial Development

1. Infancy (oral sensory): Trust vs Mistrust
2. Early Childhood (muscular-anal): Autonomy vs Shame
3. Play Age (locomotor-genital): Initiative vs Guilt
4. School Age (latency): Industry vs Inferiority
5. Puberty and Adolescence: Identity vs Role Diffusion
6. Young Manhood: Intimacy vs Isolation
7. Adulthood: Generativity vs Stagnation
8. Maturity: Ego Integrity vs Despair

As presented by Noam (1982).

such things as submersion of one's self in a closed group or clique, identification with a variety of folk heroes, such as sports figures, or the first tentative encounters with the opposite sex.

The sixth stage calls for the development of *intimacy* in relationships with others, through a new capacity for the sharing of goals and feelings and commitments, not just in boy-girl relationships but in boy-boy and girl-girl relationships as well. Failure to achieve the capacity for intimacy leads to *isolation,* social or emotional or both.

The seventh eriksonian stage is characterized by the need to develop *generativity,* which is the term Erikson has given to the stage in which becoming an adult with adult responsibilities is first accomplished. Generativity is the "concern in establishing and guiding the next generation." The alternative to generativity is *stagnation* or self-indulgence.

The final stage of psychosocial development has been termed the achievement of *integrity,* or the status of mature adult. Erikson wrote of integrity as the "acceptance of one's one and only life cycle as something that had to be . . . [with] a new and different love of one's parents" or as "a comradeship with the . . . ways of distant times and different pursuits . . .." The alternative to ego integrity in these terms is *disgust* or *despair.*

Erikson associated with each of the above eight stages a specific trait, as a basic virtue of human development. These traits, in order, are: *hope* (trust), *willpower* (autonomy), *purpose* (initiative), *competence* (industry), *fidelity* (identity), *love* (intimacy), *care* (generativity), and *wisdom* (integrity).

Greenspan

Greenspan (1981) has called attention to the difficulty in reconciling knowledge of development based on emotional experience with knowledge based on cognitive development or impersonal experience, and has attempted to bridge the piagetian and psychoanalytic views of early infant development with a scheme that he calls *developmental structuralist.* In this he draws upon elements of development that belong to the cognitive sphere and upon others that arise out of emotional experience to create a way of analyzing the behavior of infants, identifying needs, and intervening effectively.

Greenspan identifies six stages during the first 48 months: a stage for the acquisition of *homeostasis* (birth to 3 months); a stage of *attachment* (2 to 7 months); a stage of *somatic-psychological differentiation* (3 to 10 months); a stage of *behavioral organization, initiative, and internalization* (9 to 24 months); a stage of *capacity for organizing internal representations* (18 to 30 months); and a stage of *representational differentiation and consolidation* (30 to 48 months). The clinical features that belong to the infant or child who has successfully met the goals of each stage are given in Table 1–16.

TABLE 1-16. Descriptors of the Infant or Child Who Has Achieved Each of the Developmental Structuralist Stages*

STAGE	DESCRIPTION
I. Homeostasis (0–3 mo)	Relaxed, and sleeps at regular times; cries only occasionally. Is very alert; looks at one when talked to; brightens up when rocked, touched, or otherwise stimulated.
II. Attachment (2–7 mo)	Very interested in people, especially mother or father or other key caregivers; looks, smiles, responds to their voices, their touch with signs of pleasure and interest—smiling or vocalizations indicating pleasure. Seems to respond with deep feeling and with multiple sensory modalities.
III. Somatic-psychological differentiation (3–10 mo)	Able to interact in a purposeful (cause-and-effect) manner; smiles in response to smile; alerts, smiles, or looks in response to a voice; able to initiate signals and respond to signals using multiple sensory modalities and the motor system across a range of emotions; able to get involved with toys and other inanimate objects and have pleasure when interacting with a person.
IV. Behavioral organization, initiative, and internalization (9–24 mo)	Manifests a wide range of socially meaningful behaviors and feelings including warmth, pleasure, assertion, exploration, protest, anger, etc., in an organized manner. Can play or interact with parents, stringing together a number of reciprocal interactions into a complex social interchange. Able to go from interacting to separation and reunion with organized affects including pleasure, apprehension, and protest. Initiates complex, organized, emotionally and socially relevant interactions, yet also accepts limits. Can explore new objects and new people, especially when parents are available.
V. Capacity for organizing internal representations (18–30 mo)	Symbolic elaboration in descriptive and interactive contexts. Uses words or wordlike sounds to indicate wishes or intentions; can use dolls or other objects to play out a drama. Symbolic elaboration appears to cover a range of emotions including love, dependency, assertion, curiosity, anger, and protest.
VI. Representational differentiation and consolidation (30–48 mo)	Relates in balanced manner to people and things across a range of emotions (e.g., warmth, assertiveness). Is able to be purposeful, distinguishes what is real from unreal; accepts limits; can be self-limiting and feel good about self; switches from fantasy to reality with little difficulty.

* Adapted from Greenspan (1981, pp 240–243).

Freud, Erikson, Greenspan

In speaking of "stages" of development, it cannot be ignored that normal development is at the same time continuous, fitful, and punctuated by milestones of achievement, and that the word *stage* may be used with a number of meanings. Kessen (1970) discussed the various inferences to be drawn from the word or concept *stage,* and concluded that the notion of stages was useful as a way of gathering together observations or data as a basis for constructing theories of structure. In any case, however, in any schematic description of development, the processes of one stage will overlap temporally those of a previous stage or of one to follow. Indeed, in every stage there will be, along with the seeds of future stages, behaviors that belong to earlier stages, either as normal constituents or as unfinished business.

ETHOLOGIC VIEWS OF CHILD AND ADOLESCENT DEVELOPMENT

The field of ethology is scarcely 50 years old. It has been defined (Dorland, 1981) as "the study of animal behavior, particularly in the natural state, the evolution of behavior, and its biological significance." Ethologists are careful to describe behavior in objective terms, and to note or infer its causes and effects in equally objective terms; there is no immediate inference or presumption as to the inner experience of the animal or person observed.

Ethologic studies have shown that aspects of the social behavior of animals that have been presumably genetically programmed are susceptible to modification, redirection, or distortion through early environmental interventions. Particular attention has been given to the pioneer work of Lorenz, Tinbergen, Harlow, and others on such phenomena as imprinting among birds (Lorenz, 1981), and the catastrophic effect of separation of monkey offspring from their parents during the first weeks or months of life (Harlow and Harlow, 1965).

Behaviors that are of particular interest to the ethologist include earliest attachment (*imprinting* in some animals), feeding and other care of the young, nonverbal communications, greetings, separations, courting, cooperative behavior, the delineation of personal space, defense of territory, and aggressive behavior. All of these behaviors are likely to exist in one form or another in any vertebrate species.

Between behaviors in different species that appear to serve similar functions two kinds of connections may be made. The first is to find an *analogy* in behavior or in its consequences (e.g., in attachment or in the impact of separation at a critical period). An analogy compares the species-specific behavior serving a given purpose for one animal with the behavior of another species that serves the same purpose, without inferring that the mechanisms developed within one species have any evolutionary relationship to the mechanisms developed in the other. The second kind of connection has been called a *homology*, and carries the presumption that a particular behavior may be represented in the genetic makeup of two different species by identical or nearly identical genetic elements derived from a common (albeit perhaps remote) ancestor of both. There are abundant analogies between the behaviors of humans and other species, including some species that are phylogenetically remote. However, the likelihood of finding homologies in the mechanisms underlying analogous behaviors is highest between man and other primates.

Analogies have been drawn between the observations of Harlow and others with monkeys and the findings of Spitz (1965) and Bowlby (1969, 1973, 1980) on the effects of separation or loss upon the human infant or young child. Similar analogies may be derived from the studies of Provence and Lipton (1962) upon the development of infants in institutions. In some instances perhaps overzealous inferences have been drawn as to the imperative nature for human development of discovery of such analogies or homologies, and there is controversy as to which of these inferences demand revision of child-care or child-rearing practices or as to what the nature of any such revisions ought to be. Nonetheless, ethologic methods have enriched our understanding of both animal and human behavior, and when used in the studies of the behavior of infants and children, have offered new perspectives that may increasingly provide insights with clinical relevance.

So far, the principal usefulness of such analogies may be that they tell us what the proper questions are that we should ask as we seek better to understand human behavior. In addition, quite apart from the question as to whether what is observed represents analogy or homology, the ethologic method itself has an important place in the observation of human behavior.

The kinds of questions that fall within the sphere of ethology or have been advanced by ethologic studies include the following:

1. Is there a critical period for attachment of the newborn infant to a mother-figure, after which the possibility of normal socialization is irrevocably impaired? (See, for example, Klaus and Kennell, 1982.)

2. Are the human and primate forms of defense of territory and of aggression (which typically reach full strength during adolescence) built into DNA, or are they determined primarily by sociocultural forces? In either case, can they be made responsive to the creation of new systems of education and association that will make it easier to resolve conflict? (See Lorenz, 1963.)

3. How can systematic observation of the behavior of children entering an established day-care group let us know when the adjustment of a particular child newly admitted is failing to meet normal expectations, and how we may effectively intervene in support of the child? (See McGrew, 1972.)

In a discussion of the place of ethology in the study of human growth and development, Dunn (1979) suggested that the ethologic method has been particularly fruitful in addressing the question as to how differences in the early experiences of the young are related to individual differences among adults. She describes, for example, a study that showed that the handling of very young rodents had long-term effects upon their behavior and growth, with the original interpretation being that the effects were due to the handling itself. Rigorous ethologic observation of the handled animals in the setting in which they grew found, however, that the handling of the infant rodents had an effect upon the behavior of their mothers that may have been the primary determinant of the young animals' altered behavior and growth pattern. Dunn emphasizes the importance of the ethologic principle that behavior should be studied or assessed in its normal or complete context.

CONDUCT OF DEVELOPMENTAL ASSESSMENT

Developmental assessment at any age requires a review of historical data, a physical examination, and neurodevelopmental, cognitive, and psychosocial appraisal. General guidelines for history-taking and physical examination are found in many textbooks and monographs. The procedure through which the appropriate data are gathered will vary with the age of the infant or child, with his or her developmental status, and with the particular circumstances of the moment. Keys to successful data-gathering include the establishment of rapport with parents and child, and tailoring the process to the immediate needs of the family and child. A flexible approach is required.

We have a special interest here in those aspects of data-gathering (including the technique and content of the interview) that are particularly sensitive to developmental level, and knowledge of which may make the process more comfortable and productive. As we discuss each stage of infancy, childhood, and adolescence, we review these features and their implications.

In developmental assessment, it is not enough simply to measure or count physical features, such as height or weight or teeth, or to assess neurodevelopmental or cognitive level (DQ or IQ), or to appraise psychosocial landmarks. Attention should be particularly given to those aspects of the life of the child and family that reveal the *quality* of that life. For every child and family, there are many themes running concurrently through the developmental process. It will be appropriate from time to time to address each of these themes in evaluating the status and the needs of particular children and their families, and in determining their need for counseling or other help.

THEMES

Some developmental processes evolve over long periods of time without precise age-specific landmarks, and often with considerable dependency upon the experience of the individual infant or child. Both the manner in which these processes evolve and the pace of their development tend to be variable and idiosyncratic to the person. We have called these *themes*. Within their variability each contains features that are common to most infants, children, and adolescents, and that warrant description because of their clinical relevance.

Among the themes to which we give particular attention are: temperament; self-concept and body image; gender identity and sexuality; play and friendships; the role of work in child and adolescent development; aggression and violence; fears; and views of illness, death, and dying.

Temperament

It has long been evident to parents, clinicians, and others that differences between infants are apparent from the earliest days of life in their patterns of behavior and in their responses to stimulation. So far as we know, these differences appear to involve less the fundamental mechanisms of physiologic states or responses than the manner in which they are expressed. These differences impart individuality or personality to behavior. Their origins appear to reside at least partially in genetic factors, which may be modified by intrauterine experience (e.g., by maternal emotional states and other experiences that the infant may vicariously share during gestation). These constitutional factors giving individuality to behavior are thought of as defining the *temperament* of the newborn infant or older child.

Systematic study of temperament began a generation ago in the work of Chess, Thomas, and Birch (Chess and Thomas, 1986; Thomas and Chess, 1977), who found nine relatively independent elements descriptive of behavior in infants that they believed could help categorize temperament. These elements were:

1. *Activity level* (the amount of motor activity accompanying behavior)

2. *Rhythmicity (regularity)* (in sleep/wake cycles, hunger, feeding, or elimination)

3. *Approach or withdrawal* (the initial response to a *new* stimulus or experience)

4. *Adaptability* (the ease of acceptance of or adjustment to new or altered situations)

5. *Threshold of responsiveness* (the energy level of stimulus required for a response)

6. *Intensity of reaction* (energy level of the response itself)

7. *Quality of mood* (joyful, pleasant, or friendly, as contrasted with fretful, unpleasant, or unfriendly)

8. *Distractibility* (the resistance of ongoing behavior to interference)

9. *Attention span and persistence* (the time devoted to an activity and the degree to which it is maintained in the face of obstacles)

Certain clusters of relatively stable temperamental features were thought to occur with some frequency and to define groups of infants for whom these features had relevance for child-rearing and for counseling. A first cluster consists of high regularity, positive approach to the new, high adaptability to change, and predominantly positive mood. These traits were thought to characterize about 40 per cent of the infants studied, who might be regarded as *"easy"* from the standpoint of child-rearing needs.

A second cluster comprised a tendency to irregularity of functions, a negative initial response to new experiences, slow adaptability, and intense moods (often predominantly negative). Infants and children with these traits were regarded as *"difficult"* and numbered about 10 per cent of the study group.

A third cluster consisted of a somewhat negative initial response to new experiences, with a slow adaptation to changing circumstances, with relatively low intensity of response, and with a generally favorable degree of regularity of functions. Infants and children with this constellation of traits have been described as *"slow to warm up."* They made up about 15 per cent of the study group.

Suggestions have been made as to how adjustments might be made in the management of "difficult" children to compensate for their temperamental characteristics. For example, such children and their parents may be more comfortable if the general level of stimulation in the environment can be kept relatively low, and if new experiences are introduced gradually.

Chess and Thomas have shown how the behavior of older infants, toddlers, and school-aged children can be characterized with respect to the temperamental traits displayed. On the other hand, it is thought that in many older infants and children the forces exerted upon the development of the personality or character of the child by original temperament may be much less determinative of personality traits than the child's unique experiences.

Considerable attention has been given to the "goodness of fit" between the temperament of the newborn or very young infant and his or her mother's personality, needs, expectations, or child-rearing practices. For example, the confrontation between a "difficult" infant and a mother who is irritable, impatient, authoritarian, anxious, or prone to guilt feelings can set the stage for a long period of conflict and misunderstanding that may have heavy and long-term impact upon their relationship and upon the emotional and social development of the infant and child. By contrast, a very passive, "easy" infant may make so few demands upon a passive, distant, or depressed mother that the needs of the infant are not adequately communicated to nor anticipated by the mother, with the result that the infant lacks essential input for cognitive, emotional, or social growth.

Chess and Thomas have evaluated temperament in the infant and child through giving the clinical interview an orientation toward items reflecting possible temperamental factors. They and others have developed questionnaires, as well, that can be given to parents or teachers. Carey and McDevitt (1978) have constructed a questionnaire particularly designed for the evaluation of the infant.

Misgivings have been expressed (Rothbart 1981, 1982) at the possibility that "labeling" infants as "difficult" will create a self-fulfilling prophecy. Rothbart concluded, moreover, that evidence for the stability of a finding of "difficult" temperament is not very convincing prior to the age of 3 to 4 years. Other evidence (Field and Greenberg, 1982) suggests that the determination of this temperamental trait may be considerably colored by the attitudes or expectations of the person making the judgment—whether parent or teacher—as well as by the setting in which the judgment is made (e.g., home *versus* school *versus* physician's office).

Development of Self-Concept

Philosophers and behavioral theorists have long attempted to define the complex concept of "self." A recurring theme has been the duality of the self as both the "subject" (the active experience of self) on the one hand, and the "object" of one's knowledge of self on the other. Lewis and Brooks (1974) postulate that prime tasks of the infant are 1) to realize that he or she exists as a separate person from others in the environment, and as an active causal agent for events or change (the self as "subject"); and 2) to develop categories by which he or she can define him or herself (the self as "object") in relationship to that environment. We define *self-concept* as the combination of subjective knowledge and experience of one's self *(self-image)* and one's evaluation of one's self *(self-esteem)*. It is through social interaction with significant people in the environment that one develops one's self-concept.

The child's developing self-concept evolves with events and changes in the environment, especially in relationship to significant people, and with the child's ability to interpret and conceptualize these changes. Burns (1984) describes five sources of the self-concept: 1) body image (an evaluation of the physical self as a distinct object); 2) language (the ability to conceptualize and verbalize about self and others); 3) interpreted feedback from the environment (about how significant others view the person and about how the person stands in relation to various societal norms and values); 4) identification with the appropriate sex role model and stereotype; and 5) the child-rearing practices within which the child has developed.

Development of Body Image

The term *body image* (or self-image) refers to the concepts that an infant, child, adolescent, or adult may have about his or her own body. The notion embraces both anatomic and emotional elements. Ideas that are either correct or incorrect anatomically may be found satisfying or unsatisfactory, anxiety-provoking, or loathsome.

The formation of the anatomic body image may begin in utero or at the latest in very early life. We do not know with certainty what the perceptions of newborn infants may be as to the boundaries between themselves and the environment or other people. It seems reasonable to surmise that the sense of self is initially rudimentary and that it may be built chiefly around the oral area, the face, and the hands. Whether the newborn infant imitates the sticking out of the tongue because of some congruence with an innate body image is not known, and may be unlikely (see p. 152). On the other hand, hand-to-mouth activity (such as thumbsucking) occurs in utero, and contributes to the self-quieting behavior of the newborn and young infant. Any relationship of such behavior to evolving body image can be only speculative, but in any case, through the early interaction with the environment, by touching and being touched, by experiencing hunger pangs from within and their amelioration from without, and so forth, the infant in the sensorimotor stage begins to define body boundaries.

In the first months of life the progression of exploration by the hands of the infant is from predominantly facial and especially perioral activity, to touching and rubbing of the head, of the trunk, and (by 4 months) of the hands together. Later the attention of the infant is drawn to the feet (by 6 months) and (by 9 months) to the genitalia. In this way the infant discovers the sensory boundaries between his or her own body and the outer world.

Visual Recognition of Self

The most-studied aspect of development of the sense of self has been visual recognition. Recognition of one's facial features is the earliest evidence one has of one's uniqueness. Visual self-recognition during infancy follows a developmental sequence:

At 5 to 8 months: Infants smile at their images in mirrors or as captured on videotape. They may touch the image and wave, but there is no evidence that they have differentiated themselves from others (or from the image in the mirror). According to Murphy et al. (1937), it is not until after the age of 6 months that the process of discrimination between body and nonbody is clear.

At 9 to 12 months: Infants show signs of appreciating themselves as being separate from others—by touching their own bodies while looking in a mirror and by turning toward others whose reflections are seen in it.

At 15 to 18 months: The infant can now recognize a mark upon his or her own face as seen in a mirror, turning attention to and touching the corresponding point on the face. This gives evidence of the emergence of self-recognition and self-conscious behaviors. Some infants can now "label and point to pictures of themselves."

At 21 to 24 months: Infants now have a clear sense of themselves as distinct from others. Many are able to use appropriately their own names and personal pronouns. A summary of the acquisition sequence of visual recognition, as proposed by Harter (1982), is given in Table 1–17.

Motor Development and Self-Concept

With the development of motor skills (manipulation of objects, ambulation, etc.) the infant develops the ability purposefully to explore and influence the environment, and in so doing, to become differentiated from it. As he or she begins to ambulate, there are contacts with an increasing number of significant other persons, all of whom help in this process of differentiation.

Language Development and Self-Concept

The process of development of self-concept is greatly aided by the development of language. Some theorists believe that the most crucial event in the infant's development of a sense of self is his or her realization that he or she has a name different from that of significant others. At around the age of 2 years, the child begins to use personal pronouns such

TABLE 1–17. Summary of Stage Models Related to the Infant's Development of Self*

APPROXIMATE AGES	VISUAL RECOGNITION STUDIES	MAHLER'S PHASES OF SEPARATION-INDIVIDUATION	AINSWORTH'S PHASES OF ATTACHMENT	SANDER'S STAGES OF MOTHER-INFANT INTERACTION
0–5	(1) No self-other differentiation	(1) Normal, autistic and symbiotic phases	(1) Preattachment phase	(1) Initial regulation
5–10	(2) Awareness of bodily self as cause of movement	(2) Differentiation	(2) Attachment in the making	(2) Reciprocal exchange
10–15	(3) Differentiation of self as active agent from others	(3) Practicing	(3) Clear-cut attachment	(3) Initiative (4) Focalization
15–20	(4) Featural recognition of self	(4) Rapprochement		(5) Self-assertion
18+	(5) Verbal labeling of the self	(5) Resolution and consolidation	(4) Goal-corrected partnership	(6) Recognition (7) Self-constancy

* From Harter S: Developmental perspectives on the self-system. In Mussen PH (ed): *Handbook of Child Psychology*, 4th ed, vol IV. New York, John Wiley & Sons, 1983, p 291.

as "me" and "mine"—another step in defining individuality. At approximately 3 years youngsters become interested in "name games" and in having their names placed on possessions; this is viewed by some as evidence of "identity-uncertainty" at this age. At approximately 5 years of age, first-person plural pronouns begin to appear in the vocabulary, as the child has more experiences as a member of a group.

With language acquisition, the child gradually becomes able to define previously amorphous feelings and moods, and in so doing further defines him or herself as an individual separate from those around.

Gender Identity

One of the first self-defining factors to which the infant is exposed is his or her sex. From the moment of birth (and even earlier, when amniocentesis reveals the fetal sex), the cultural and psychologic significance of the baby's biologic sex will influence parental expectations and his or her name, dress, and toys. The gender label is learned by the end of the second year. It is not until the age of 5 to 7 years, during the stage of concrete operational thinking, however, that the concept of gender constancy is internalized. Before that time, the youngster, although knowing his or her gender, finds it plausible that this might change.

Development of Self-Esteem

The terms *self-image* and *self-esteem* are often used interchangeably, but they really reflect different dimensions of the developing self. The nearly 100-year-old definition of William James (1890) captures the distinction:

$$Self\text{-}Esteem = Success/Pretensions$$

Physical Attributes and Self-Esteem. As children grow up, physical attributes play an increasingly important role in determining their sense of adequacy and value. It is not unusual to find that children with major deformities have excellent self-image until they enter school and get exposed to nicknaming and negative feedback from classmates. As the individual begins to interact with an ever-widening circle of friends and significant others, language serves another function in forming self-concept, in that it provides the vehicle for feedback from them. A common and often derogatory manifestation of this is the assignment of nicknames that reflect features of physical appearance (e.g., "Four-eyes," "Slim," "Tubby," or "Twiggy").

Richardson et al. (1964) studied the effects of having a *physical disability* on self-concept in 10- to 11-year-old children. They found that the handicapped children were realistic in descriptions of themselves in that they were aware that they could not live up to the peer values, which they shared, about the importance of participation in physical activities. They reported being more restricted physically and socially, both within the family and within the peer group. Sex differences were noted in children's coping styles with respect to disabilities. For example, girls were found more likely to choose nonphysical recreation, whereas boys indicated more problems with interpersonal relations, were more concerned about aggression, and made more use of humor in their attempts to win peer acceptance.

As early as 6 years of age boys have stereotypic behavioral expectations of their peers that are based on *somatotype*. Those with mesomorphic builds are clearly regarded as having the most favorable attributes, being characterized as outgoing and leaders. Since it appears that boys are able to describe accurately their own body type from the age of 7 years, it is likely that dissatisfaction with one's own body arises at about this time. The desirability of having a mesomorphic build increases during adolescence for boys, with early maturers being greatly favored (see p. 300).

The Role of Feedback. Feedback from significant other persons in the caretaking or social environment is viewed as one of the most important bases for development of self-esteem. The conventional impression has been that parents are most important in this regard during childhood, and peers during adolescence. On the other hand, when Kirchner and Vondraek (1975) asked children from the ages of 3 to 5 years to identify people who liked them, more of them cited peers and siblings than parents as sources of esteem. Mothers were mentioned more often than fathers when parents were cited, and girls were more likely to include parents than were boys.

In preadolescence the concept of self continues to be modified by an increasingly wide circle of social relationships that includes peers and teachers, whose feedback assumes great import. Achieving scholastically, socially, and athletically, and living up to standards set by parents and teachers, become the benchmarks of success and the basis for high self-esteem at this age.

The literature supports the notion that peer influences are greater during middle adolescence than before or after. "The crucial arena for arriving at a clearer and realistic picture of one's assets and liabilities does seem to be that of peer interaction. Peers are approximately the same in size and age, whereas at home there exists an age hierarchy, even brothers and sisters being older or younger. Accordingly, differences in competence are expected at home, but within the peer group the child need only show he is at least equal with others. At home he must be love-worthy, within the peer group he must be respect-worthy, competitive and competent" (Burns, 1984).

Cognitive Development and Self-Concept. The implications of cognitive development for the developing self-esteem must also be considered. In piagetian terms, older infancy and young childhood (2 to 7 years) is the time of preoperational thought, greatly aided by the acquisition of language, as indicated above. At this stage, the child acquires the ability to label concrete characteristics of him or herself, with a repertoire of categories of such characteristics that grows rapidly at this time. During the stage of concrete operations (7 to 11 years), with growing orientation to reality, the ability to classify hierarchically and logically further influences self-perception. The child now develops the ability also to take the perspective of the other person and as a result, to consider how he or she may be viewed by another person. In the stage of formal operations achieved during adolescence, the youngster develops the capacity for introspection, the powers of deduction, and often, a preoccupation with things hypothetical. As a result, adolescents typically develop a "theory of self."

The Content of Self-Concept

Just as the process of development of self-concept evolves with time, so does its content. For example, 6-year-old children focus more on differences between themselves and others than do 16-year-olds, who appear more interested in identifying similarities. Studies of children from the ages of 7 to 14 years also reveal that with increasing age there is less emphasis on objective factors such as physical appearance and more on those that relate to interpersonal relationships, personal attributes, attitudes, and philosophy. At the age of 15 years, however, the importance of physical appearance and attractiveness is again apparent. Sex differences in content of self-concept have also been noted: girls appear more concerned with relationships with the opposite sex and within families, and boys more with hobbies.

The concept of the ideal self changes during childhood, as well as the relationship between the perceived and the idealized selves. In studies of the developmental sequence of the ideal self Havighurst et al. (1946) found that until the age of 8 to 10 years, primary identification is with a parental figure; that there is next a stage of romanticism and glamour in which the idealized person is a movie star, teacher, or even a physician; and that in late adolescence a composite emerges of desirable characteristics representing the idealized self. Lynch (1981) suggests that the idealized self does not begin to be developed until the ages of 6 to 9 years; he attributes such a finding to the fact that younger children have not yet acquired rules for setting expectations.

Antecedents of Self-Esteem

With the recognition of the importance of high self-esteem in our society has come the search for parental characteristics associated with desirable outcomes. According to Maccoby (1980), parents of boys with high self-esteem were more likely to have been: 1) accepting, involved, and affectionate; 2) consistent in their setting and enforcement of rules and in encouraging high standards for their children's behavior; 3) noncoercive disciplinarians; and 4) democratic, in allowing the child to be heard when decisions were made concerning issues that affected him. In general, it is accepted that an important prerequisite for developing positive self-esteem is "unconditional positive regard" on the part of parents (Rogers' term [1951]).

Adolescence and Self-Concept

The ericksonian view holds that adolescence, at least in our culture, is the time when the self-concept is revised in reaction to the physical, emotional, and social changes that have taken place with the onset of puberty. The weight of evidence has suggested, however, that one's self-concept is relatively stable from early to late adolescence and even from late childhood through adolescence (Piers and Harris, 1964). On the other hand, Simmons, Rosenberg, and Rosenberg (1973) found changes in self-image over this period of time: that early adolescents had lower self-esteem, increased self-consciousness, and greater instability of self-image than younger children. They attributed many of their findings to the environment, and particularly the transition from elementary to junior high school. Other investigators report that those who enter junior high school with higher self-concepts appear to have the greatest decrement in self-concept in this setting.

As indicated above, the physical self in adolescence again becomes an important factor in self-concept, but in addition to the desirability of possessing a fashionable body, it is important that the timing of pubertal change be in synchrony with that of the peer group. Particularly for boys in our culture, to mature late (in relationship to the peer standard) is associated with adverse social, educational, and psychologic sequelae. The self-esteem of girls appears to be adversely affected by the fact that the onset of puberty is associated with increased adiposity and broadening of the pelvic girdle, with the resultant feeling that they are fat. The desire to be thinner is a common finding among adolescent women, to which in recent years has been added the desire to be taller, and even more muscular! (The latter desire appears to be in response to the changing image of women in our society, with its increasing emphasis on involvement in athletics.)

The Development of Sexuality

The community does not generally regard "sexuality" as a developmental issue prior to adolescence, yet its foundation is clearly laid down throughout the preceding years, beginning in earliest infancy, or even earlier in the experiences and attitudes of parents. Developing sexuality represents an amalgam of biologic, psychologic, social, and cultural contributions.

Biologic Sex

The infant's biologic sex is determined by his or her chromosomal makeup; that is, by the presence or absence in fetal life of the testicular differentiating factor, which is carried on the Y chromosome and transforms the undifferentiated gonad into a testis; in the absence of this factor the gonad differentiates into an ovary. The testis, in turn, through the action of dihydrotestosterone, stimulates the formation of the male external genitalia. The appearance of the genitalia will determine the sex assigned to the baby at the time of birth.

When amniocentesis permits examination of the chromosomes during fetal life, the biologic sex of the fetus may be revealed prior to birth. On the other hand, errors may occur at the time of birth in the assignment of the infant's sex.

In the newborn infant, the hypothalamic-pituitary-gonadal axis is structurally identical to that of the pubertal adolescent, but it is functionally dormant owing to inhibition of production or release of hypothalamic gonadotropin-releasing factor, possibly by the action of melatonin. In the first few days of life estrogen passively transferred from the mother is responsible for breast enlargement in infants of both sexes and for a milky and occasionally blood-tinged vaginal discharge. These findings rarely are misinterpreted, but the appearance of clitoral hypertrophy may cause erroneous assignment of gender. Such hypertrophy occurs rarely, as the result of stimulation by androgenic hormones taken by the mother or because of congenital adrenal hyperplasia, in which exposure to excessive levels of androgens may produce marked enlargement.

Biologic differences between the sexes in infancy include greater muscular strength and lower basal skin conductance in males. Females are more advanced than male infants in neurologic development at birth, spending more time asleep and less crying.

Gender Identity

Ehrhardt and Money (1967) have written: "Gender identity [is] the sameness, unity and persistence of one's individuality as male, female, or ambivalent, in greater or lesser degree, especially as it is experienced in self-awareness and behavior; gender identity is the private experience of gender role, and gender role is the public expression of gender identity." More simply stated, gender identity reflects the individual's sense of being feminine or masculine.

From the time of determination of the infant's sex, whether through amniocentesis during pregnancy or at the time of birth, boys and girls are treated differently, in accordance with the sex assigned. It is the assigned sex that will be the most important factor in determining the infant's and child's own view of his or her sexual identity. It is this view that defines the gender identity. Name, color and type of clothing, and selection of toys will all reflect and reinforce societal stereotypes and expectations based on assigned sex. Fortunately, there is usually congruence between the biologic sex, the assigned sex, and the ultimate gender identity.

The factors that determine gender identity are not fully known. The behavior of caretakers undoubtedly plays an important role. Mothers provide more stimulation to female babies than to males. The fact that newborn male infants are awake more and cry more than female infants often results in a more intense, but potentially less satisfying interaction between mother and son than between mother and daughter. It has been postulated that this phenomenon may be responsible for a difference in the focus of socialization between the sexes, with behavioral control emphasized in males and comfort in females. In support of this view is the finding that boys receive more physical punishment than girls, which may partly explain the ultimately heightened aggressiveness of the former. It has been observed that by the time infants are 3 months old, their mothers interact more with and speak more to female than to male infants. Kagan (1971) suggested that mothers may find easier rapport with daughters than with sons, the latter being less easily identified with.

Bower et al. (1979) reported that as early as the age of 9 or 10 months, the infant is able to recognize in pictures the portrayal of other infants of his or her own sex, even when the infant in the picture is dressed in the clothing of the opposite sex. Jacklin et al. (1973) found that as early as 13 months of age, the infant is likely to choose toys consistent with his or her own sex. The same study found that this preference was not the result of mothers offering different playthings to sons and daughters, and suggests that the infant's sex-stereotyped preferences were already established by this young age. It is not until the age of 5 to 7 years that one recognizes his or her gender identity as unchangeable.

There is considerable information regarding the relationship of later sexual behavior to exposure of young animals to hormones, but relatively little is known about the contribution of hormones to the development of gender-specific social roles in humans. Some studies of girls in whom adrenogenital syndrome led to prenatal exposure to elevated levels of androgens have found that, despite surgical correction of their masculinized genitalia within the first 2 years of age, they are more likely than normal sibling controls to be "tomboyish," are less interested in dolls as play objects, and show preferences for male playmates rather than female (Ehrhardt et al., 1968). In such studies, it is difficult to assess the possible impact of confusion concerning the child's ambiguous genitalia at birth on the parents' manner of rearing the child or upon their report of subsequent behavior. Another study found that the administration of estrogens and progestins to infant boys was associated with less "rough and tumble" play, less aggression, and diminished athletic prowess (Ehrhardt, 1981).

Psychosocial Theories of the Origin of Gender Identity. Freud theorized that sexual behavior involves a complex interplay between excitation and satisfaction, and that neonatal sexual impulses are not different in principle from those of adults. In the newborn infant, for example, excitation results from the need for nourishment and satisfaction from the meeting of this need through feeding. Freud postulated that the satisfaction derived from feeding generalizes to the process of sucking, which, through conditioned reinforcement, becomes endowed with elements of pleasure. Freud viewed the child's first sexual object to be his mother's breast, the source of both nourishment and pleasure. He acknowledged that sexuality is transformed during the course of development, but argued the case for continuity between infantile and adult sexuality.

Classical psychoanalytic theory held that boys and girls are relatively undifferentiated in their sexuality during the first years of life, having much the same experiences in nourishment and other care. Their courses in development of sexuality parted company with the discovery of anatomic differences at about the age of 4 years, with the discovery leading to *penis envy* in girls and to *castration anxiety* in boys. Female sexuality was regarded as being driven by the need of the girl to recapture the penis by union with the father (a taboo) or by having a baby. The effect was to define female sexuality as born out of a deficiency.

These early constructions were derived mostly from retrospective analysis of clinical problems of adults, in an age when little was known of the early development of infants and young children. More current psychoanalytic views, informed by what we now know of the elements that go into the formation of gender identity, give much less importance to a notion of penis envy, and would regard major evidence of penis envy in an adult woman as a sign of psychopathology.

There is now ample evidence that both girls and boys come to the discovery of their anatomic differences with their femininity or masculinity already well established as a result of the climate of parental and cultural attitudes within which they have lived for the first months and years of their lives. The discovery of anatomic differences, moreover, begins to be elaborated as early as the second year, and Bower et al. (1979) have found evidence, as indicated above, that an appreciation of differences between boys and girls may be shown as early as 9 to 10 months of age in the preferences of infants to look at the pictures of other infants of their own sex. In any case, the turning of the little girl toward the father and the wish to have a baby may well antedate the discovery of anatomy, and be integral to the early formation of gender identity.

The above comments are not to say that the discovery of anatomic differences is irrelevant. It is not uncommon for the little girl who has discovered the penis to wonder if her mother has one or why she herself does not, or to attempt to urinate in a standing position, with predictable consequences. In situations, however, where there is a good and free relationship between mother and daughter, "penis curiosity" presents no problem of penis envy. For boys the discovery seems more likely to enhance feelings of masculinity than to create castration anxiety.

Erikson's contribution to understanding of the child's development of sexuality rests in his delineation of the importance of identity formation as an element in each of the psychosocial crises that he has described (pp. 80–81). Erikson has held that adult sexuality depends upon the mastery of the stage that sets *intimacy* against *isolation,* and that true psychosocial intimacy, in its capacity for shared feelings and purposes, is not to be confused with sexual intimacy or experiences. The latter may considerably antedate that mastery.

Sexuality in Infancy

Biologic Aspects. Infants possess the capacity for penile erections from the time of birth. These may be associated with a variety of circumstances, including crying, thumbsucking, fullness of bladder and bowels, or voiding. Spontaneous erections also occur during sleep, and those that occur during rapid eye movement (REM) sleep are often accompanied by smiling. Direct genital stimulation may result in erection, with smiling and cooing, in older infants of both sexes.

By the age of 3 years, both sexes are capable of orgasm. This typically consists of a rapid arousal to climax, without ejaculation, followed by a brief refractory period of several seconds in length.

Sexual Behavior in Infancy. Masturbation often follows the infant's discovery, in the course of bodily exploration, of the pleasurable nature of genital touching. Between 60 and 90 per cent of 1-year-olds appear to engage in masturbation, its onset being somewhat later in girls than boys (means ages 10 and 6 months, respectively). A sex difference is also seen in frequency of masturbation, male infants engaging in self-stimulation twice as often as females.

After its accidental initiation, masturbation becomes intentional and systematic by the age of 5 years in many children of both sexes. The emotional impact of such experiences on young children is still unclear, as are its implications for later masturbatory behavior. It appears, however, that such activity is harmless if it is kept private and if parents accept it as normal and do not punish it.

Psychosocial Aspects. Cognition is a major factor in the development of sexuality, both as to content and process. The content includes the child's developing gender identity and increasing factual knowledge about sex. By the end of the second year of life, the child often knows that his or her genitalia differ from those of the opposite sex.

Sexuality in Childhood

Biologic Aspects. The finding that serum levels of melatonin decrease after the age of 7 years has been viewed by some as accounting for the lessening of inhibitory control of hypothalamic gonadotropin-releasing hormone that eventuates in the onset of puberty. While this change of level of melatonin is occurring, the growth of the average child involves a steady increase in height and weight, with no change in body habitus or in secondary sex characteristics. In some children, however, precocious puberty or some component of it, occurs.

> Premature thelarche refers to the isolated growth of breasts in a girl before the age of 8 years. It has its onset most often before the age of 2 years, but may appear at any age thereafter. It is not associated with elevations in serum hormone levels, nor are other manifestations of puberty apparent. The natural course is spontaneous regression.

> Premature adrenarche refers to the appearance of sexual hair, without other secondary sex characteristics, before the age of 8 years in girls or before 9 years in boys. It generally has its onset after the age of 6 years, and may be associated with elevated serum levels of 17-ketosteroids and mild acceleration of height and bone age. There is no associated enlargement of genitalia and treatment is usually not necessary.

> In isosexual precocity, there is development of all secondary sex characteristics before the usual lower limit of normal ages of 8 years in girls and 9.5 years in boys. This condition may be benign and of unknown cause or the result of ingestion of exogenous hormone, lesions of the central nervous system, hypothyroidism, or tumors of adrenal, gonad, or gonadotropin-producing tissue.

> Heterosexual precocity occurs when there is development of sexual characteristics of the opposite sex, the result of adrenal or ovarian androgen secretion in girls or estrogen production by teratomas or adrenal tumors in boys.

Sexual Behavior in Childhood. Masturbation during childhood may or may not be continuous with earlier similar activity. The prevalence figure of 38 per cent for males between the ages of 4 and 14 years is much lower than for infancy, suggesting that infantile masturbation is often not continued. The majority of boys indicate that they began to masturbate between the ages of 3 and 7 years, with one third indicating that it was discovered by themselves and most of the others reporting having heard about it or watched a companion masturbate before they themselves initiated it. Of females in the sample studied by Kinsey et al. (1948), the majority began to masturbate following accidental discovery and typically at an older age (some not until adulthood). Among those women who began autoerotic behavior during childhood, the frequency diminished with approaching adolescence, a pattern quite different from males.

Masturbation in the young child is a self-quieting activity, not unlike thumbsucking in its effect. It is typically performed in private, at night and usually in bed. When it becomes more frequent and particularly if it occurs in public, parents should be aware that it should be discouraged and perhaps be considered an indicator of the need for professional consultation. It should never be punished. In the older child, as in the adolescent, masturbation may serve as a means of exploring a growing curiosity about sex.

Sex Play in Childhood. By the age of 2 to 3 years children typically first begin to investigate the genitalia of playmates and expose their own in return. "Playing house" and "playing doctor" are common games among older preschool children and often include elements of genital exploration or apposition. In cultures in which children are permitted to observe adult lovemaking, such play may include attempts at copulation.

Psychosocial Aspects. Kreitler and Kreitler (1966) found that nearly all of the 4- to 5½-year-old boys they studied knew that their genitals were different from those of girls.

Bernstein and Cowan (1975) evaluated developmental changes in understanding of sexual information in middle-class children from the ages of 3 to 12 years. They asked them: "How does the baby happen to be inside the mother's body?" A five-step developmental sequence was observed:

At the first level, the responses of 3- to 4-year-old children were considered to correspond to Piaget's preformist stage. They believed that a baby who now exists has always existed. Prior to being in the mother's body, it must have existed some other place.

At Level 2 (ages 5 to 6 years), children now attribute causality to the existence of babies and believe that they must be assembled, as are inanimate objects.

At Level 3 children are in transition from the stage of preoperational to concrete operational thinking in the piagetian schema. They have become aware of the necessity of contributions from social relationship, sexual intercourse, and genetic material but are unable to organize these into a coherent system.

At Level 4 children (ages 8 to 9 years) at the stage of concrete operations have constructed a coordinated system of biologic causality.

By Level 5, children tend to believe that the union of gametes releases a preformed embryo, a notion not unlike the homunculus theory of the past.

A final Level 6, representing full understanding, is not reached until early adolescence.

Sexuality in Adolescence

Biologic Factors. As indicated above, there is, after the age of about 7 years, a gradual diminution of the forces (probably mediated through melatonin produced by the pineal gland) that had previously inhibited hypothalamic production of gonadotropin-releasing hormone (Gn-RH, which appears to be responsible for the release both of follicle-stimulating hormone [FSH] and of luteinizing hormone [LH]).

Gn-RH is first detected in early adolescence, with rising levels produced in a pulsatile manner. Pulsatile secretion appears necessary for stimulation of the anterior pituitary's production of the gonadotropic hormones LH and FSH, which are also released in pulses, in association with each sleep cycle. LH and FSH are responsible for stimulation of the ovaries and testes to produce estrogen and testosterone, respectively. The development of the secondary sex characteristics and reproductive capability that characterizes puberty is the result of these dramatic endocrine changes (see pp. 231–236).

Early adolescence also sees enhanced production of pituitary growth hormone, which, in conjunction with somatomedin-C produced by the liver, is responsible for the spurt in linear growth in puberty. (see p. 236).

Physical Manifestations of Puberty. Only the transformation in size and shape of the human body that occurs during fetal life is as dramatic as the changes that occur with puberty. These changes are most apparent in growth of the skeletal system, in the soft tissues (emphasizing muscle and fat in males and females, respectively), and in the reproductive organs and development of secondary sex characteristics. Less obvious growth occurs elsewhere in the body; this is least manifest in the central nervous system, whereas the lymphatic system actually undergoes involution during puberty.

Secondary sex characteristics *in males* result from increased production of testosterone with the onset of puberty. There is growth of hair in the genital area, the axillae, on the face, and eventually on the chest and trunk; the voice changes; acne appears; and there is growth of the external genitalia. *In females,* production of estrogen by the ovaries, as well as some androgen secretion by the adrenals, is responsible for growth of the breasts and of pubic and axillary hair. Because many of these changes occur in an orderly and predictable pattern, their appearance forms the basis for a system of categorizing pubertal development (see Figs. 8–12 to 8–14).

The average age at *menarche* (the onset of menstruation) is currently 12.4 years, with a normal range of 10 to 16 years. The occurrence of menarche coincides with the peak of the weight velocity curve. Many factors determine the timing of menarche and the normal patterns of menstrual cycling that follow. They include genetic, familial, nutritional, chemical, and psychologic factors. Ten per cent of girls have their menarche when they are at SMR 2, 20 per cent at SMR 3, 60 per cent at SMR 4, and 10 per cent at SMR 5.

The timing of the onset of pubertal changes and the pace of their evolution are quite variable within any population as the result of genetic and familial patterns. Moreover, illnesses and other events can alter the timing. Acceleration in time of onset of puberty is associated with obesity, acquired hypothyroidism, myelomeningocele, and blindness. Delay may result from nutritional deprivation, secondary either to physical or to psychologic illness; to hypoxia (such as may occur in cyanotic congenital heart disease or cystic fibrosis); to participation in endurance athletics; to chronic administration of medications, such as corticosteroids; or to gonadal damage by chemotherapeutic agents, radiation, or hemo-chromatosis.

Orgasm. Orgasm in postpubertal males is different from that of younger children because of the occurrence of ejaculation, with discharge of semen. The capacity for ejaculation typically first appears within 1 year of onset of testicular growth. In Kinsey et al's sample, 90 per cent of 11- to 15-year-olds had experienced ejaculation, with the economically advantaged group reporting earlier onset than those who were from the lower socioeconomic group. Orgasm was most often accomplished through masturbation among those in the higher socioeconomic group. Young adolescents (under the age of 15 years) reported the largest number of orgasms, an average of 2.9 per week. First nocturnal emissions typically occur 1 year after achievement of ejaculatory ability.

Less information is available about orgasm in female adolescents. Kinsey et al's retrospective and now outdated study (1953) found that females 15 years of age or younger reported an average of one orgasm every 3 weeks, with masturbation the most frequent source. A more recent survey (Sorensen, 1973) of adolescents and their sexual beliefs and behaviors, likely also outdated, reaffirmed the frequency with which adolescent females reach orgasm as a result of masturbation (71 per cent). An additional finding of interest was that more than half of those who had experienced intercourse reported that they had rarely or never had an orgasm during intercourse.

Reproductive Capability. In females, reproductive ability awaits the establishment of ovulation, which may or may not commence with menarche. In general, monthly ovulatory cycles are not established until between 12 and 18 months after menarche. Pregnancy may, however, occur after the first ovulatory episode. In males, spermarche (the production of mature sperm capable of impregnation) may occur at any stage of puberty, though it is most likely to appear with SMR 5.

Developmental Problems of Adolescent Sexuality. Certain normal aspects of pubertal development may, despite their normality, present problems to young adolescents and have negative impact on their feelings about their developing sexuality. Because they are misinterpreted or misunderstood, they are common sources of worry and doubts about sexual adequacy. Breast development in girls, for example, may be unilateral or asymmetric for a while, an occurrence that the girl may find unexpected and anxiety provoking. *Gynecomastia* occurs in 30 to 50 per cent of normal boys around SMR 3 and resolves within 18 months. It usually consists of a round and commonly tender disk of tissue located directly under the nipple. The condition may be unilateral and sometimes recurrent; it rarely lasts more than a few months, and needs no treatment other than reassurance. In both sexes *acne* is produced by the elevated levels of androgens, which produce an increase in size and secretion of sebaceous follicles. Acne is considered to be unattractive among adolescents, who resent it but are often reticent to discuss it. *Myopia* often has its first appearance with puberty, and the need to wear eyeglasses, like acne, often has a negative impact upon self-image.

Development of Interpersonal Sexual Behavior

Mutual Masturbation (Same Sex). Parents who discover their children, boys or girls, engaged in mutual masturbation are often concerned that this activity signifies homosexuality, but it most often represents simply rehearsal for future heterosexual experiences, and a means of self-exploration, experimentation, comparison, and reassurance. Glasser (1977) describes the early adolescent male as becoming narcissistically self-absorbed, selecting friends (with whom he may masturbate) who possess characteristics he would himself like to possess. It is only when the partner is an adult that mutual masturbation may suggest homosexuality.

Development of Heterosexual Relationships. Chess et al. (1976) described a developmental sequence in the sociosexual behavior of adolescents. The youngsters they studied progressed from having friends of the same sex, to having friends of both sexes, to heterosexual dating with a number of friends, to dating one individual as a "steady," and finally, but not inevitably, to having sexual intercourse.

Schofield (1965) found that even within the steady dating relationship, there appears to be a developmental progression. Among the British 15- to 19-year-olds whom he studied, he found the first stage of the dating relationship to be limited to shared social activity without kissing. In stage 2, there is kissing and possibly stimulation of the fully clothed breasts. In stage 3, there may be touching of unclothed breasts, genital stimulation, or apposition. Stage 4 was defined by sexual intercourse with a single partner, and stage 5 by intercourse with multiple partners.

In a study of American youth Sorensen (1973) found a similar sequence. Among approximately one quarter of the 13- to 15-year-olds interviewed (20 per cent of males and 25 per cent of females) heterosexual activity was limited to kissing. An additional 17 per cent (14 per cent of males and 19 per cent of females) had experienced touching each other's bodies and exposing one's body to another for pleasure. Among adolescents mutual caressing (petting) appears to represent more than foreplay to intercourse. It serves to teach teenagers about each other's bodies as well as about their own emotional and sexual feelings. Besides providing pleasure and satisfaction, it also functions to socialize the adolescent as to rules and customs of sexual behavior.

In the United States, approximately 6 per cent of females and 18 per cent of males have engaged in sexual intercourse by the age of 13 years. By the age of 19 years, this prevalence increases to approximately 60 per cent for females and 79 per cent for males. During the past decade there was a 66 per cent increase in sexual activity among 15- to 19-year-old females, with most of the increase accounted for among white teenagers. The average age of onset of intercourse appears, however, to be remaining fairly constant. The home has replaced the automobile as the most common site for adolescent intercourse.

The determinants of the transition from virginity to initiation of sexual intercourse have been examined by Jessor and Jessor (1975b), in a prospective study of a large sample of youth followed from the time of junior high school. The Jessors found that when compared with virgins, non-virgins tended to be those who valued independence more and achievement less. The nonvirgin group seemed to be more influenced by the views of friends than those of parents, to be less religious and more tolerant of drug usage, and to have poorer records of scholastic achievement than those who had remained virginal. The consequences of the experience of sexual intercourse are discussed later (pp. 302–304, 315–316).

Psychosocial Aspects

Effect of Variations in Timing of Pubertal Maturation. Despite the evident wide range of age at onset of pubertal development, adolescents in our society who perceive their maturation to be discrepant from that of their peer group (that is, their age group) are often put at a psychologic and social disadvantage by this perception. This is especially true of boys who are late maturers, albeit within the normal range. Even youngsters whose tempo of growth during earlier childhood portended delay experience, nonetheless, a number of problems in adolescence when they fail to grow in height and muscle development at the same pace as their peer group. Both cross-sectional and longitudinal studies, recent as well as those 50 years ago, show these boys to have poor self-image. They tend to be less popular, which is understandable given the generally earlier maturation of girls and the consequent difficulty for the late-maturing male of finding for a close friend either a girl or a boy shorter than he. Affected boys tend to be less athletic than their earlier maturing friends and their academic status often suffers as well.

Girls who are late maturers tend to do as well, in general, as their "on-time" peers. Early-maturing girls, on the other hand, may experience difficulties under certain circumstances. The effect of early maturation on girls is modified by socioeconomic status. Those from the lower socioeconomic status groups experience more parental restriction than do girls who mature later. They are, as a result, more likely to be given stricter curfews, as well as less choice in choosing friends. If such restrictiveness is viewed by the girl as a sign of distrust of her by her parents, acting-out behavior, including sexual promiscuity, may follow.

A longitudinal study in the Midwest (Blyth et al., 1981) found that when an early-maturing female continued through the first eight grades in the same school, her adjustment was likely to be good, whereas early-maturing girls who moved in the seventh grade from elementary to junior high school experienced a fall in their self-image, had a lower grade point average, and had more dates than did later maturers or early maturers who remained in elementary school. These findings suggest that the environment is an important mediating force on the effects of biologic variability. Being a late maturer can in certain circumstances be advantageous. Late maturation is associated with having longer legs and a shorter upper-to-lower body ratio. Such a body habitus is considered desirable in activities such as ballet dancing and running.

Effects of Puberty on the Family. The social context within which puberty takes place includes both the peer group and the family of the adolescent. Peer group relationships provide a reference standard against which a given adolescent measures his or her growth pattern. The family plays a more subtle but very important role. The status of the family at the time of the adolescent's pubertal onset may be critical in understanding the family's reaction and the adolescent's adjustment to pubertal events and changes. Important questions include: Have the parents prepared the youngster for puberty, and how? Have there been siblings who have already gone through puberty? What is the status of the parents' marriage and their adjustment to middle age? These issues are all relevant to the adolescent's adjustment to puberty.

It has been shown (Hill, 1980; Steinberg, 1988) that the boy's puberty, as evidenced by his height spurt, is associated with a change in the familial homeostasis in terms of authority relationships. Whereas prior to puberty the hierarchy of authority was likely to be father > mother > son, after puberty it becomes father > son > mother.

The appearance of breasts is a signal to parents that their daughter is becoming reproductively capable. Depending on the meaning of such a transformation to the parents, they may react by imposing curfews and other restrictions that adversely influence a previously trusting relationship between daughter and parents. Fathers who were previously affectionate in physical ways often retreat from contact and are reluctant to show affection. Daughters who do not understand the basis for the change may misinterpret this and imagine that they have done something wrong. Conversely, the advent of puberty is associated with modesty and a need for privacy on the part of a young woman, whose normal behavior may be misinterpreted by her father as a sign of rejection.

Pleasure, Play, and Friendships

Pleasure

The infant first exhibits pleasure at the mother's breast, in the suckling that relieves hunger. Self-quieting behavior, such as thumbsucking or other self-touching or self-exploration, extends the experience of pleasure to other areas of the infant's own body. Through touching and bodily exploration the baby achieves gratification through stimulation of self. Pleasure is soon associated with interpersonal exchanges and is fostered by the smile of the infant, the response of the mother, and the vocal and somatosensory and kinesthetic avenues of interaction that are opened by normal maternal care.

Play

Play is a complex activity of childhood, with no universal agreement as to its nature, content, or purpose. It is imbedded in the neurodevelopmental, cognitive, and social aspects of development, and seems (Gottfried, 1985) to have the following general characteristics: 1) it is intrinsically motivated; 2) its focus is on the activity itself rather than upon some goal or outcome; 3) it is not simply exploratory with respect to objects, but involves what can be done with objects; 4) it may derive or impose novel meanings upon objects and events; 5) it is not governed by normal rules of behavior, especially with regard to "pretend" play; 6) it involves the child actively, not as a spectator; and 7) it has an obvious component of pleasure.

Play in infants and children can be seen as a way of learning more about the environment, and as a form of rehearsal for the activities of older children or adults. Ethologists have been interested in apparent analogies between human and primate or other feral play, with opinions differing as to how tight may be the analogies that can be drawn. The role of aggression in play has been under particular study (Blurton Jones, 1967, 1972).

Play in Infancy. During the first months of life, with the infant's increasing motor and cognitive development, the domains of pleasure and of play are expanded. Play first involves the simple manipulation of objects (e.g., "playing" with a mobile in the neonatal period). The infant grasps objects at 3 to 4 months of age, transfers them at 6 to 7 months, and will bring two objects together at 9 months (40 weeks). These activities are spontaneous, of consuming interest, and give the infant apparent pleasure. They belong to the piagetian stages of primary (1 to 4 months) and secondary (4 to 8 months) circular reactions. By 5 to 6 months initiation of play with objects is followed by repetitions of actions, accompanied with growing delight at their predictable results. Such activities as shaking a rattle to produce sound, or hitting a bell and having it ring, are sources of continuing joy at this age, as will later be the sound produced by banging the spoon on the tray when the infant is learning to feed him or herself.

Social play grows out of the imitation of gestures and facial expressions, and may have its beginning in the neonatal period, so far as the readiness of the infant's equipment is concerned. By 4 to 6 months the infant will respond with laughter to tickling and to repeated approaches and withdrawals of a parent, in a "game" from which both derive pleasure.

Infants begin to imitate the movements of others between 4 and 8 months, beginning with such simple gestures as patting a table or banging an object after seeing a demonstration. The movements that can be reproduced become more complicated, and by 9 months will include a simple game of patty-cake. By the age of 12 months, there may be the intermediation of objects in imitative play (a ball, for example, may be pushed in turn by the infant and a parent).

With the development of separation anxiety between the ages of 6 and 8 months, and with the growing sense of the permanence of objects that follows, by 9 months the imitative game of peek-a-boo played with the mother serves to reassure the infant not only that the disappearing mother may return, but that the infant herself or himself can control this phenomenon.

Before the age of 9 months, other infants may be investigated as if they were other physical objects. At 9 to 10 months, however, other infants begin to be of interest, and with the second year comes awareness that other children present the potential for *social* interaction.

Play in the Second Year. In the second year of life, youngsters become fascinated with the workings of toys and the interrelationships of objects to each other. A "busy box," with its buttons, cranks, knobs, and so forth, may become the favorite plaything. At this age, the wrappings of gifts often hold more fascination for the child than the toy itself, sometimes to the dismay of a doting grandparent donor. With increasing maturity, the child becomes more imaginative in the exploitation of toys and play situations.

The intensity of involvement with toys and the duration of the infant's attention span in playing with them may provide useful developmental information; deprived or developmentally delayed children may fail to react with sustained interest to situations in which playful activity would be expected.

The earliest acts of pretending begin to be seen at about 12 months of age, and consist of the infant simulating things he or she normally does, such as pretending to eat or to sleep. Toys serve increasingly as catalysts for solitary play, as well as for social interactions of a playful nature.

At around 18 months, the forms of play with objects are likely to involve single actions, such as feeding or dressing a doll; by 24 months serial activities may be seen, such as feeding and then putting to bed (Fenson, 1985). By 24 months the child is projecting the action into other persons or dolls and making them responsible for the simulations (involving the mother in play with the telephone, for example, or the doll feeding the doll's baby, rather than the child feeding the doll).

After 12 months infants begin to initiate interpersonal actions and to respond to overtures. A toy often generates this interaction when it attracts the attention of two youngsters, who become forced to coordinate their behaviors so that both can make use of it or compete for it. During the second year the toddler spends most of his or her time with parents or caretakers, or engaged in object-centered contacts with one other child. Two children may play side by side at this age, but there is often little interaction between them, other than the occasional grabbing of toys. Interchanges involving more than two children at a time are rare before the age of 2 years.

Play in the Third Year. Between 24 and 36 months the interactions in play among children are likely to involve pairs rather than larger groups, with the nature of the play being parallel rather than reciprocal. Notions of property rights ("mine") emerge at the end of the second year, and may become the source of conflict.

Play in the Preschool Child. Interactive play, first seen at the beginning of the third year, sets the stage for future social relationships. After 36 months play begins increasingly to involve children in role-playing and in taking turns and following the rules. Blurton Jones (1967) has described *rough-and-tumble* play as a typical form of interaction in preschool children. It consists of laughing, running, jumping up and down, hitting *at* (usually without contact or injury), and wrestling. Roles may change from chasing to being chased, with the play element being underlined by the smiling or laughing that Blurton Jones believes distinguishes this behavior from truly aggressive behavior.

Play at this age is greatly enhanced by verbal communicative abilities. Toddlers with older siblings develop peer relationships more easily than those who are only children. Play serves to enhance self-concept when it is associated with a sense of mastery and accomplishment or when it results in approval from playmates or adults. On the other hand, the experience of rejection by a playmate may provide an early lesson about popularity and competition. Toddlers show preferences for playmates who are similar to themselves in temperament and level of development, as well as for children of their mothers' close friends.

Preschoolers typically begin to include fantasy in their games and often play roles that are familiar to them, notably in such games as "house" and "doctor." These games provide an opportunity to explore gender role identity, as well as to learn about anatomic differences between the sexes. The roles played are generally true to gender identity at this age. It is of interest to note that boys who consider themselves to be homosexual in later life have often in the preschool years taken the feminine role, preferring dolls as playthings in these sorts of games.

Favorite playthings for preschoolers include vehicles that can be ridden (trucks, tricycles, etc.), puzzles, and puppets; the last are often incorporated into stories. Children who use toys in a nonconventional way may be either particularly creative or developmentally delayed.

Studies of social class differences have found among children from middle class families more variety in themes and more cooperation in play situations during the preschool years than was found when such children were compared with those from lower socioeconomic classes.

Parental Roles in Play. The role of play in the life of the infant and young child will be heavily dependent upon the manner in which parents and others participate, both in the material and in the emotional resources they bring to the stimulation of the infant or interaction with the child. Their expectations of the infant or child will be important in determining both the quantity and the quality of interactions. Resources and expectations will vary with the socioeconomic level of the family, and with the expectations also of the culture within they live. Parents from the lower socioeconomic strata apparently play less often with their children and speak less often when playing with them. There is evidence that in cultures in which much is expected of children in the way of contribution to the work of the family and community, children will nonetheless find ways to play.

In the ways in which parents establish or maintain an environment conducive to exploration and play opportunities, sex differences as well as class differences have been described. For example: mothers are more likely than fathers to follow the baby's lead in developing a play situation and more often use toys; fathers are more likely to involve their youngsters in physical play. Overstimulation with toys can be counterproductive, dampening the infant's curiosity and initiative.

Older Children and Adolescents. The elaborate games of older children and adolescents are more clearly preparation for adult roles. The learning and the following of rules, and the achievement of skills and of positive self-image are prominent features. Preadolescents enjoy "kissing games," and there is increasing emphasis upon individual prowess in such games as baseball or in such sports as tennis or swimming.

The games of adolescents, and particularly of male adolescents, often involve groups in competition for dominance of territory, in the form of traditional games (football or baseball, for example), either supervised or casual, or in the less structured and sometimes more physical defense in groups of areas of the city or countryside with which each group identifies and which each will defend as off-limits to other groups. The similarity of this behavior to the territorial orientations of other animals (and of primates, in particular) is striking, and has begged the question as to what extent its biologic roots are genetic and therefore physiologic, rather than the expression simply of social and cultural forces.

Friendships

Between 3 and 5 years of age, despite their engagement in the kinds of play described above, children do not have the concept of an enduring relationship that transcends the here and now. Accordingly, friends are "momentary physical playmates," whose salient characteristics involve physical, rather than psychologic, attributes.

The literature on friendships focuses on two main issues: the changes that occur from childhood through adolescence that reflect social and cognitive development; and the sex differences in the structure and function of friendship.

Friendships provide children with the opportunity to learn social skills, facilitate social comparisons in the service of developing a sense of their own identity, and promote a sense of belonging to a group rather than the family. Absence of close childhood friendships has been linked with both psychopathology and social isolation in adulthood. On the other hand, Rubin (1980) points out the need to recognize the importance of privacy and solitude for some children. He also points out potentially negative aspects of intimate childhood relationships: "[They] give rise not only to self-acceptance, trust, and rapport, but also to insecurity, jealousy, and resentment."

During the ages from 5 to 9 years friendships among boys are largely based on competition. Rubin found that in experimental situations, in contrast to girls or to older children, boys of these ages shared less with their friends, presumably out of the desire not to appear inferior to them.

Sullivan (1953) found in studies of fourth to eighth graders (9- to 13-year-olds) that it was not until early adolescence that students behaved in a more helpful and mutually responsive way toward a close friend than toward another classmate. This change from competition to equality or cooperation with onset of adolescence appears to parallel changes in cognitive level, with development of a new concept of reciprocity. In early childhood, reciprocity is viewed as action exchange; in later childhood, the concept becomes more idealized, reflecting the youngster's desire to treat others as he or she would wish to be treated.

For early adolescent girls the typical structure of social interaction is a dyadic relationship or a threesome, whereas the typical relationship for boys at this stage consists of crowds or gangs. It has been suggested that these different forms for peer interaction reflect the different needs of the two sexes at this time of life, boys needing a context for manifesting achievement and independence, and girls an opportunity to develop interpersonal skills and emotional support. A more cynical view of the need for different structures for the sexes is offered by Savin-Williams (1980): "The preadolescent and early adolescent years for the girls was a time for cattiness, jealousy, and antagonisms—making large groups unfeasible."

The activities of early adolescent girls in their small peer groups are summed up by the phrase "hanging out together," meaning joking, confiding, relaxing, teasing, and talking about fashion. In a study of the function and ontogenesis of groups among early adolescent females in a summer camp, Savin-Williams found the more popular and dominant girls to be those who were more advanced in their pubertal development and more athletic. The finding is rather similar to what has been reported by others for male adolescents. What is different, however, is the finding that, in contrast with boys, who "assert their status by utilizing such power-related acts as physical contact, verbal argument, physical displacement, and verbal-physical threats, . . . the adolescent girls . . . expressed their status by recognizing others, shunning, ignoring requests, and giving unsolicited advice."

It is of interest that the above pattern of movement of female adolescents toward increased peer interaction with the onset of puberty is not universal, nor is it seen in certain nonhuman primates. Cross-cultural studies, albeit some quite old, indicate that the adolescent female peer group structure currently typical of the United States is not found in any other society. In the Far and Middle East, middle Europe, and the South Seas, the puberty of girls is associated with abandonment of earlier play or social groups in favor of assuming additional household responsibilities or having a single girlfriend. In the same cultures, on the other hand, adolescent males behave much as they do currently in this country.

Savin-Williams points out that in four different monkey species, as adolescence begins, the female adolescent decreases her contact with peers of either sex, while there is an increase in her interaction with adult females and their infants. Male conspecifics, on the other hand, continue at the onset of puberty to interact with and travel with their male peers.

The ages of 14 to 16 years represent the time of transition from same-sex to mixed-sex friendships. These are discussed later, with the stages of adolescence.

The Role of Work in Child and Adolescent Development

The passage of child labor laws in the United States had a profound effect on the role of children in the family. According to Zelizer (1985) the role shifted from their "being seen as 'economically useful,' with a value that could be assessed in terms of the money value of their labor, to being 'priceless', treated as 'sacred' and greatly sentimentalized." The effect was that the world of the child was "regulated by affection and education, not work or profit" (Zelizer, 1985, p. 209). With this change, household work has been assigned to children for its presumed developmental value, the impression being that assigning such tasks will foster a sense of independence and instill the work ethic.

Contrary to popular expectation, English studies have found an inverse relationship between the socioeconomic status of the family and the amount of work assigned to children, especially to boys (Newson and Newson, 1976). In the United States, on the other hand, White and Brinkerhoff (1981) found that "children's work in households, together with the rationale of developmental value, have been described as a cultural norm . . . cutting across families of diverse compositions and socioeconomic status." There are variations based on ethnicity, gender, and age, according to Goodnow (1988). These differences obviously reflect views about the nature of children.

In their study of families in the Midwest, White and Brinkerhoff found that "by the age of 9 or 10 well over 90 per cent [of children] are involved in regular chores. Participation begins to fall off slightly in the late teens as adolescents reduce their participation in all family activities, but chores remain a near universal" (p. 792). Regardless of the actual age of initiation of chores, the first category assigned appears to relate to self-care, and later to "family work" (Goodnow), or moves from helping parents to assuming full responsibility for certain tasks previously performed by the latter.

As early as 1 year of age, children show an interest in participating in household tasks, but such interest appears to wane by about 30 months. This has been attributed to parental attitude, rather than to any developmentally determined characteristic of the child. By the time of adolescence, it is the youngster, rather than the parent who appears to be the determinant of decreased involvement in chores.

Interestingly, in surveys of U.S. adolescents spanning a 30-year period, "jobs around the house" were cited more frequently than sex, drugs, religion, or politics as the cause of conflict with parents (Montemayor, 1983). Rejection of maternal authority at this time has been cited as one explanation.

In addition to age, gender is important in determining the nature of the chores done by children, as well as the rewards they receive. According to Goodnow, chores assigned to younger children are not sex stereotyped and consist largely of those centered around the kitchen. By the age of 10 years, work assigned at home becomes more gender specific, with girls working inside and boys outside. Girls put in more than twice the number of hours of work, however, and are most often rewarded by praise for doing what is generally construed as "womens' work." Boys, on the other hand, are more likely to earn money as a reward for work learned at home and done outside. According to Goodnow, "mothers do not get paid in money, and their daughters seem to be socialized into a similar pattern of work that is 'for love'."

The common assumption that the responsibility for chores enhances the child's social and cognitive development has been challenged by a number of investigators. For example, Kohlberg in 1964 stated: "Strong training demands which serve the parents' convenience (cleanliness, chores, neatness) . . . are, if anything, negatively related to moral response." One study found no relationship shown between children's sense of responsibility as shown at school and their involvement in household chores (Harris et al., 1963). On the other hand, studies by Whiting and Whiting (1975) demonstrated a clear relationship between altruism (defined as being helpful to others or making responsible suggestions to them) and the amount of work done at home. Similar findings are apparent in studies of other cultures.

In exploring the effect of children's household work on psychosocial development, Goodnow suggests that a child's construct of friendship is "likely to be influenced by the extent to which children are called on to interweave work and play and to look on other children as potential partners in a round of current and future chores rather than only as playmates or sharers of intimacy."

There is some suggestion that youngsters apprenticed to adults may acquire certain cognitive skills, if work is assigned with clear goals and if support is provided as to how to structure tasks in time and sequence. Greenberger and Steinberg (1986) have studied the role of the adolescent's work outside the family (specifically part-time work during the school year) in affecting psychosocial development. Exploring first the widely held notion that such an experience will enhance the youngster's sense of personal and social responsibility, they found in fact that such work presented the teenagers with few opportunities for taking initiative or becoming involved in decision-making.

Their longitudinal study found that increased self-reliance resulted from working, but only for girls. For boys, scores on self-reliance actually fell after undertaking work. In this context, they point out that the nature of jobs available to adolescents may be a factor in thwarting creativity or the enhancement of self-reliance. Nor did they find many opportunities for learning in what they call the "new" adolescent workplace. They found little evidence of job-related skills training, that most jobs involved simple tasks, and that the adolescents themselves indicated that they needed "a grade school education or less' to perform their duties.

In follow-up Greenberger and Steinberg found no evidence of increased practical knowledge when teenagers in the work force were compared with those who had not taken jobs. They did feel that certain jobs did enhance social understanding, specifically those "having to deal with strangers, or people from different social backgrounds or age groups." In exploring the relationship of working to school performance, they found that working longer hours led to decreased grade point averages.

Greenberger and Steinberg also challenge the widely held notion that working during adolescence will lead to an enhanced sense of financial responsibility, inasmuch as they found that the majority of teenagers use their money for their own purposes, rather than contributing to support of the family. This is consistent with other studies, including the national study of Johnston et al. (1982a), who reported that only 1 per cent of youth turned over their entire paycheck to help the family. The same study found also that in boys working led to development of more materialistic attitudes, evident once they joined the work force, though an initial cross-sectional study had found no difference in this respect between teenagers who sought jobs and those who did not.

Another important finding of research in this area is that working may be associated with an increase in frequency of delinquency rather than any anticipated decrease. This observation is explained by Ruggiero (1986) as follows: "Characteristics of the jobs adolescents generally hold, and characteristics of middle class youth themselves, might lead to increases in four types of deviance among youngsters who work. In view of the fact that most middle class youngsters do not need their earnings to buy the necessities of life, some of their earnings may be channeled into deviant activities that require money: e.g., buying and selling drugs and gambling. Moreover, because jobs may be stressful and because adolescence itself is a stressful period of life, employed youngsters with money to spare may engage in illegal and or unhealthy forms of stress-reduction: e.g., smoking cigarettes, drinking alcohol, and using marijuana and other drugs . . . [which may also] confer signs of adult status. Third, because the demands of working may interfere with the demands of school, working may elevate certain forms of school-related deviance: being absent from school, cutting classes, and coming to school late; and cheating, copying others' homework assignments, and lying about having turned in assigned work."

The above perspective was supported by the findings of the longitudinal study by Greenberger and Steinberg, who reported that "working per se leads to more frequent gambling among boys," "more money-related deviance among girls; more overall school-related deviance among boys," and increased use of alcohol among boys and more use of marijuana among girls. A significant relationship emerged in this study between use of alcohol and marijuana and exposure to job stressors (poor work environment; boring, meaningless tasks; conflict between work and other obligations; supervision by autocratic management; impersonal setting; poor pay without opportunity for advancement). Interestingly, job stress was not associated with increased incidence of physical or psychologic symptomatology.

Aggression and Violence

Aggression in children, adolescents, or adults represents the *need* to overpower or to hurt some one in order to achieve some end, or the *act* of doing so. The need to hurt may be exhibited immediately in hitting, pushing, or name-calling; or indirectly, through destruction of property, tattling, and the like; or unconsciously, in dreams. Such behaviors as temper tantrums or disobedience may also be regarded as forms of aggression. *Aggressiveness* is the propensity to choose aggression to try to solve interpersonal (or intergroup or international) problems.

The sources of aggression are by no means fully understood. It is clear that some children are more aggressive than others. There is ample evidence, for example, that boys are from early infancy more prone than girls to use aggression in problem-solving. They cry more than girls in early infancy, and have a generally higher level of activity. Later, the typical behavior of boys toward such creations as sand castles or houses of cards will be to destroy them when they are done playing with them, whereas girls will be more likely to try to preserve them. Whether or to what degree such behavior is driven by innate biologic urges and/or evolves out of experience (socialization and acculturation) is uncertain. On the other hand, Kagan et al. (1988) have presented evidence that *shyness,* an emotion and behavior antithetic to violence, may, like aggression, be built in at birth, as a manifestation of temperament.

Studies in animals have shown that exposure of the newborn animal to sex hormones can modify adult behavior. For example, Bronson and Desjardins (1968) found that injection of 3-day-old male mice with estradiol reduced the amount of aggression displayed as adults, as compared with controls. Conversely, female newborn mice manifested increased aggressive behavior as adults after having been injected with either testosterone or estrogen.

Studies of children who have had congenital adrenal hyperplasia (adrenogenital syndrome, which exposes them to increased androgen levels in fetal and neonatal life) display similar effects (see p. 96). This and other evidence indicates that both the intensity and direction of aggressive behavior in children are driven in part, at least, by biologic imperatives, either structural or hormonal.

How an innate aggressive disposition becomes translated into specific behavior is not fully known. The earliest origins of aggressive behavior are likely to be found in infancy. It has been postulated, for example, that if the response of the mother to a hungry or otherwise needy infant is generally postponed until the infant must *hurt* her by *screaming* to get her attention, then the seeds may be sowed for aggressive behavior. If, on the other hand, the mother always responded to the need of the infant before there was any exhibition of aggression, then there might develop a nonaggressive, but possibly dependent child. If the mother's response were delayed until the child *stopped* crying (especially, stopped upon request), then there might develop a submissive child.

No parents are completely consistent in their child-rearing practice, but some comfortable balance must be found between those parental behaviors that allow aggression to appear in the children and those behaviors that direct this aggression into useful channels. Children need to develop enough aggressiveness to be able to direct their behaviors constructively against difficulties or impediments and to protest against mistreatment or injustice.

Unfettered aggression in older children creates bullies. Horne (1988) believes that the roots of this are likely to be found in the family, rather than in the innate biologic makeup of the bully. He finds that parents of bullies do not use as much humor, praise, or encouragement in dealing with their children as other parents, but are more prone to use put-downs, sarcasm, and criticism. When they touch their children, it is to control them rather than to show affection.

Hughes (1988) finds that bullies view the world as threatening, and misinterpret accidents (e.g., jostling) as intended affronts, to which they react with violence. She feels that bullies do not outgrow their aggressive impulses, but are destined to have school problems, and are at risk of becoming involved in criminal behavior. Patterson (1988) holds that the best results in dealing with bullies is through work with their parents, with the teaching of new child-rearing and problem-solving techniques.

The victims of a bully need reassurance that they are not the cause of the assaultive behavior, to which they often react with self-blame, shame, and loss of self-esteem.

Violence is the exercise of aggression in behavior that hurts or injures persons, or defaces or destroys property. Bullying is a form of violence, whether it consists of hitting, name-calling, or the stealing of lunch money at school.

Some forms of violence are institutionalized in our society, in the forms of war, capital punishment, torture, or other indignities (including the banal and mindless dramatization and exploitation of violence in cinema and on television [see pp. 221–225]).

On the other hand, for many animals some forms of violence serve the preservation of the species, and are integral to an evolutionary process that depends upon the "survival of the fittest." For many species, these forms of violence are written in the genetic code, as DNA. The studies of ethologists, anthropologists, sociologists, and others have brought new perspectives to the ways in which we look at animal and human behavior, and particularly at the analogies between human and other primate behavior. A question has come to the fore as to the extent to which human aggressive and violent behavior is written in DNA.

The question is not easily answered, except to say that it would be astonishing if humans and primates did not share in DNA some of the essential physiologic and behavioral ingredients that lie behind patterns of socialization, care of the young, and defense of territory. On the other hand, Kaye (1982) has presented evidence that the infant is born not only with innate equipment directing behavior, but also into a social setting that is in its own process of evolution. As parents and infants learn from each other, the behavior of the infant evolves also in accordance with traditions of the society into which he or she is born.

Various social and cultural groups give quite different places in their lives and assign widely disparate values to violence as an instrument of personal, social, or political power. These differing views may owe something or much to DNA, but there is no reason not to hope that aggression may find acceptable outlets on Earth.

Lorenz has suggested (1963) that a variety of ritualized nondestructive competitions might serve as acceptable outlets for exercise of aggression. He believes that the space race (for example) may in some respects be serving that function in international competition (albeit at great expense).

It is likely that football, baseball, and other contact sports may serve similar functions for the individual, and for the groups that identify themselves with the teams involved. Even these rituals, however, may become distorted in the execution, with uncontrolled violence the consequence of emotions that may represent either exhilaration at winning or frustration at losing.

Even for young children contests (Little League baseball, for example) take place too often in climates so competitive that losing performances may unleash unbridled frustration, anger, and violence. The need and effort to win may be so imperatively felt that notions of fair play and sportsmanship are discarded, and superiority is pursued at any cost. The opportunity for admiration of excellence is lost. In such a climate the cost of losing for some children can be very heavy in shame, in loss of self-esteem, and sometimes in depression.

Fears

To know the nature and the content of the fears of infants, children, and adolescents is to have some insight into the ways in which they perceive and comprehend reality, and into their assessments of the relationships, risks, and dangers that they attribute to the world of their perception. "Reality" is, in any case (for adults as well as for children), largely a construct born out of the relationship between genetic potential, physiologic mechanisms, level of cognitive development, and experience, unique for each person, rather than an objective entity with features upon which all would agree.

The fears of infants and children vary with their ages (Table 1–18). As the "real world" is formed out of his of her experience, the infant, child, or adolescent builds an evolving understanding of the world out of both pleasant and unpleasant confrontations. For as long as the young child's knowledge remains fragmentary, fantasy has ample opportunity to invent pseudorealities provoking fears or anxieties, as well as to gain insights into the "true" nature of things.

TABLE 1–18. Age Specificity of Fears in Normal Children*

	AGE (YR)							
	0–½	½–1	1	2–4	5–6	7–8	9–12	Teens
Loss of support/noise	X	X	X					
Strangers/heights/looming		X	X					
Separation		X	X	X	X			
Animals/masks				X	X			
Darkness				X	X	X	X	
Bodily harm					X	X	X	
Fantasies (ghosts)					X	X		
Media events						X	X	X
Reality (tests in school, etc.)							X	X
Death							X	X
Social performance								X
Sexuality								X

* Adapted from Morris and Kralochwill (1983).

Sensations of fear that are generated by internal stimuli, without any evident external precipitant, are often referred to as *anxieties,* particularly when they do not respond to factual explanations that they have no basis in reality. Feelings of anxiety may be generated by unconscious or repressed memories or emotions. Both fears and anxieties are normal in infants and children unless they are particularly persistent, interfere with normal activities, or are inappropriate to the developmental stage of the child. *Phobias* are fears that persistently keep the child from engaging in normal activities. They will generally require medical or psychologic intervention and generally respond to desensitization; they may require exploration of the psychodynamics of the entire family.

Certain universal and basic fears have their roots plainly in the psychosocial aspects of development. Of these the most primitive is the fear of *abandonment,* which we see first as separation anxiety in the last half of the first year. The next is fear of the *loss of love,* which is generated particularly during the second year, as the infant adapts his or her behavior to the demands and expectations of parents and others. The third basic fear is that of *bodily mutilation,* which has a complex origin in notions of body image. It may, in the preschool child, involve growing awareness of differences in anatomy among boys and girls, or may be derived from experiences with injury, illness, or surgery, in self or others. Experiencing or observing in others the effects of abnormal growth or anomalies may threaten body image.

Fears in Infancy

Very young infants react to loss of physical support or to loud noises with the physiologic changes we associate with fear. For example, when the Moro response is produced by such stimuli, the infant may show tachycardia, an increase in motor activity and tone, and a cry. Young infants attempt to avoid looming objects by turning the head or averting the gaze. By the age of 6 to 8 months these reactions evolve into evident fear at the approach of such objects, and by this age the reactions of fear may be elicited by other changes in visual, aural, or other sensory input that indicate or imply that the infant is in danger of suffering pain, injury, or loss of security or protection. Fear reactions to loss of support are elaborated into fear of heights or of falling, fear no longer being just the result of the immediate physical circumstances, but beginning to be called forth by the anticipation of possibly dangerous situations. Fear at the approach of strangers begins to be manifest at this age.

Fears in the Young Child

During the second year of life, there are continuing fears at the approach of unfamiliar persons ("stranger anxiety"), with growing evidence of fear of separation from parents, of injury, and of other special circumstances, such as noisy or large objects (thunder, alarms, trucks, etc.) or the toilet (which has a disconcerting way of making products of the body disappear). In the second and third years, as the child begins to be able to imagine what might be lurking in shadows, fear of the dark is common, and often associated with sleep resistance. Fear of animals becomes common, particularly if the child has had an unpleasant experience or if the approach of an animal has been too noisy, intrusive, or precipitous.

To the above, the child adds after the second year fears of changes in the personal environment, of physical abnormalities in others, of masks, and the like. The growth of the child's fantasy life after the second year may make for creative daytime play, but at night the child's fantasy may become relatively uncontrolled, and fears may be generated by experiences of the day, including images derived from books or from television (see pp. 208, 221–225). Fears of the dark become common, and the darkness may begin to be occupied by animals, monsters, ghosts, and other images. Nightmares become relatively common.

Exploitation of the child's capacity for fantasy may sometimes do him or her a disservice, particularly when it is associated with attempts at control of behavior. Santa Claus, for example, is perceived by many preschool children as a fearsome creature, as much the mediator of punishment as a messenger of love. For example, Santa Claus "knows when you're asleep, knows when you're awake, knows when you've been good or bad, so be good for goodness' sake!" Other distortions of the child's fantasies may occur when parents evade reality in dealing with such events as pregnancy, birth, sickness, or death. Sleep disturbances may occur in the child who has been told that a family member has "gone to sleep" or "died in his or her sleep," rather than simply "died."

Nightmares occur during REM sleep, and often awaken the child in panic. He or she is frightened, can give a description of what the frightening experience was, and may need consolation and reassurance before sleep comes again. The content of nightmares may be clearly related to events of the day. For some children residual anxiety from nightmares may carry over into the day. Wittmer and Crouthamel (1986) give the following suggestions for parents in dealing with nightmares:

> Provide the child with a flashlight to keep under the pillow. It can be used to probe the corners, ridding the room of monsters.
>
> Use "magic" to help drive monsters or ghosts away. The child can make the creature disappear by pretending to spray it with water. The child might even keep a spray bottle filled with "pretend water" by the bed.
>
> Tell the child, "You can be the boss over the ghost. It is not real and you can tell it so!"
>
> Encourage the child to draw a picture of the creature and tell the picture, "I am mad at you." Then, have the child tear up the picture and throw it away.
>
> Give the child a list of things he or she can do when feeling frightened—for example, turning on the radio, playing lullabies on a cassette player, turning on the light, stomping the floor three times.

Night terrors (pavor nocturnus) have their onset during deep rather than REM sleep. The affected child awakens suddenly, often with a cry or scream, and is found agitated, crying or talking wildly, often with the eyes open, though not awake or responsive. Night terrors differ from nightmares in that the child is inconsolable and has no memory for the episode the following day. The child may return to sleep after a period of being held, with no indication of having been fully awake. The origin of night terrors is unclear. They may respond to medication, but usually no therapy is necessary.

Fears of Older Children

With the ages of 5 to 6 years and the entry of the child into the educational arena and a wider sphere of experience, the content of fears may begin to include such things as "bad" people, and dangers discussed in the news media (such as of nuclear war or accident, other accidents, kidnapping, and the like). Earlier concerns with the supernatural, with separations, and with bodily injury or death are continued in some degree, albeit evolving with the changes that reflect the child's growing cognitive maturity.

At the time of entry into school some children manifest fear of separation from the parent (school refusal or school phobia). The underlying cause is often a joint anxiety of child and parent at the separation that must take place. School refusal generally responds to counseling, with insistence that the child attend school, fears notwithstanding.

Later, schoolchildren may develop fears of failure, often because the expectations of their parents are excessive or are considered unachievable. Tests and examinations may be approached with considerable or much anxiety, and the need to make a solo performance may be approached with misgivings or dread.

School-aged and adolescent children may develop fears of rejection by their peers, or that their personal appearances may be unattractive. As adolescents enter the period when they are forming new personal and social and sexual alliances, they may normally have fears and anxieties as to the quality of their behavior or its acceptance. Risk-taking in adolescents is often their means of denying their fears.

Health Care and Hospitalization

Each of the basic fears of children is likely to be brought to the surface in the medical care setting. When the infant or child must be separated briefly from the parent for examination or for a painful procedure, the loss of parental shelter and protection may be viewed as a kind of abandonment, and the pain reinforces the fear of major injury.

Recognition both by health personnel and by parents that such fear is understandable, and that it is all right to protest or to cry, is critical to management. There is no place for shame or punishment of the fearful or struggling child for his or her loss of control, nor for anger on the part of either parents or health workers. Such responses could only reinforce the child's sense of having lost the love of parent or the respect of the health worker. Other steps that health personnel can take to minimize the anxiety and fear of the child are discussed elsewhere (see pp. 178, 188, 200, 217).

When hospitalization becomes necessary, the experience may be particularly frightening for young children who are incapable of understanding the reasons for their removal from familiar surroundings and persons, and for those older children for whom surgery or serious illness threatens to alter their concept of their own body image. For the adolescent who is making gains in a struggle for independence, hospitalization may be viewed as a threat to his or her new status.

Recognition that hospitalization is not only a medical but a *social* event, and safeguarding its social qualities, may be crucial to patients' or families' perception of the experience as restorative, reassuring, or growth-promoting on the one hand, or as irritating, frightening, agonizing, demoralizing, or devastating on the other. Their perceptions may profoundly affect the ways in which patients or their families use health services in the future.

Pain in Children and Adolescents. For many children and adolescents, an integral part of their feelings about visits for health care or hospitalization is the fear of painful procedures. Opinions have differed as to whether infants or young children felt or remembered their experiences of pain. Recent studies support the view that even premature infants feel pain, and that it is likely that circumcision and other procedures produce in the newborn or young infant reactions to pain that are physiologically like those of older children, adolescents, and adults.

Memory for circumstances associated with pain appears to have been established by the age of 6 months, as indicated by the tendency of the infant to cry, resist, struggle, or, in the second year, to have a tantrum in anticipation of a painful procedure. These reactions reach their peak between the ages of 6 months and 2 to 3 years of age (Kassowitz, 1958).

Infants and children vary considerably in their responses to painful procedures. The differences have been attributed to temperament, but there have been few systematic studies of these differences. The emotional climate within the family of the child experiencing pain may also contribute to the child's perception of the circumstances under which pain is felt, and to the nature or the intensity of the child' reaction.

Gaffney and Dunne (1986, 1987) have studied childrens' definitions of pain and their understanding of its cause. The development of these notions appears to follow the piagetian scheme of cognitive development, moving from preoccupation with the pain itself as the central experience (preoperational), to pain as having certain qualities or producing certain feelings (concrete operational), to pain as having a reason and serving a purpose in identifying illness or being tolerable in the service of therapy (formal operational).

Brown et al. (1986) have studied the coping strategies of children faced with the possibility of a dental procedure. They identified two categories of response: coping strategies and catastrophising strategies. Among the former were: positive self-talk, diversion of attention, relaxation, and thought stopping. Among the latter were: focusing upon negative aspects, thoughts of escape or avoidance, concerns about unlikely complications, concerns about the dentist (Is he mean?) or negative feelings toward the dentist (I hate him). The proportion of copers increased with age.

Olness and Gardner (1988) and others have studied the role of hypnosis in helping children to cope with pain. The technique employs relaxation imagery and is strikingly successful with some children, including for such procedures as dental extraction.

Infants and young children often appear to tolerate operative procedures with less complaint than might adults who have had comparable surgical procedures, but these young patients are limited in their capacity to describe what they feel, or to complain about pain and ask for help.

Inasmuch as it is sometimes difficult to know whether a preverbal or verbal child is having pain, or what the intensity of the child's discomfort may be, there has been concern that children in postoperative pain may receive less than the appropriate or required amount of analgesic help to control either subjective distress or physiologic stress due to pain.

McGrath and Unruh (1987) summarize the evidence that children need help with postoperative pain just as adults do, and offer the following suggestions (abridged) for management:

1. [E]nsure adequate analgesia during surgery.
2. Eliminate unnecessary surgery.
3. Select appropriate analgesic medications . . .
4. Avoid p.r.n. schedules . . . [that] guarantee that the child will suffer pain . . . before . . . relief . . . . Regularly scheduled medication can prevent pain from emerging.
5. Avoid injections . . . [which children] fear . . . and may deny pain to avoid. . . . [Substitute] intravenous, sublingual, rectal, or oral medication.
6. Titrate dosage.
7. Consider . . . regional blocks . . . in circumcision . . .
8. Provide an interesting and supportive environment . . .
9. Provide preoperative teaching . . .
10. Educate parents to use analgesics when the child goes home . . .

Humanizing Hospitalization. In the past quarter-century great strides have been made in understanding the needs of hospitalized patients and their families. For each age of patient there are predominantly social measures through which the experience of hospitalization can have reassuring, educational, or growth-promoting potential. In the case of infants or young children, the rooming-in of a parent with a child who is sick or needs surgery may be reassuring to both child and parent, and may substantially improve the response to medical care. For both infants and older children the provision of play facilities and recreational therapy under professional leadership may be crucial to the child's favorable perception of the experience and of the institution.

Whenever an uncomfortable or possibly painful or anxiety-provoking procedure is to be carried out, the child should be moved from his or her crib or bed to a treatment room or other designated facility for the procedure. The child's bed or the ward's or hospital's recreational facilities should be regarded as *sanctuaries* to be kept inviolate. Hospital personnel should not enter the play room even to read a tuberculin test, but only to share in the recreational activities when that might be appropriate.

In recent years attention has been increasingly given to the possibility that participation of parents in the care of the hospitalized child or preadolescent can allay anxieties of both. This sharing of responsibility for care with parents may help make illness and hospitalization more likely growth-promoting for all concerned.

Children scheduled for surgical procedures should have an opportunity to visit the hospital beforehand and become familiar with the places where they will be, the persons whom they will meet, and the experiences that they are likely to have. The surgical experience should be described only in the most general terms, except as the child asks for more detail.

Following illness or surgery, children can be given opportunities in supervised recreational settings to discharge some of the emotions that they may have with regard to what has happened to them, with opportunities both to learn and to relieve tension. They may be encouraged to review in play with dolls what they have experienced. The reliving of the experience in this way is often helpful.

The fears of adolescents regarding illness and hospitalization are likely to focus upon alterations in body structure and function, and may be confused by the intrusion of concerns and misperceptions with respect to normal aspects of changing body image and functions. Adolescents admitted to hospitals for care are often deeply involved in defining their evolving status as independent or autonomous persons in the family, and to have thrust upon them the dependency of illness or the need to submit to surgical or other medical interventions can be deeply distressing. The threat to the social self can be particularly intensely felt, for example, by adolescents undergoing genitourinary or gynecologic or renal manipulations, who may need explicit reassurance as to their structural integrity and that their future sexual adequacy is not at risk.

Adolescents are neither children nor adults, and their needs with hospitalization can often be best met in adolescent units within which they can be reassured that they have not lost touch with their adolescent peer culture. The support of a peer sharing the same room may achieve the same. Providing the teenager with age-appropriate activities will also help to maintain newly achieved identity and independence.

Many hospitals now have adolescent units with ample provision of adolescent technology in music, fast foods, video or video games, and the like, and with formal arrangements made for keeping up with schoolwork through hospital teachers and classrooms. These opportunities to remain in touch with normal interests may for some adolescents be crucial to their feeling about the use of needed health care facilities in the future.

When a separate adolescent unit is not available and the adolescent is hospitalized on a pediatric ward, his or her emerging maturity can sometimes be harnessed and promoted by delegation of responsibility to the adolescent for some aspects of the care of younger patients, willingness and circumstances permitting.

Other Fears

Many professionals and other citizens are concerned that the world is increasingly regarded by children and adolescents as a dangerous place, with a growing sense of menace. The media (press and television, particularly) are given to highlighting and dramatizing violence and terrorism, as well as accidents and natural catastrophes. Children are warned to keep their distance from strangers, lest they be kidnapped. Rape, sexual abuse, and mutilation have become reportorial commonplaces. Shapiro (1988) has suggested that "these days we raise our children to be fearful, in contrast to the way in which I was raised, which was to be brave."

Children's fears of *nuclear catastrophe* have been particularly well studied. There is evidence that by the age of 8 years children have begun in large numbers to think about the problems posed by the nuclear threat, and that their concerns and perceptions evolve and mature as they enter and complete adolescence.

In 1962 Escalona (1965) asked a group of youngsters ranging in age from 10 to 17 years what they thought about "the world 10 years from now," how it will be changed, and what they would like changed, and what three wishes they might have regarding the future. In response to these questions 70 per cent of children mentioned war and a wish for peace. In the same year, around the Cuban missile crisis, Schwebel (1963, 1965) asked junior high school students if they thought there would be a war, whether they cared, and what would happen if there were a war. Forty-four per cent of these children expected war, and 95 per cent of them cared deeply about this danger.

By contrast, in 1981, after the nuclear accident at Three Mile Island, Schwebel and Schwebel (1981) asked a group of children whether there would be another nuclear accident, whether they cared, what would happen if there were another nuclear accident, and what should be done about nuclear plants. Seventy per cent of these children felt that there would be a nuclear accident, and 85 per cent of them cared deeply about the possibility. Girls were more pessimistic than boys.

The Schwebels note that between 1962 and 1981 there appeared to be a rising sense of risk, with a lower sense of fear and outrage than they encountered in 1962. They offer six possible reasons: first, a nuclear accident seemed to offer more chance of surviving injured than of being annihilated; second, there appeared to be less threat of separation from family; third, there had already been a major nuclear accident; fourth, the accident could be ascribed to human carelessness, and was therefore "avoidable"; fifth, it seemed that escape from a nuclear accident might be possible; and sixth, there might be a feeling of resignation about the inevitability of accident, with a feeling of powerlessness in the face of it.

Chivian and Snow (1983) have recorded the thoughts of schoolchildren of various ages regarding the nuclear menace. Their videotape recording shows the following with respect to the preoccupations of children of various ages:

> Children of 8 and 9 years of age expressed concern that they might die, not grow up, be left alone, not know what to do, be better dead, or die of sadness (themes of death and isolation).

> Children of 10 and 11 years discussed themes of injury and not growing up, with "no more life left in the universe."

> Children of 12 and 13 years felt that there was no place to go ("The target might be me"), and began to examine the issues ("What are we fighting about?").

> Children of 14 to 16 years expressed frustration and anger at the possibility of having no future, with hope dampened, and their lives resting in the hands of a few crazy people or a mistake of some kind. Some saw no winners, and would not want to

survive a nuclear war. Some expressed concern that nobody seems to be doing much about it, and believe that it is their generation that will have to find solutions.

Mack (1982) has questioned whether growing up in the nuclear age is changing the structure of personality itself. Is it becoming more difficult, for example, for children to develop stable ideals or a sense of continuity between past and future? How much can hedonistic or impulsive behavior be traced to a belief that a future is no longer secure? How much do children share in the sense of "psychic numbing" or sense of powerlessness that has been thought to characterize the reaction of many people to the menacing nature of the times?

The findings of Chivian and Snow suggest that the emotional and cognitive responses to the nuclear menace may be more or less specific to the developmental stage of the child. The responses will vary also, of course, with the circumstances of the individual child, and will need to be examined in the contexts of developmental and cognitive levels, emotional adjustment, and family, school, and community situations.

Overby et al. (1989) found that among a group of adolescents with hemophilia, most of whom had evidence of past exposure to the human immunodeficiency virus (HIV), the fear of acquired immunodeficiency syndrome (AIDS) was by no means a dominant force among their concerns, ranking well behind more mundane concerns, and only a little ahead of nuclear catastrophe. We cannot know to what extent these results represent psychic numbing, denial, ignorance, naiveté, or a healthy preoccupation with day-to-day needs and activities.

Development of Perceptions of Death and Dying

About 5 per cent of children will experience the death of one or both parents before the age of 15 years. Accordingly, it is inevitable that the physician caring for children and adolescents will be called upon at this crucial time or be in a position to have an impact on the child's adjustment to the event. He or she will be best able to be supportive of the child and family if armed with knowledge of the development of the child's understanding of death and the grieving process.

It is important to note that little is yet known about these processes in children from low socioeconomic status groups or from minority groups, or from other than Northern European or American backgrounds. In addition, most studies have failed to consider the interactive effect of the grieving of other surviving loved ones on that of the child at various stages of development. It is also of interest that the concepts and reactions of adolescents have been rarely studied. Attention has only recently been given to developmental differences in the child's conceptualization of his or her own death.

Death was long considered a forbidden subject for discussion with children, the erroneous assumption being made that they would be unable to comprehend its meaning and would be harmed as a result of participating in or hearing conversation about it. It was not until 1940 that Anthony described a developmental sequence in the child's understanding of death. He suggested that the child's interpretation of the word "dead" grew from an "initial ignorance, through personal associations, to an ultimate biologic understanding of the concept." Nagy in 1948 delineated three stages in the development of understanding of death: under the age of 5 years, children conceived of death as a reversible aspect of separation; between the ages of 5 and 9 years, death was personified as a "boogeyman"; and after 9 years of age, it was understood to be a universal and irreversible process.

Koocher and O'Malley (1981) found the level of understanding of death to be correlated with the stage of cognitive development. The child at the stage of preoperational thought (2 to 7 years) tends to view death in an egocentric way and to express magical thinking about it. When the stage of concrete operations is reached (at about 6 to 7 years), the child's ability to assume the role of another person facilitates the development of a sense of permanence about death. Thinking about the causation of death is still immature, however. When the stage of formal operations is reached during adolescence, a realistic and biologically based understanding of death is finally reached.

Reactions to death vary with the developmental level of the child's view of death; Table 1-19 lists typical reactions.

Under Six Months

For the very young infant, the concepts of grief and mourning have no clear meaning, but their precursors are discernible. At this age, inasmuch as the sense of time is not yet developed, separation may have potentially the same meaning as death; absence is its equivalent. If the infant's mother dies during the first few months of life, evidence of distress, such as crying, may result from the withdrawal of vital supplies, but according to Raphael (1982), good mothering care by a surrogate may settle this quickly. After the age of 5 months, the child may manifest nonspecific indicators of distress in specific reaction to his or her mother's absence, likely the earliest of grief reactions.

From Six Months to Two Years of Age

Grief and mourning as we know it are first seen at this age. Although it is not yet possible for the infant to conceptualize the permanence of death, he or she is able to respond to his or her mother's absence by looking for her in places where she was previously or last seen. Those who are verbal will inquire as to her whereabouts. Failing to find her, the infant will react initially by shock, and then by angry screams. Since crying brought mother in the past, it has been suggested that crying is now designed to bring her back and to "punish" her for having left. Finding crying to be in vain, the child may lapse into a withdrawn state, to protect him or herself from pain, or may become manic or aggressive. Eventually, the infant gives up the search, and despair and sadness become dominant.

Bereavement in this age group may be manifested by a range of responses, including exaggerated separation responses, especially clinging,

TABLE 1–19. Reactions to Death at Different Developmental Stages*

Infants and toddlers
  Fearfulness
  Food refusal
  Failure to thrive
  Sleep disturbance
  Loss of toilet training
  Irritability
  Developmental delay
  Loss of speech
Preschool children
  Bowel disturbances (constipation, encopresis)
  Hyperactivity
  Enuresis
  Nightmares
  Temper tantrums
  Crying spells
School-aged children
  School avoidance
  Poor school performance
  Poor concentration
  Somatic complaints (headaches, abdominal pain, fatigue)
  Antisocial behavior (lying, stealing)
  Crying spells
Adolescents
  Truancy
  Poor school performance
  Depression
  Suicide attempt
  Acting-out behavior (sexual promiscuity, drug use, delinquency)
  Somatic complaints

* Adapted from Green (1986).

screaming, and sleep or eating disturbances. Older infants often regress by curling up in the fetal position and becoming mute, perhaps in an effort to return to the security of an earlier time.

Terr (1981) describes the unsuccessful attempts of children after the age of 15 months at dealing with their trauma by playing "forbidden games" with themes of death. Often the surviving parent, in an attempt to suppress painful memories, may deny that the child is affected by the loss. According to Raphael (1982), the cries of anguish of the unconsolable child reawakens the pain of the parent's own inner experiences of separation and fear, and comforting does not ease the pain, at least initially, for the child wants only the absent parent. "Yet it is only with our comforting that the pain will eventually ease and he will be supported to accept his loss, to relinquish the bond. This same pattern applies to bereavement throughout the life cycle, but never so poignantly as at this early stage."

Bowlby (1980) found three stages of mourning in children as young as 15 months of age: stage 1 is characterized by *protest* (hope, clinging, anger); stage 2 by *despair* (hope relinquished, tears, depression); and stage 3 by *detachment* (disinterest).

From Two to Five Years

Whereas death is experienced as a profound separation prior to the age of 3 years, preschool children tend to view it as a reversible "sleeplike" state. The child's earliest encounters with the concept of death may be seen in the "peek-a-boo" games of infancy, in the period during the first year when things are "all gone," and in the increasing recognition in the second year that things that are "all gone" may not return. In the play of 4-year-olds, one may see the projection of death onto others with such games such as "cowboys and Indians," as well as by the killing of insects and other creatures. Furman (1974) believes that normal children above the age of 2 years are capable of understanding the meaning of the altered and permanent state of death if they have first experienced the phenomenon in birds and animals, before experiencing the death of a loved person. If the latter does occur, the child can be helped to better understand the event through provision of clear and realistic information and support. It has been noted that 2-year-olds may approach death with fascination and curiosity, rather than terror.

Rochlin (1967) found that 3- to 5-year-olds were very curious about death and thought a lot about it. Lacking receipt of accurate information at this age, magical thinking is common. Among those in this age group who have experienced death of a loved one, fantasies of omnipotence and egocentricity are defenses against feelings of helplessness.

The same egocentricity may, on the other hand, be the basis for the child's feeling responsible for the death by having thought or said that he or she wished the parent dead (e.g., after having been punished). Bowlby (1980) suggests that parents may inadvertently reinforce such fantasies in advance of the death by comments such as "You'll be the death of me." Although not feeling vulnerable to death at this age, the child may become fearful of sleeping when told that death is like going to sleep, or when sick if he or she learns that someone has died as a result of illness.

In Nagy's (1948) sample, one group of children denied death, viewing it as a process of "going away," with the departing individual remaining intact in the process. The other group recognized death as an entity that was somehow continuous with separation. Children at this stage of understanding concretely envision the dead person as being in another room or place from which he or she will come back. On the other hand, Raphael's (1982) prospective study of 2- to 8-year-old bereaved children found in some the tendency to think that the dead parent was either being kept away or not wanting to return to them. Many of the parental deaths in her study had been sudden and unanticipated and the children, either because of what they were told or because of the level of their understanding, were extremely confused about the dead parent's state or location, or about the finality of the event. Seemingly inappropriate questions are common, much to the irritation of the surviving parent, who often views the child as being relatively unaffected by the loss.

As with younger children, the distress of the bereaved 2- to 5-year-old may be manifested by regression in toilet training or by wanting to drink from breast or bottle, in an attempt to elicit the caring response he or she so desperately needs. Others in this age group, whose experience of feelings of omnipotence may have led them to feel responsible for the death, may test environmental control of misbehavior, in order to receive reassurance that they are not really "that" powerful. Sleep, appetite, and bladder or bowel disturbances may be misinterpreted by a grieving parent as symptoms of illness. The physician who is contacted at this time has an opportunity to explain their meaning and to assist the parent in the difficult task of trying to meet the child's needs. If the child is not given accurate information, the magical thinking that can surround death at all stages of the life cycle will be most prominent. If told that the deceased has gone to Heaven, the child may concretely view this as a star in the sky.

From Five to Eight Years

At this stage, the child begins to view death as irreversible, albeit irrelevant to his or her life. In a study of a child's concept of death in relation to piagetian theory, Field (1979) found that the two were, not surprisingly, highly correlated. The concept of death was less well developed in 5- and 6-year-olds than in those who were older, and tended to lag slightly behind the concept of physical causality, as indicated by the child's understanding of the origin of night.

Most researchers agree that by the time the child is 8 years old, his or her concept of death is adultlike, death being viewed as a natural process, as irreversible, and as likely to happen to anyone, including him or herself. The further development of the child's conscience at this age makes the child more apt to consider him or herself responsible for a parent's death. Nagy (1948) and Kastenbaum (1965) found that death at this age is often personified (for example, in the form of the "Skeleton Man").

The power of denial as a coping mechanism at this age may render the bereaved child manic or nonchalant, misleading loved ones into thinking that he or she is not in need of comforting. Boys at this age have considerable difficulty in revealing sad emotions and may hide them by becoming aggressive. Concern about being different from his schoolmates may lead a boy to hide the fact of death from those at school. Girls, on the other hand, according to both Bowlby (1963) and Raphael (1982), may become "compulsive caregivers," showing their need to be cared for by caring for younger siblings in an exaggerated and intense way. Children in this age group typically will have returned by the end of the first year following the death of a parent to a more normal emotional state (one in which the deceased is remembered with sadness), provided that family continuity and support have been sustained. It is not uncommon for the child to begin to fear loss of the surviving parent at this age. When the child is not allowed opportunities for mourning and resolution of guilt, psychopathologic responses may be seen.

When a child in this age group is suffering from his or her own terminal illness, anxiety regarding death is expressed in terms of separation and fears of mutilation and/or castration; 3- to 7-year-olds, prone to fantasizing, often become afraid of their fantasies and need reassurance that they will not come true. Parents are the most appropriate source of reassurance but are often unable to provide it because of their own grief at the impending death. Indeed, many parents do not want the child told of the seriousness of his or her illness. Nothing, however, can be more terrifying to a child of this age than to see parents in distress and not understand its origin. Under such circumstances, it is natural for them to imagine that they have done something to upset their parents.

Another counterproductive behavior of well-meaning, grief-stricken parents is overindulgence. This is frightening to the child and often results in him or her becoming demanding, often to the point of causing parents and hospital staff to become angry and to withdraw from the dying child, despite their wish to be compassionate and supportive.

From Eight to Twelve Years

Kastenbaum (1965) found that children of "this age are better able to recognize the difference between animate and inanimate on a logical thought basis (Piaget), egocentricity is less, and concepts of time, space, quantity and causality are set. By this age children have had sufficient experience in learning what it means to be alive and can appreciate and understand not being alive." As a result the child at this age has an understanding of death that is similar to that of an adult. Death is viewed as a fearful experience, because of the new-found realization that their own deaths and those of loved ones are clearly possible. Because children at this age are more future oriented than younger children, their sense of future loss, as well as of present loss, is emphasized in the mourning process.

Reactions of preadolescents (and early adolescents) to loss of a loved one may include behaviors seen in younger children (such as denial, and feelings of helplessness and of vulnerability). Boys are more likely than girls to appear unaffected by the loss and to be in control of their emotions. More than in younger children, one sees in children of this age expressions of anger and rage, particularly directed at the surviving parent. The anger may be manifested in aggressive play and in bullying of younger children.

Difficulty in accepting the finality of the loss may cause preadolescent children to "hold on to the relationship with the parent in fantasy, as may the younger child, imagining in many scenes the return of the parent, his own virtue in the rescue, the love all will give him, the magic of things being right again and the way they were before the death. This fantasy relationship is often idealized, creating further problems in the child's relationship with the surviving parent" (such children often become withdrawn from friends and at school, with schoolwork suffering as a result.)

The child needs encouragement to express his or her grief and despair in quiet, protected, settings. A caring schoolteacher may provide this support if the emotional atmosphere at home is too charged to be comfortable. As with younger children, compulsive caregiving or pseudoadult behavior may appear; such behavior may often turn away needed potential nurturance.

Enhanced feelings of vulnerability to death in children of this age commonly breed phobias (e.g., of the dark and of sleep) and hypochondriasis. Fears of imagined disease may be so intense that the child is unable to express them, which creates increased anxiety. The physician must be sensitive to this possibility in the grieving child of this age who has no complaints. Counseling may be indicated to help the child express and resolve his or her death-related fears.

Children at this age should be allowed to attend the funeral of a parent, relative, or friend if they so desire. This may help them accept death's finality. Before attending the funeral, the child should be prepared for what will happen and get his or her questions answered. It is recommended that someone close to the child be designated his or her caretaker, prepared to leave if the child requests it. Mention during the service that the child was a source of joy and pleasure to the deceased may be comforting and may help to counter feelings of guilt or of responsibility for the death.

When a child in this preadolescent or early adolescent age group becomes himself or herself fatally ill, his or her response will depend on stage of development, as well as upon the reactions of loved ones and of health care professionals. The major fear of children over the age of 8 years is of suffering pain. Reassurance that they will be protected from pain is necessary. When at all possible, the patient should be offered control over his or her experience of pain, through instruction in self-hypnosis and/or by having input into decisions as to the timing and conditions of painful procedures. Children at this age are often protective of their parents and collude in a conspiracy of silence about their fears. Without professional intervention to encourage communication, such children are destined to die a lonely death.

The Adolescent

Because many adolescents are considered to be in the piagetian sense capable of formal operations, it has been assumed that their understanding of death is comparable to that of adults, but little research has been done to confirm this. Kastenbaum (1965) examined features of adolescent psychosocial development in respect to thinking about death, and concluded that because the adolescent lives in the intense present, and sees the remote future as risky and devoid of meaning and the past as confusing and unpleasant, he or she considers death a remote possibility. If actually confronted with a fatal illness, the adolescent becomes angry at the prospect of being deprived of the experience of life, which is so intense and important at this time. This view must be reconciled with the fact that adolescence is a time of spiritual thinking and fascination with the mysticism of death. Jersild and Holmes (1935) remind us of a common adolescent fantasy about death, which is the expectation of rescue at the last minute. These factors may combine to lead a vulnerable teenager to attempt suicide.

It has been assumed, but is not well documented, that adolescents who have fatal illnesses will deal with them in the same way as adults, in the successive stages described by Kübler-Ross (1969):

Stage 1: The stage of shock and denial ("not me")
Stage 2: Irritability and anger ("why me?")
Stage 3: Attempts at bargaining ("perhaps me, but . . .")

Stage 4: Anger, with beginning acceptance ("it's me")
Stage 5: True acceptance, with ability to separate from loved ones (it's "OK")

The depression that invariably accompanies the acquisition of a fatal illness during adolescence may have an etiology different from that in the adult. When the adolescent male realizes that the illness will prevent him from participating in an activity that has previously provided an opportunity to excel, he will become profoundly depressed, and may need specific help. For example, the depression of a 16-year-old star pitcher with aplastic anemia unresponsive to therapy was improved when he was encouraged to swim in the hospital pool, as he learned that his prowess as an athlete could have another outlet.

According to Weinberg (1970), the adolescent female with a fatal illness may experience profound depression if she feels that the illness has been the reason for the loss of a loved one (parental separation, breaking off with a boyfriend, or even failure of a girlfriend to visit while she is hospitalized). Hospital personnel who are aware of these age-specific bases for depression may find ways for prevention or intervention.

Chapter 2

FETUS AND PREMATURE

FETAL GROWTH AND DEVELOPMENT

The normal duration of human pregnancy is about 266 days from the time of fertilization, or 280 days (40 weeks) from the first day of the last menstrual period. The "period of gestation" generally refers clinically to the 40 weeks that follow the last menstrual period. The World Health Organization has defined any pregnancy that ends before 37 weeks' gestation as *preterm*, weight alone being no longer a criterion determining "premature" delivery. In the United States about 7 per cent of pregnancies end before 37 weeks (the percentage is higher in black and other socioeconomically deprived groups). Preterm infants have increased morbidity and mortality for a variety of reasons. Infants born after 42 weeks gestation are regarded as *postterm*; those born after 43 weeks have increased mortality. About 12 per cent of pregnancies end after the 42nd week, and 5 per cent after the 43rd week.

Intrauterine life comprises two principal phases: *embryonic* and *fetal*. The embryonic period is usually considered to be the first 8 weeks of growth, during which the ovum differentiates into an organism with most of the gross anatomic features of the human form. Organogenesis in some systems continues beyond 8 weeks, so that some prefer to designate the embryonic period as the first 12 weeks of pregnancy, or the first *trimester*. The period between the 12th and the 26th to 28th weeks of gestation (second trimester) is marked by rapid growth in size and progressive elaboration of function. These may permit the survival of infants born at 24 to 26 weeks. Before this time the fetus is generally considered *previable*.

Physical Growth of the Fetus

The first week of embryonic life is *germinal*, and consists of active cell division. During the second week the tissues differentiate into two layers (ectoderm and entoderm); during the third week mesoderm is added. During the fourth week the somites appear, and between the fourth and eighth weeks there is rapid differentiation into an essentially human form. At 8 weeks of age the fetus weighs about 1 g and is about 2.5 cm in length;

131

at 12 weeks it weighs about 14 g and is about 7.5 cm long. By the end of the *first trimester* the sex of the fetus can be distinguished on external examination.

By 16 weeks the fetus weighs about 100 g and is about 17 cm long, at 20 weeks it is about 300 g and 24 cm, and at 24 weeks about 600 g and 30 cm. By the end of the *second trimester* (28 weeks) the fetus weighs about 1000 g and is about 35 cm (14 in) in length.

During the *third trimester* the further increase in size of the now-viable fetus involves especially skin, subcutaneous tissue, and muscle mass. The body content of fat is about 0.5 per cent until the fifth month of gestation; it increases to about 16 per cent by the time of full-term delivery. Fat is the principal element in subcutaneous tissue.

The mean weight of normal full-term newborn infants is about 3200 g, with girls weighing a little less than boys. Many factors affect the size and birth weight of the fetus, both genetic and environmental. Among the genetic are 1) normal genes selecting for various characteristics of growth, 2) abnormal genes that may modify or distort growth, and 3) chromosomal abnormalities that involve many genes. Environmental factors may begin to play their roles very early in intrauterine life, and include the mother's nutritional status, her exposure to environmental modifiers of fetal growth (hypoxia, smoking, infection, radiation, and chemicals, for example), abnormalities of the placenta, and number of fetuses (twins are generally smaller than singleton infants).

About 5 per cent of infants weigh less than 2500 g at birth, and about 5 per cent more than 4000 g. Infants weighing less than 2500 g at birth are classified as *low birth weight* (LBW) infants, those weighing less than 1500 g as *very low birth weight* (VLBW) infants. These weights correspond to those of normal fetuses at gestational ages of about 36 and 32 weeks, respectively.

When the weight of the infant at birth is substantially less than that which is appropriate for the gestational age (arbitrarily, below the 10th percentile), the infant is said to be *small for gestational age* (SGA). The impact of some of the factors indicated above (maternal smoking, for example) will be to retard intrauterine growth and lead to the birth of infants who are SGA. Mothers under the age of 15 years have an increased incidence of SGA infants. Similarly, when the birth weight of the infant is above the 90th percentile of that expected for gestational age, the infant is termed *large for gestational age* (LGA). Mothers who have diabetes mellitus or who are prediabetic tend to have infants who are LGA.

It is often helpful to be able to estimate the gestational age of the newborn infant when the duration of pregnancy is uncertain. Crude assessment of gestational age and fetal growth prior to delivery can be made from such indicators as the time of quickening, or the height of the uterine fundus above the symphysis pubis. More precise estimates can be obtained from ultrasonographic examination (see later in this chapter).

The weight of the infant is an unreliable index of gestational age, owing to its wide variation. More accurate estimates are given by an examination of details of the physical state and neuromuscular or neurologic behavior of the infant delivered in late fetal life. Dubowitz and Dubowitz (1977) have brought together into a scoring system 21 indices to gestational age (11 clinical and 10 neurologic) that can estimate the gestational age within an error of ±2 weeks. The features and some elements of the scoring system are illustrated in Table 2–1 and Figure 2–1. The conduct of the examination is described in Table 2–2. The total scores for the neurologic and clinical examinations are added, to give a score that is related to the gestational age by the formula:

$$\text{Gestational age (wk)} = (0.2642 \times \text{score}) + 24.595$$

The relationship is shown in Figure 2–2. For the gestational age of 40 weeks the 21 items of the examination generate an average score of about 58 (2.8 per item); at 36 weeks about 43 (2.1 per item); at 32 weeks about 28 (1.3 per item); at 30 weeks about 20 (1.0 per item); and at 28 weeks about 13 (0.6 per item). The infant of 42 weeks gestation scores an average of about 66 (3.14 per item). The clinical findings that would correspond to such average scores can be inferred from the descriptions in Table 2–1 and Figure 2–1.

More accurate assessment can be made by ultrasonography, with the biparietal diameter (BPD) of the head giving good correlation with the gestational age in normal infants, and serving as an indicator of abnormal growth (growth failure or hydrocephalus, for example) in infants in whom the length of gestation is known with some precision. The use of sonography in the estimation of fetal age is most helpful in midgestation (12 to 20 weeks' gestation), when the gestational age may be approximated by the formula:

$$\text{Gestational age (wk)} = (\text{BPD [cm]} + 1.65)/0.3$$

After 20 weeks the slope of the growth curve of BPD averages about 0.21 cm/week, a little higher initially, decreasing as gestation nears 40 weeks. Variability is high near term, and the measurement less reliable than earlier.

For the newborn infant, estimation of maturity may take advantage of a brief review of developmental features that will be adequate for most circumstances. Useful signs include the appearance of the *creases of the sole*, which consist prior to 36 weeks' gestation of only one or two transverse creases on the anterior third of the sole (more will appear by 37 to 38 weeks); and complex criss-crossing of creases over the entire sole by 40 weeks. The *breast nodule* of the newborn infant is not generally palpable prior to 34 weeks, and its diameter does not usually exceed 3 mm at 36 weeks; it measures 4 to 10 mm in full-term infants. The *auricular cartilage* appears mainly after 36 weeks. Before 36 weeks *scrotal rugae* are few, and anterior and inferior only; by 40 weeks rugae cover the entire scrotum.

Although during the second trimester there is rapid acquisition of new functions in many systems, for the infant born at the end of this trimester some functions are likely to be marginal, and they will be critical for survival in the respiratory and gastrointestinal systems and in some metabolic areas. The most dramatic changes that take place with delivery of

TABLE 2–1. External Characteristics of the Dubowitz Examination*·†

EXTERNAL SIGN	SCORE				
	0	1	2	3	4
Edema	Obvious edema of hands and feet; pitting over tibia	No obvious edema of hands and feet; pitting over tibia	No edema		
Skin texture	Very thin, gelatinous	Thin and smooth	Smooth; medium thickness; rash or superficial peeling	Slight thickening, superficial cracking and peeling, especially on hands and feet	Thick and parchmentlike; superficial or deep cracking
Skin color (infant not crying)	Dark red	Uniformly pink	Pale pink; variable over body	Pale; only pink over ears, lips, palms, or soles	
Skin opacity (trunk)	Numerous veins and venules clearly seen, especially over abdomen	Veins and tributaries seen	A few large vessels clearly seen over abdomen	A few large vessels seen indistinctly over abdomen	No blood vessels seen
Lanugo (over back)	No lanugo	Abundant, long and thick over whole back	Hair thinning, especially over lower back	Small amount of lanugo and bald areas	At least half of back devoid of lanugo
Plantar creases	No skin creases	Faint red marks over anterior half of sole	Definite red marks over more than anterior half; indentations over less than anterior third	Indentations over more than anterior third	Definite deep indentations over more than anterior third
Nipple formation	Nipple barely visible; no areola	Nipple well defined, areola smooth and flat, diameter <0.75 cm	Areola stippled, edge not raised; diameter <0.75 cm	Areola stippled, edge raised; diameter >0.75 cm	
Breast size	No breast tissue palpable	Breast tissue on one or both sides <0.5 cm diameter	Breast tissue both sides; one or both 0.5 to 1.0 cm	Breast tissue both sides; one or both >1 cm	
Ear form	Pinna flat and shapeless, little or no incurving of edge	Incurving of part of edge of pinna	Partial incurving whole of upper pinna	Well-defined incurving whole of upper pinna	
Ear firmness	Pinna soft, easily folded, no recoil	Pinna soft, easily folded, slow recoil	Cartilage to edge of pinna, but soft in places, ready recoil	Pinna firm, cartilage to edge; instant recoil	
Genitalia Male	Neither testis in scrotum	At least one testis high in scrotum	At least one testis down in scrotum		
Female (with hips half abducted)	Labia majora widely separated; labia minora protruding	Labia majora almost cover labia minora	Labia majora completely cover labia minora		

* From Dubowitz L, Dubowitz V: *Gestational Age of the Newborn*. Reading, MA, Addison-Wesley, 1977.
† Physical criteria are recorded and a final score is obtained following addition of each category's score.

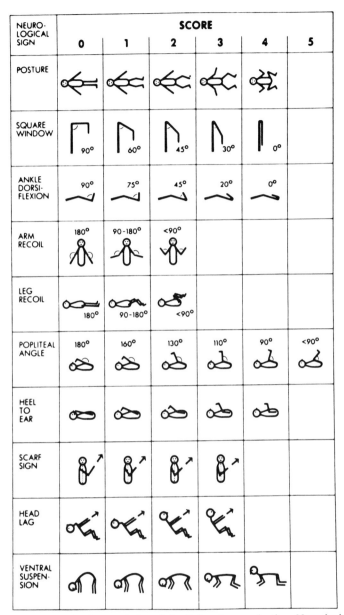

Figure 2–1. Neurologic characteristics of the Dubowitz examination. Neurologic criteria are recorded and added to a final score as performed for the physical assessment. From Dubowitz L, Dubowitz V: *Gestational Age of the Newborn.* Reading, MA, Addison-Wesley, 1977.

TABLE 2–2. Conduct of the Neurologic Assessment*

POSTURE: Assessment of posture is done with infant quiet and in supine position. Grading of posture is done according to position of legs and arms in resting state.

SQUARE WINDOW: Infant's hand is flexed between examiner's thumb and index and third finger. Angle between hypothenar eminence and ventral aspect of forearm is measured; this measurement determines grade.

ANKLE DORSIFLEXION: Ankle is flexed with thumb of examiner placed on infant's sole, and examiner's other fingers behind tendo Achillis. After maximal dorsiflexion, angle is measured between dorsum of foot and anterior aspect of leg; this angle determines grade.

ARM RECOIL: With infant in supine position, arms are first flexed, then fully extended, by pulling on forearms, and released. Angle at elbow is assessed after release of forearm and grade is given according to this angle.

LEG RECOIL: With infant in the supine position, legs are first fully flexed, then extended, by traction on the feet, and released. Score is based on amount of flexion of hips and knees after release.

POPLITEAL ANGLE: With infant in supine position and pelvis flat on examining couch or in incubator, thigh is held in knee-chest position with examiner's left index finger and thumb supporting knee. Leg is then extended by gentle pressure from examiner's right index finger behind ankle. Popliteal angle that can be maintained against this index-finger pressure is measured. Grading is done according to angle at knee.

HEEL-TO-EAR MANEUVER: With infant in supine position, baby's foot is grasped gently and is drawn toward his head until foot tends to slip out from examiner's fingers. Distance from foot to infant's ear is assessed as well as popliteal angle. Note that in this maneuver knee is left free and might draw down alongside abdomen. Grading is done according to position of foot and angle at knee.

SCARF SIGN: With infant in supine position and head central, hand is drawn across to other shoulder as far as it will go without resistance. Maneuver may be assisted by pushing elbow across body at same time. Assessment is based on position of elbow.

HEAD LAG: Infant is pulled toward sitting position from supine position by his hands. Position of the head in relation to trunk is assessed as infant moves through range of about 45°. In small or ill infants, head can be supported during this maneuver. Grading is done according to position of head.

VENTRAL SUSPENSION: Infant is suspended in prone position with examiner's hand under chest. Assessment is based on position of back, degree of flexion of arms and legs, and position of head.

* From Dubowitz L, Dubowitz V: *Gestational Age of the Newborn.* Reading, MA, Addison-Wesley, 1977.

the infant from the intrauterine environment are those that involve the circulatory and respiratory systems.

The Fetal Circulatory System

The circulatory system of the fetus attains its final form between the eighth and 12th weeks of gestation. From then until the delivery of the infant, blood returning to the fetus from the placenta by way of the umbilical vein enters the inferior vena cava through the ductus venosus. On entering the right atrium, this blood is preferentially shunted through the

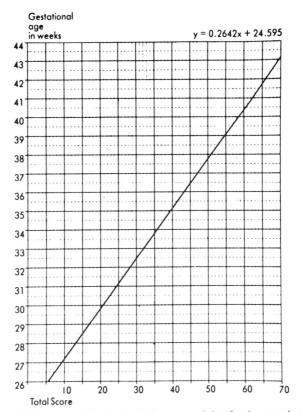

Figure 2–2. Both the external physical criteria score and that for the neurologic criteria are added together and gestational age ($\pm$ 2 weeks) may be read off this graph.
From Dubowitz L, Dubowitz V: *Gestational Age of the Newborn*. Reading, MA, Addison-Wesley, 1977.

foramen ovale into the left atrium, from which it passes through the left ventricle into the aorta, providing the head and brain with the most highly oxygenated blood in the body. Blood returning from the head by way of the superior vena cava tends to cross the right atrium into the right ventricle and pulmonary artery, and to pass by way of the ductus arteriosus into the descending aorta, whence a portion is returned to the placenta through the umbilical arteries.

Shortly after birth there is closure of the ductus venosus, the ductus arteriosus, the foramen ovale, and the umbilical arteries and vein. Functional closure of the foramen ovale likely occurs within the first few minutes, owing to the fall in pulmonary arterial pressure that accompanies aeration of the lungs and establishes a lower pressure on the right side of the heart than on the left. During the first few days of life, crying may lead to reversal of the flow through the foramen ovale, with mild cyanosis. Closure of the ductus arteriosus probably occurs somewhat later, though usually within the first 10 to 15 hr of life. The stimulus for this closure is probably the establishment of a high oxygen level in arterial blood. Closure can be delayed or reversed by administration of prostaglandin E_1, which is the substance that maintains the patency of the ductus in fetal life. Umbilical arteries undergo spasm with the cutting of the umbilical cord, and are ultimately reduced to fibrous cords. The changes in blood flow at birth transform the circulatory system from one in which the two ventricles act in parallel, with shunts adjusting unequal outputs, to a system in which the two pumps act in series, which demands that their outputs be equal.

The Respiratory System of the Fetus

Respiratory movements of the fetus may be seen as early as the 18th week of gestation, and in the fetus delivered at 22 weeks there may be weak phonation, but the development of the alveolar structures will usually not be sufficient to permit survival until the 26th to 28th weeks. The tidal flow of amniotic fluid into and out of the developing lung may contribute to pulmonary arborization. Respiratory movements may be intensified by hypoxemia. Late in pregnancy, when amniotic fluid contains more cells and may contain meconium and other debris, aspiration may deposit these materials in the airways and lead to respiratory difficulties following delivery.

An important element in the development of pulmonary function in the fetus is the production of the pulmonary surfactant that normally lowers the surface tension of the fluid that lines the alveolae. The lowered surface tension permits the alveolae to remain open against the tendency of a higher surface tension to collapse them. The surfactant is composed of lecithin, phosphatidylglycerol, and other ingredients. The formation of surfactant normally begins at about the 20th week of gestation in the type II alveolar cells, but does not reach the alveolae until later, and does not reach mature levels until after 35 weeks, with considerable variation among fetuses in the timing and quantity of production.

In the absence of adequate levels of surfactant the prematurely born infant is at risk of hyaline membrane disease (respiratory distress syndrome of the newborn), which is a consequence of the collapse of the alveolae, with the development of atelectasis, respiratory distress, pulmonary edema, and the appearance of a proteinaceous alveolar exudate. The exudate is seen microscopically at postmortem as the hyaline membrane. Hyaline membrane disease accounts for about 50 per cent of all neonatal deaths in the United States.

The *hemoglobin* of the fetus is predominantly fetal in type (Hgb F). Hgb A is produced in late fetal life and represents about 30 per cent of the hemoglobin of the mature newborn infant. Hgb F carries more oxygen than adult hemoglobin (Hgb A) at a given oxygen tension; this difference favors the transport of oxygen across the placenta to the fetal erythrocyte. The fact that Hgb A gives up more oxygen than Hgb F at a given oxygen tension gives it an advantage over Hgb F in the transfer of oxygen from the erythrocyte to fetal tissues.

Gastrointestinal Development in the Fetus

Bile begins to be formed by about 12 weeks of gestation, and digestive enzymes soon thereafter. Meconium, the distinctive intestinal content of the fetus, is present by 16 weeks; it consists of desquamated intestinal cells and intestinal juices, and of squamous cells and lanugo hair swallowed by the fetus in amniotic fluid.

The fetus makes swallowing movements as early as the 13th week of gestation; at 17 weeks it may protrude the upper lip on stimulation in the oral area, and by the 20th week it may protrude both lips on stimulation. At 22 weeks the lips are pursed upon stimulation, and by 26 to 28 weeks the fetus may actively suck in attempting to gain nourishment.

Placental Function and the Fetus

There is evidence of renal function with the production of urine as early as 10 weeks, but this likely contributes little to the fetal economy. The *placenta* is the chief route of metabolic exchange between mother and fetus. Its most urgent function is to provide for gas exchange; for this, adequate perfusion is needed on both sides. The placenta elaborates hormones and enzymes that participate in the regulation of pregnancy, and effects the selective transfer of nutrients and metabolites between mother and infant. Hormones and drugs may also be transferred to the infant.

Placental permeability is selective even for such closely related substances as antibodies against viruses and bacteria, the former being more readily transmitted (as immunoglobulin [Ig] G) than the latter (as IgM). Much of the transfer of calcium, iron, and IgG to the infant occurs in the last trimester, with the result that the infant born prematurely may have greater need then the full-term infant for calcium and iron and greater susceptibility to infection.

Neurodevelopmental Aspects of Fetal Life

The brain of the fetus appears to be electrically silent during about the first 6 weeks of life. After this time intermittent slow wave activity of low intensity occurs. Neuromuscular activity in the fetus is first seen by about 7 to 8 weeks of gestation, when isolated muscular contractions occur upon local stimulation. By the eighth week the first reflex activity can be elicited by light stroking of the upper or lower lip or alae nasi, which produces contralateral flexion of the neck and trunk. By 9 weeks contralateral flexion on stimulation may be followed by ipsilateral flexion, and some spontaneous movements may be seen. By 9 weeks' gestation the palms and soles have also become reflexogenic; by 13 to 14 weeks graceful flowing movements may be produced by stimulation of all areas except the back, the back of the head, and the vertex. At this time the movements of the fetus may first be felt by the mother.

Finger closure on stimulation of the palm may be seen as early as 10 to 11 weeks, and closure is complete at 14 weeks. By 17 weeks the grasp reflex is evident; it is generally well developed by 27 weeks. By 25 weeks the earliest signs of the Moro response can be elicited.

After the 28th week the activity in the electroencephalogram (EEG) becomes continuous rather than intermittent, as it was until mid-pregnancy, and begins to show greater hemispheric synchrony, rhythmicity, and responsiveness (as evoked potentials) to auditory and visual stimulation. The fetal EEG of late gestation is dominated by sleep activity of the rapid eye movement (REM) type.

The fetus is capable in late pregnancy of *habituation* to certain sensory stimuli; for example, the fetal movement and acceleration in the fetal heart rate that occur in response to noise transmitted through the mother's abdomen are blunted on repetition of the noise (see discussion of orienting response, pp. 155–156).

In addition to habituation, the fetus is capable of some form of *memory*. It has been found that if during the third trimester the mother of the fetus will vocalize repeatedly some words or recitation, the newborn infant will indicate a preference for those words over other sounds (DeCasper and Spence, 1986). Moreover, the infant will within the first hours of life indicate a preference for the voice of his or her mother rather than for a voice not previously heard.

Psychosocial Aspects of Fetal Life

Fetuses differ in levels of activity, and fetal activity may be responsive to maternal emotions, possibly as a result of placental transfer of epinephrine or other substances. Little is known about how the activity of newborn infants or the quality of the infant's demands during the first few weeks of life may reflect aspects of gestation that are dependent upon maternal emotional states. The comfort that some newborn infants receive from rhythmic motion or sound may stem from similar sensations imparted by maternal motion, breathing, heart sounds, or voice.

The mother's experience of pregnancy and of the gradual differentiation for her of the fetus as a separate person, with not only her hopes and expectations but those of the father and family as well, contributes substantially to the emotional climate into which the infant is born. Maternal bonding (see p. 156) is normally well advanced by the time of delivery. The infant has in turn stored up a potentially rich store of experiences (kinesthetic or auditory, for example) that may give direction to later responsiveness or activity.

PROBLEMS OF EMBRYONIC AND FETAL LIFE

Mortality during the *embryonic* period is probably higher than at any other time of life. Causes include abnormalities of genes and chromosomes and alterations of maternal health. These may be interrelated;

advanced maternal age, for example, disposes to certain chromosomal abnormalities. Maternal infection during the first trimester may alter the differentiation of the fetus to produce congenital anomalies. In general, environmental factors responsible for defects in differentiation must exert their effects within the first trimester, before differentiation is complete.

Morbidity during the *fetal period* may result from many causes, including: interference with oxygenation, through disturbances of the placenta or umbilical cord; infections of bacterial, viral, or protozoal origin; injury by radiation, trauma, drugs, or noxious chemicals; immunologic disorders due to maternal immunization and transfer of isoantibodies; or maternal nutritional disturbances.

The effects of *intrauterine malnutrition* upon cerebral structure or function in later life are not fully understood. The rate of increase in the number of neurons is high during gestation, and the number of neurons probably continues to increase at a decreasing rate until about 18 months of postnatal age. In this postnatal period there is also an increase in the number and complexity of dendritic connections, in the number of neuroglial cells, in the sizes of neurons and glial cells, and in myelinization. The effects on the central nervous system of malnutrition occurring after this time can be much more readily reversed than those that have occurred during the periods of increase in cell number.

ASSESSMENT OF THE FETUS

Assessment of the developmental status of the fetus can be made at a number of levels. A steadily increasing number of metabolic errors can be identified by chemical examination of amniotic fluid. Chromosomal analysis of the cells in amniotic fluid or of cells of the chorionic villi (in biopsy material) can detect structural defects of chromosomes (trisomies, deletions, or translocations, for example). Analysis of DNA by recombinant technology can identify genetic markers (restriction fragment length polymorphisms) that will identify carriers of a variety of genes in family studies.

Some structural defects of the fetus give clinical evidence of their presence during pregnancy. Intestinal obstruction or neural tube defects, for example, may produce polyhydramnios or diminished fetal activity, respectively. Oligohydramnios, on the other hand, may be the clue to renal agenesis or hypoplasia, or another renal anomaly. Some structural defects can be detected by sonography or by roentgenographic examination, sometimes effectively supplemented by amniocentesis or amniography.

Occasionally, genetic and environmental factors interact in producing deleterious effects upon the fetus, as in the case of the mother with phenylketonuria whose normal infant may be harmed if her diet contains enough phenylalanine to lead to an elevated serum level of phenylalanine during pregnancy, with mental retardation in the infant as the result of transplacental transfer of phenylalanine.

Preterm delivery and intrauterine growth retardation often interact in producing problems for the newborn infant, though their effects may differ. For example, characteristic problems of preterm infants whose weights are appropriate for gestational age (AGA) include respiratory distress syndrome, immaturity of enzyme systems, and difficulties in temperature control and in feeding, whereas problems more characteristic of full-term infants who are SGA would be hypoglycemia, pulmonary hemorrhage, evidence of perinatal asphyxia (such as meconium aspiration), polycythemia, and hyperirritability.

DEVELOPMENTAL FEATURES OF THE INFANT BORN PREMATURELY

The infant born prematurely begins to have substantial chance of survival at about 26 to 28 weeks of gestation, at a weight of 800 to 1000 g and length of about 33 to 35 cm. The experiences and demands of extrauterine life alter the pace of acquisition of some postnatal behavior patterns. By the time he or she reaches the expected date of delivery, a small premature infant who has made normal progress may seem more alert and active than a full-term baby born on that day, but by the age of 4 to 8 weeks the actual developmental level reached will correspond to gestational age rather than postnatal (chronologic) age and will generally be lower than that of a full-term infant of the same chronologic age. The deficit in level tends to correspond to the level of prematurity. Accordingly, a correction for prematurity will need to be made in assessing the developmental level during the first year of life. These differences will generally have disappeared by the end of the second year of life, so long as no complicating factors occur.

Neurodevelopment

Infants whose birth weights are from 800 to 1500 g (VLBW) tend to be predominantly atonic and to lie in a tonic neck attitude, often with little motion of the extremities. Vocalization is weak, as are the grasp and Moro responses. These infants may show little hunger on deprivation of food, and their sucking responses may be weak, with a need for gavage feeding.

It is difficult to tell whether these small infants are awake or asleep, though they can be stimulated to greater alertness. For the first time at about 7 to 8 months of fetal life the EEG begins to show sleep patterns that supplant earlier patterns of slow frequency and low voltage that typify midgestation (see earlier in this chapter).

Among LBW infants, those weighing from 1500 to 2000 g have good muscle tone when stimulated, more vigorous grasp than earlier, and complete Moro responses. A sleep pattern is easily discernible; the EEG and the behavior of the infant indicate that the predominant form of sleep is that accompanied by REM. These infants are able visually to fixate some objects in their environment. The more vigorous of them are able to manage breast feeding.

LBW infants weighing between 2000 and 2500 g generally have the appearance of small full-term infants, from which they cannot usually be differentiated in the neonatal period by developmental examination. They have good cry and sustained muscle tone.

Physiologic Problems

The premature infant faces difficulties from failure of adequate maturation of enzymatic, respiratory, renal, metabolic, hematologic, and immunologic mechanisms. Developmental defects are more common in premature infants than in full-term infants and often include impairments of motor or intellectual function. The latter are commonly due to residual damage from anoxia or infection.

Respiratory problems are the most common causes of death in infants born prematurely. The most important of these is hyaline membrane disease, or respiratory distress of the newborn (see earlier in this chapter).

Metabolic problems of the immature infant include increased susceptibility to hypoglycemia, hypocalcemia, and other disturbances. On the other hand the newborn infant is relatively tolerant of hypoxia, when compared with the older child or adult, owing to the predominance of anaerobic metabolism. Immaturity of hepatic enzyme systems is present in many infants. For example, the activity of the enzyme (glucuronyl transferase) that is responsible for the glucuronidation of bilirubin (and of some drugs, such as chloramphenicol) does not reach mature levels for some days after birth; the delay is prolonged in the premature infant, with the result that hyperbilirubinemia is more common and more prolonged in the premature infant than in the full-term infant. There is evidence, moreover, that in instances of hyperbilirubinemia the immature infant is more susceptible to the occurrence of kernicterus, owing to greater permeability of the blood-brain barrier.

Neurologic Problems

With the growth of high technology in the care of the premature infant, it is clear that many infants now survive who would have succumbed to the problems of immaturity in past years. Concern has been expressed that a significant number of surviving infants of very low birth weight who have required strenuous intervention for the prevention or control of hypoxia now survive with neurologic deficit or chronic respiratory problems.

Residual conditions include mental retardation; cerebral palsy with or without mental retardation (complications of hypoxia, intracranial hemorrhage, infection, etc.); bronchopulmonary dysplasia or retinopathy and blindness (complications of oxygen therapy); or more subtle sequelae (deafness, learning disabilities, etc.). Current data indicate, however, that even among the smallest infants, those who weigh under 1000 g at birth, the likelihood is high that survivors will have adequate future functional and coping skills. Such infants appear to be at highest risk of delays in the development of language functions, these delays becoming evident by the age of 2 years. The ultimate implications for the future development and function of these infants as adults cannot yet be known with certainty, since the survival of a large proportion of them is as yet a relatively new phenomenon.

With care of high quality most infants of birth weight 1500 g or more, or of 32 weeks' or more gestation, will survive with no residual problems. Their development appears to be rapid following delivery; and with the stimulation that is a consequence of delivery, they may appear more alert and active when they reach a gestational age of 40 weeks than will a full-term infant born on that day. As indicated earlier, however, the appearance is illusory, for when the performances of the two infants at the same *chronologic* age are compared, the prematurely born infant will be found to lag behind the full-term infant by a number of weeks of development corresponding to the degree of prematurity.

Psychosocial Problems

The premature infant is particularly vulnerable to the effects of *sensory* or *social deprivation* in the neonatal period, owing to the restrictions imposed by illness and by the sometimes prolonged period of relative isolation in intensive care, often in incubators impeding touching and holding. Recent studies emphasize the importance of involving the mothers of even the smallest babies in some aspects of their care as early as possible in order to enhance the opportunities for mutual emotional bonding and attachment. Fears that such involvement of parents would expose the infant to increased risk of infection or in some other way frustrate or complicate care have proved groundless, so long as reasonable care is taken in handwashing and in excluding from such contact those persons who are known to have active infection.

The premature infant is at increased risk of becoming the central figure in the *vulnerable child syndrome*, particularly if the neonatal period has been marked by need for prolonged hospital care or by stormy illness. Parents often are left in such instances with the conviction that the infant has been rendered permanently fragile and needs more care and protection than the usual amounts required by all infants and children. Chronic anxiety and overprotection may be life-long consequences. In support of the parents of premature infants, health care workers must follow a fine line between overoptimism and sober realism in assessment of the infant's status at any moment and in sharing with parents their appraisal of that status and its prognosis.

Chapter 3

THE NEWBORN INFANT

INTRODUCTION

The *neonatal* (or newborn) period has been defined for statistical purposes as the first 28 days of life. (The perinatal period is less sharply defined as the period from 20 or 28 weeks of gestation to the seventh or 28th day after birth.) Neonatal mortality is higher than at any other period of life, owing primarily to immaturity and its complications, with congenital defects and neonatal infections also prominent. Mortality is highest on the first day of life, the majority of neonatal deaths occurring within the first 3 days. A lower limit to neonatal mortality is set by the frequency of congenital defects that are incompatible with survival.

A nation's neonatal mortality rate (deaths within the first 28 days per 1000 liveborn infants) affords a good measure of the adequacy of general health services. Rates have fallen dramatically in recent years among the industrialized nations as a result both of improvements in health care systems and of technologic advances. More than a dozen countries have better records than the United States, where the rate (about 8 deaths per 1000 liveborn infants) is particularly high among ethnic minorities and other socioeconomically deprived groups.

The newborn period is a time of adjustment to extrauterine life, with a need to set homeostatic mechanisms, to begin to adapt internal rhythms to the diurnal pulses of the surrounding life, and to begin to form those social relationships that will be essential to survival and to psychosocial development.

PHYSICAL FEATURES OF THE NEWBORN INFANT

The weights of newborn infants average about 3.2 kg (7.5 lb), with boys slightly heavier than girls. About 95 per cent of full-term newborn infants weigh between 2.5 and 4.5 kg (5.5 and 10 lb). Lengths average about 50 cm (20 in), approximately 95 per cent of infants being between 45 and 55 cm (18 and 22 in). Head circumferences average about 34.5 cm (13.5 in), with 95 per cent of measurements between about 32.5 and 36.5 cm (12.5 and 14.5 in) and boys slightly larger than girls.

Body proportions of newborn infants differentiate them sharply from older infants, children, or adults (see Fig. 1–8). The head is relatively

145

larger, the face rounder, and the mandible smaller than in older children or adults. The chest tends to be rounded rather than flattened anteroposteriorly; the abdomen is relatively prominent; and the extremities are relatively short. The midpoint of stature of the newborn infant is near the level of the umbilicus, whereas in the adult it is at the symphysis pubis.

Examination of the newborn infant may show the effects of stresses of delivery (edema of the scalp or scrotum, overriding cranial sutures, etc., that tend to correct themselves with a few days). There may also be minor anatomic variants of little or no significance (such as the transient changes in the skin that include milia, small sebaceous cysts, cutis marmorata, erythema toxicum, or residual lanugo). More persistent variant features include mongolian spot and hemangiomata.

Other anatomic features differentiating the newborn from the older child include external auditory canals that are relatively short and straight, with thicker drums placed more obliquely to the canal. The middle ear contains a mucoid substance that may be mistaken for an exudate of infection. The eustachian tube is short and broad. There is usually a single mastoid cell in the antrum; maxillary and ethmoid sinuses are small, and the frontal and sphenoidal ones undeveloped. The liver and spleen are commonly felt at or just below the costal margins, and the kidneys are often palpable.

The posture of the newborn infant tends to be one of partial flexion. It is often possible to establish what the predominant intrauterine posture of the infant was by determining the most comfortable pattern into which the extremities can be placed to make the infant assume a more or less ovoid shape. Sometimes minor and occasionally major orthopedic abnormalities of the infant will reflect the effect of intrauterine posture on the growing fetus. For example, club feet may develop in the fetus with a neural tube defect and neurologic impairment, owing to the inability of the paraplegic fetus to vary intrauterine posture.

NEONATAL PHYSIOLOGY

Respiratory

The prime need of the newborn infant is for the establishment of adequate respirations and the exchange of gases. The rate of established respirations ranges generally from 35 to 50/min, with brief excursions well outside this range relatively common.

Cardiac

Cardiac adjustments of the neonatal period are often associated with transient murmurs. The heart rate ranges from 120 to 160/min. Blood pressure varies modestly with birth weight (Fig. 3–1). The heart of the

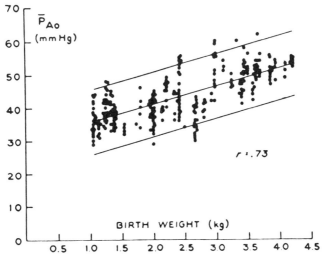

Figure 3–1. Linear regression and 95 per cent confidence limits of mean aortic blood pressure in infants between 2 and 12 hr of age.
(From Kitterman J, Phibbs R, Tooley W: Pediatrics 44:959, 1969.)

newborn infant seems large in proportion to the thorax when assessed by adult standards.

Gastrointestinal/Nutritional

Activity of newborn infants addressed toward the meeting of nutritional needs includes crying when hungry, a tendency when hungry to turn the head toward and to "root" about for the nipple or another stimulus placed close to the oral area *(rooting reflex)*. Sucking, gagging, and swallowing reflexes are active. The newborn infant is capable of nausea and of vomiting.

The digestive enzymes are usually adequate for the diet of the newborn infant, though fat is handled somewhat less well than protein or carbohydrate.

The infant initially expresses hunger at irregular intervals, but during the first week will fall reasonably comfortably into patterns of feeding at intervals ranging from 2 to 5 hr. No arbitrary schedule of feedings will meet the demands or needs of all infants; if infant and mother are close to each other during the immediate postnatal period, as in a rooming-in arrangement, the opportunities for comfortable meeting of the baby's needs are optimal.

The first stools will generally be passed within 24 hr and will consist of meconium. With milk feedings established, these will begin to be replaced on the third to fourth day by *transitional* stools, which are greenish brown and may contain milk curds. The typical yellow milk stool of the older infant follows after an interval of 3 to 4 days.

The frequency of stools in the newborn infant seems closely related to the frequency of feeding and the amount of food obtained, averaging 3 to 5/day by the end of the first week. On any given day during the first week about 1 infant in 50 will have no stool at all; it is unusual for an infant to have as many as 6 to 7 stools/day after the second day. Breast-fed infants have fewer stools than formula-fed infants.

Metabolic

At delivery the body temperatures of mother and infant are virtually the same. The infant's temperature falls transiently, with restoration usual within 4 to 8 hr. The caloric need of the newborn infant to maintain body heat and basal activity is usually about 55 kcal/kg/24 hr. By the end of the first week the caloric needs will be approximately 110 kcal/kg/24 hr, of which 50 per cent supplies basal metabolic needs, 40 per cent is invested in growth and in activity, 5 per cent is for the specific dynamic action of protein, and 5 per cent is lost in feces and urine.

In the newborn infant the extracellular fluid compartment may constitute up to 35 per cent of body weight. During the first few days there is loss of fluid that (in the absence of unusually large intake) generally averages about 6 per cent of body weight and may occasionally exceed 10 per cent. When this loss is excessive, there may be dehydration (or "inanition") fever on the third to fourth day. With the establishment of an adequate milk supply, this loss is usually restored by 10 days of age (more slowly in premature infants).

After the first week the need for water will range between 120 and 150 mL/kg/24 hr. About half of this will be devoted to formation of urine and the rest to insensible loss by lungs and skin and to other losses. Insensible loss is in a relatively fixed relationship to the calories metabolized by the infant (about 40 mL/100 kcal). Losses in stool are variable, those in sweat minimal.

Metabolism in newborn infants favors the anaerobic or glycolytic pathway, so that they are more tolerant of periods of hypoxia than older infants, children, or adults. This tolerance for anoxia is only relative, however. If oxygenation of the infant is not quickly established, there may be a rapidly progressive metabolic and respiratory acidosis (from accumulation of lactic acid and carbon dioxide) and hypoxic tissue injury.

At the cellular level a number of *enzymatic deficiencies* may have important clinical consequences. The red blood cells of the newborn infant have relatively low levels of reduced glutathione, which may contribute to increased hemolysis under a variety of circumstances. A deficiency in capacity of the liver to conjugate bilirubin with glucuronic acid leads to hyperbilirubinemia, often with no evidence of hemolysis. A diminished capacity for the metabolism of certain drugs (e.g., chloramphenicol) may place the newborn infant at increased risk when drug therapy is needed.

Renal

Glomerular filtration rate (GFR) and urine output are low in the first days of life and rise rapidly in the first 2 weeks. Failure of the infant to urinate within the first 24 hr will require investigation of the possibility of an obstruction or other anomaly. The GFR does not approach adult standards until the end of the first year. During the first week proteinuria is common, and the urine may contain an abundance of urates, which may give the diaper a pink stain. Urea clearance is low, and the ability to concentrate urine limited. Production of ammonium ion is limited, and phosphate clearance is low. The blood urea nitrogen level may rise transiently.

Hematologic

The hemoglobin level of the newborn infant ranges from about 17 to 19 g/dL, and mild reticulocytosis and normoblastemia may be observed for the first day or two of life. Blood leukocytes number about 10,000/cu mm at birth and generally increase in number for the first 24 hr, with a relative neutrophilia. Counts as high as 25,000 to 35,000 may be encountered. After the first week the total white cell count is likely to be below 14,000, with the characteristic relative lymphocytosis of infancy and early childhood. Stressful situations in the newborn infant, including overwhelming infections, may be associated with little or no leukocytosis and even with leukopenia.

There is little or no transfer of certain clotting factors from mother to infant. Establishment of normal hemostatic mechanisms depends upon the acquisition of normal intestinal flora and its elaboration of vitamin K. Vitamin K must be administered to the newborn infant to protect against hemorrhagic disease. The breast-fed infant is particularly susceptible.

Endocrinologic

Placental transfer of maternal hormones produces temporary changes in the breasts and genitalia of the newborn infant and possibly in other tissues; and the withdrawal of maternal hormones or other metabolites may contribute to temporary hypofunction of the parathyroid. Maternal hyperglycemia will dispose the infant to hyperinsulinemia and hypoglycemia. Blood levels of glucose and of calcium are normally relatively low in the newborn infant (30 to 60 mg/dL and 7.0 to 10.6 mg/dL, respectively), and further decreases (to below about 20 mg/dL of glucose or below 7.0 mg/dL of calcium) may cause convulsions.

Immunologic

The gamma globulin level of the newborn infant (almost entirely maternal immunoglobulin [Ig] G) is slightly higher than that of the mother, owing to an active transplacental transport mechanism. The IgG affords protection against many viral and some bacterial diseases. On the other hand, antibodies against certain antigens of gram-negative enterobacteria are, like isohemagglutinins, found in the IgM fraction of immune globulins; these do not cross the placenta in substantial amounts, leaving the newborn infant susceptible to infection with those organisms. IgM antibodies may be formed by the fetus, however, in response to intrauterine infection. IgA antibodies and IgE do not generally cross the placenta. T lymphocyte functions are somewhat reduced in newborn infants.

The gamma globulin level of the infant falls to a low level by about 3 months of age, as maternal antibody disappears; a rise then occurs to the levels that characterize older children and adults, as the infant produces his or her own immunoglobulins. Responses to immunization are relatively sluggish in term newborn infants and markedly so in premature infants. Antibodies of the major blood group system (ABO) usually appear by the second month of life.

NEURODEVELOPMENT

The behavior and neurologic responses of the newborn infant will depend upon the level of maturity of the infant. The traditional neurologic examination has focused upon the Moro response, postural reflexes, stepping and placing and rooting behavior, sucking and swallowing, grasp reflex, and tests of vision and hearing and of stretch and sensory reflexes.

The *Moro (or startle) response* can be elicited when the infant lying supine with the head supported in the examiner's hand has that support suddenly withdrawn, permitting the head to fall back by 10 to 15 degrees. Loss of support is followed by extension of the trunk and extension and abduction of the arms; these motions are followed by flexion and adduction of the arms, often with closure of the fists. The response is often partial, and may habituate rapidly to a repeated stimulus. An asymmetric response is abnormal, and may indicate neurologic or orthopedic injury (trauma to the brachial plexus or to the clavicle, for example). The Moro response may be elicited by other sudden sensory inputs, such as loud noises or mechanical shock to the infant's crib. It is generally not elicited in its typical form after the age of 3 months in normal infants.

Postural reflexes include the *neck-righting* and *tonic neck reflexes*. Neck-righting refers to the tendency of the infant to turn the trunk in the direction to which the head is passively turned. The full-term newborn infant is often rather stiff in the first days after delivery, and may turn the trunk with the movement of the head. At this time the tonic neck response may be not easily elicited; it consists of extension of the arm and leg on the side to which the head of the supine infant is rapidly turned, with contralateral flexion of the limbs (adoption of a "fencing" posture). The infant becomes more supple within a few days, and may then often fall spontaneously into this posture, which has been termed the *tonic neck attitude* (TNA).

The *stepping reflex* is elicited when the infant is held upright and inclined forward with the feet touching the surface of the examining table; walking movements occur as the infant is gently moved forward. The *placing reflex* is seen when the infant is held upright and the dorsum of a foot is brought to touch the undersurface of the edge of the table; the infant will flex and then extend the leg, as if to put it on the table's surface. Stepping and placing reflexes are not generally obtainable after the age of 6 weeks, but if the mother of a newborn infant is encouraged to exercise the stepping behavior for a few minutes each day, the behavior may persist and the infant may integrate it into walking without support some weeks earlier than would normally be expected.

The *rooting reflex* consists of turning of the infant's head toward a stimulus on the cheek, as when the cheek is gently touched by a fingertip or is brought to touch the mother's nipple. Sucking movements may be associated. This reflex may frustrate the efforts of the nursing mother to turn the head of her infant toward the nipple when she puts the pressure on the wrong cheek.

Stretch reflexes vary in their activity, but should be symmetric.

Sensory reflexes may not be easily elicited. The Babinski response (dorsiflexion of the toes on stimulation of the sole) has been said to be normal in the newborn and young infant until about 18 months of age. On the other hand, when the procedure used to elicit the response is precisely defined and controlled, it appears that the response of most newborn infants is usually plantar flexion. Any response that appears abnormal must be interpreted with care at this age.

The *visual* apparatus of the newborn infant is organized and complex. The newborn infant will close the eyes and turn the head away from a strong light. Estimates of the visual acuity of newborn infants vary with the techniques used (instrumentation, distances examined, and other criteria). The visual acuity of the infant is thought to be optimal at a distance of about 30 cm (1 ft).

It is clear that the infant will look for a visual stimulus with saccadic movements of the eyes, and that these movements are controlled both by internal mechanisms and by the nature of the stimulus. A moving stimulus is particularly "interesting," but it must move more slowly for the infant to follow it than will be necessary later. Movements are at first jerky, becoming smooth by 6 weeks of age.

The mechanisms are complex through which infants hold fixation of faces or of points of contrast, movement, or changing intensity of light within their visual fields. During the first week they are able to maintain these fixations against passive movements of their bodies *(doll's eye reflex),* and responses originally partly vestibular become increasingly oculomotor alone.

Contour density seems to be an important factor in attracting the attention of the newborn. For example, a checkerboard stimulus with small squares is more attractive than one with large squares. Circles are preferred to lines by the newborn infant, and by the age of 2 months vertical lines will be preferred to horizontal ones.

Such observations make it seem likely that some preference for patterns may be "prewired" (as visual schemata) into the construction of the nervous system of the infant, possibly even into DNA. This may be most clearly demonstrated by the studies of Fantz, Goren, and others that showed that the newborn infant prefers to look at an array of identical elements that resembles the human face, rather than at an arrangement of the same visual elements that is asymmetrical or bizarre. Goren et al.'s demonstration (1975) of this was particularly dramatic. They found the preference for features of the face in infants who had never seen a human face and were between 2 and 9 min old.

We have other reasons to wonder if the infant may not have built-in genetic schemata that inform him or her as to the features and functions of the face. The newborn infant is able, for example, to imitate the facial gestures of others, such as sticking out the tongue, fluttering the eyelids, or opening the mouth. We do not know whether this is written in DNA, or whether it is possible that through intrauterine exploration of his or her own face, the infant has formed in darkness some map that could be superimposed upon the retinal image of the face of the mother.

In neonates such imitation is limited to things that the infant can do anyway, there being no evidence that the newborn infant can imitate an unfamiliar act. The usual sequence of behaviors is often that the infant first produces the behavior, which is imitated by the adult, whereupon the infant repeats the behavior, possibly because it is positively reinforced. Bower (1977) has suggested that this behavior on the part of the infant appears to be enjoyed by him or her, and that it is both for the infant and for the mother a satisfying form of interaction fostering socialization.

Other evidence suggests either that the infant has built-in schemata or that he or she is capable of unexpectedly sophisticated analysis of the environment at a remarkably early age. Within the first days of life, for example, the infant responds to looming objects with reactions of avoidance or recoil that are sensitive to their distance and direction. A looming object at a distance is not so scary as an object that subtends the same visual angle but is closer, and if the object is coming at an angle that promises a miss, the infant finds it tolerable. The speed of a looming object is an important factor in such decisions; if a looming object comes too fast, there is no response, there having not been enough time given for analysis of the situation and for decision-making. The infant can distinguish an object from an aperture in an object, and appears able to differentiate between solidity and hardness of surface.

Bower (1979) has reviewed the evidence for *intersensory coordination* in the newborn infant. It begins early; Wertheimer (1961) found, for example, that before the infant is fully delivered from the birth canal, when the head is delivered and a sound is made at one side or the other of the head, the infant's eyes will turn toward the sound as if he or she already knows that something is to be seen there.

Beyond the reflexology of the newborn infant lies a capacity for *interaction with the environment* that was unappreciated until recently, and that gives further evidence of a complex neurologic organization.

An important discovery of Prechtl and Beintema (1975) was that the behavior of the newborn infant is critically dependent upon his or her *state of arousal*. There are now defined six stages of arousal: deep sleep; light (REM) sleep; drowsy; quiet and alert; awake and restless; and crying intensely. Prechtl and Beintema found that it is in the quiet and alert state (state 4) that newborn infants are capable of their most complex interactions with the environment.

The behavior of normal infants whose behavior has not been modified by anesthetic or other agents, and who have been examined in the quiet, alert state (state 4), has shown us: 1) that from the moment of birth infants are capable of visual fixation on objects and of following the movements of these objects; 2) that they are capable of visual scanning of simple geometric figures; and 3) that among somewhat similar and rather complex figures they will give preferential attention to figures that resemble the human face.

Within the first hour or two after normal delivery of an unanesthetized and unsedated infant, the infant will commonly spend a good deal of time in state 4. Within the next few days the amount of time spent by the baby in this state will constitute about 10 per cent of the day, increasing with age.

In the case of the crying newborn infant, Korner and Thoman (1972) found that the infant can usually (in 75 per cent of cases) be brought to state 4 by being picked up and held upright against the shoulder. The crying stops and the eyes open, and the infant becomes ready for input from the environment. This manipulation both soothes and alerts. The vestibular input associated with bringing the baby to an upright position seems to be responsible for the visual alerting, whereas it is the bodily contact that seems to be more important for the soothing effect on crying.

During the first 3 days of life the infant generally sleeps 14 to 17 hours/ day, with a range from 10 to 23. This sleep consists typically of about half REM sleep and about half deep sleep. By the age of 3 months, the proportion of REM sleep will be reduced to about a third, as compared with about a quarter in adults. Duration of the REM cycles averages about 47 min in infants, as compared to about 90 min in adults (Parmelee, et al. 1974). Sleep patterns of newborn infants begin to change as early as the second day from the predominantly REM sleep of the older fetus toward the patterns of older infants and children.

COGNITIVE DEVELOPMENT

Not long ago the infant was regarded by many psychologists and other scientists as having been born into the world not just physically naked but pretty bare also with regard to experience and personality, and it was believed that upon this relatively clean slate (tabula rasa) life was about to begin to be written. Mothers and grandmothers may have always doubted this, but a relatively recent explosion of interest in the behavior of the newborn infant on the part of scientists in many fields has begun to reveal to others the complexity and potential of that behavior.

A number of factors have contributed to renewed interest in the behavior of the newborn. These include: 1) animal studies that show that the experiences of young animals in the first hours or days of life may have profound effect upon their capacities to learn and to make social adjustments in later life; and 2) the re-creation of childbirth as a primarily social, rather than medical, event. The latter has led to much-reduced use of analgesics and anesthetics in labor, with the result that the opportunities have been increased for the observation of the truly normal newborn infant, unimpaired in function by drugs.

We have referred earlier to the ability of the fetus to learn in utero, as he or she reacts to the sound of a buzzer placed against the mother's abdomen. The first experience of this novel sound will produce acceleration of the fetal heart rate, with fetal movement, and these responses abate with repetition of the sound. The abatement is not the result of fatigue. Substitution of a new sound will show that the fetus is fully capable of producing the original acceleration of heart rate and muscular activity. This phenomenon represents the earliest evidence of cognition, or "knowing," and is an example of habituation (see later in this chapter).

It is easily shown that a newborn infant in the quiet and alert state of arousal (state 4) can learn rapidly; and it is very likely that most neonatal learning takes place in state 4.

Within the first week of life the infant is capable of learning to distinguish between the voices of his or her mother and other persons, and may react differentially to the sound of his or her own name spoken in the voice of the mother. By 2 weeks of age the infant will associate the voice of the mother with her face. If the voice of the mother is associated with some other face, the infant is made unhappy by the observed discrepancy.

Infants are capable within the first week of life of identifying breast pads containing the odor of the milk and breast of their own mothers, turning their heads toward those pads more readily than toward the pads of other nursing mothers.

Even on the first day of life the infant can solve complex problems. If an apparatus is designed that presents an infant with milk when the head is turned to the right at the sound of a bell, whereas the head should be turned to the left if the sound is that of a buzzer, the infant can solve this problem within 10 trials. Moreover, he or she can reverse the procedure rapidly if the rules of the game are reversed. We once thought the human infant to be relatively less mature at birth than other primate infants, say monkeys, who can move about rather freely by 2 or 3 days of age; but in situations such the above, the human infant displays a more rapid pace of learning than is found in any other primate infant.

Besides auditory and visual stimuli, prenatal and postnatal experiences involve kinesthetic, somesthetic, thermal, olfactory and proprioceptive stimuli, such as those associated with the intrauterine position. The baby is exposed in utero to the regular rhythm and rate of the maternal heart beat; and it has been shown that sounds having the quality, rhythm, and rate of a normal heart beat can sometimes comfort fretful infants. It has been noted that more mothers carry their infants on the left side, close to the heart, than on the right.

The infant can carry into extrauterine life other things learned in utero. Fifer (1987) has found that infants nursing at an apparatus that measures the intensity of and times the duration of sucking activity will respond to the recorded sound of their mothers' voices with sucking behavior that clearly distinguishes between their mother's voice and that of a stranger. Further, he has found that when sucking during the presentation of a certain tone produces the mother's voice and during the presentation of a different tone the voice of a stranger, infants between 24 and 60 hr of age will learn in 5 to 10 min to suck in such a way as to maintain the mother's voice. It seems virtually certain that some qualities of the maternal voice are learned in utero, and that it is familiarity with these that governs this later behavior. (We are reminded that some birds learn the typical call of their species *in ovo*. If they have not heard that call or if they have heard the taped call of another bird played to them before hatching, they may never produce the sounds that were once thought probably to have been built into DNA.)

Other evidence of learning resides in the phenomenon of *habituation,* through which it is easy to show that the infant can quickly recognize old experiences. Habituation is related to the *orienting response*. When an unfamiliar stimulus is received in the auditory or visual fields or through some other sensory input, the infant becomes more alert, with suppression of spontaneous movement, with a likely turning of the head toward the stimulus, and with physiologic changes, including an acceleration in heart rate. When a new stimulus becomes repetitive, the orienting response rapidly habituates, even in a few seconds: there is less startle reaction or cardiac acceleration, and as the stimulus becomes familiar, cardiac deceleration may supervene.

Habituation is not a matter of fatigue, as might be thought when an effort to induce a Moro response becomes less successful on the third or fourth try than on the first. A new stimulus can recreate the response immediately in its original intensity. The cleverest demonstration that habituation rather than fatigue is the cause of the increasingly blasé response of the infant was devised by investigators who showed that when an infant, after stimulation by a mixture of several odors to behavior that displayed rapid habituation, was then stimulated by a second mixture identical to the first except that one of the odors had been removed, the original response returned in full intensity.

Neonatal habituation as a form of learning must be regarded as distinct from memory. Such responses as learning how to control the flow of milk from an apparatus must be relearned the next day. The memory for these skills appears to last a few minutes at most. Memory for his or her own name may last for 15 to 42 hr by 2 to 4 weeks, for 2 weeks by the age of 8 weeks, and for 1 month by the age of 12 weeks.

Brazelton (1973) has brought a number of observations together to form a *Neonatal Behavioral Assessment Scale* that may provide a more precise and predictive assessment of the newborn infant than a traditional neurologic examination or the Apgar rating (see later in this chapter). The Brazelton scale assesses the behavior of the infant in four dimensions:

Interactive processes (orientation; alertness; consolability; cuddliness)

Motor processes (muscular tone; motor maturity; defensive reactions; hand-to-mouth activity; general activity level; and reflex behavior);

Control of physiologic state (habituation to a bright light, a rattle, a bell, and a pinprick; self-quieting behavior)

Response to stress (tremulousness; lability of skin color; and startle reaction)

The Neonatal Behavioral Assessment Scale has been used to identify deficits in neurobehavioral function; to describe the level and quality of normal behavior; to assess the impact on behavior of injury, drugs, or other interventions; and to attempt prediction of future development and function. As late as 1 week after delivery the use of this examination has detected changes in the infant's behavior as a result of drugs given to the mother (such as phenobarbital). The demonstration of some of the items in the scale to parents may foster healthy attachment as they reveal the infant's complexity and early evidence of the infant's personality and individuality.

In summary, the newborn infant has an impressive capacity for learning and his or her perception of the world has unexpected complexity, far from the fuzzy quality that has been fantasized in the past. For example, the psychologist William James 100 years ago (1890) regarded the newborn infant as functionally blind until the age of 6 weeks. We now know not only that the infant can see geometric forms during the first week of life but that analysis of these gives particular attention to angles (Salapatek, 1971). Fifty years ago Gesell and Amatruda (1941) set as a standard to be achieved first at 4 weeks that the infant follow an object a few degrees from the visual midline; we now know that for the proper stimulus for the infant in the proper state, this is possible to nearly 90 degrees within the first 10 min of life. Gesell also set 3 months of age as the time when infants should first be expected to reach for a dangling object and miss it. Bower (1977) has found that infants well within the first month of life will move their hands and arms in response to a moving object in what has been termed a *larval* form of reach, and that they will be able to contact the object rather than miss it if it is simply placed within their arm's reach.

PSYCHOSOCIAL DEVELOPMENT

The most important implications of the discovery of the sophistication of the equipment of the newborn are surely social. The infant is born into a social structure and setting of which he or she has already for some time been an important part, represented in the hopes and fears of parents, and particularly in the mother's experience of pregnancy. To this earlier experience of the mother and father are added the events surrounding the mother's labor and the delivery of the child. These experiences have the effect of *bonding* the participants in greater or lesser degree to the child.

Bonding consists of those emotional ties and commitments that bind the parents or other participants in the social events of pregnancy and childbirth to the child that becomes the central figure. During the next hours, days, weeks, and months the infant matches bonding with his or her *attachment* to the significant persons in the environment to whom he or she will turn in the future for protection, nurturance, and love. Analogues of bonding and attachment have been studied in animals, and the animal studies, such as those of *imprinting,* have greatly enriched the study of socialization in infancy.

The equipment that the infant brings to bonding and attachment is striking in its complexity, beginning with the observation that the infant in the first minutes of life responds visually preferentially to figures that resemble the human face. Such behavior may be important in facilitating or eliciting those interactions leading to the formation of social bonds. For example, the steady gaze of the newborn infant into her eyes is often experienced by the mother as a powerful stimulus to her emotional involvement. Moreover, newborn infants give attention preferentially to high-pitched or female voices, and can be shown within the first week of life to turn their heads more readily toward the sounds of their own mothers' voices than to voices not previously heard, and even to be able to distinguish a familiar sound (his or her own name) in that voice (Hammond, 1970).

A subtle aid to socialization was first described by Condon and Sander (1974), who showed that the motor activity of the newborn infant is not random, but that the infant moves in cadence with his or her mother's voice or that of another person engaging him or her in a social relationship. This translation of sound into body movement is a lifelong characteristic of conversations between people. It becomes modified by experience and by social and cultural forces and its forms may become typical of certain social or cultural groups. It begins in the neonatal period, in any case, with the infant ready from the start to respond to the cadences of whatever language is spoken to him or her with behavior that has importance for social bonding. Mothers and others may have an intuitive expectation of this, and some mothers will know very early that something is amiss with their infant and will seek help for the unknown for some time before it becomes apparent to them or to their physicians that the infant is deaf.

There is new appreciation of the role of the infant in initiating and driving the interactions that contribute to his or her care. It is now clear that about half if not the majority of the caretaking episodes that mark the relationship between mother and infant are initiated by the infant (through crying, fussing, or movement), rather than by the mother. And it is likely that the *responsiveness* of the mother or other caretaker to the infant's signals is more critical to the behavioral development of the infant than her *initiation* of interaction.

We have already seen that newborn infants will use environmental signals to make decisions as to how they will use their bodies to sustain a socially significant relationship—that is, with movements that are in cadence with the voices of their mothers. They will use their bodies also to shape their environments in other ways. With the appropriate apparatus they will learn how to turn on a picture, to make lights brighter, to sharpen the focus of pictures projected on a screen, and to make mobiles turn.

There is much evidence that the opportunity to produce such changes in the environment is an important growth-promoting and socializing force in the infant. It is speculated that this control is important to the growing sense of self even in very young infants, and even in prematures. Brazelton has reported (in personal communications) instances in which the opportunity given a premature infant who was not thriving to move a mobile by means of a string tied to a toe seemed to be a turning point in the recovery of the infant from a previously downhill course. Mobiles are not just to look at but to move, even in the bassinet or incubator. If they are to be maximally useful as objects of interest to or stimulation of the infant, they should probably be placed within reach of the infant (with appropriate safeguards), or some other arrangement made through which they can be exploited by the infant.

Besides the imitation of expressions in the maternal face, referred to above, another piece of equipment that the infant brings to the needs of socialization is the smile. The first facial expressions that deserve the name "smile" may be seen even in premature infants. They have been attributed to the passage of gas or to other events or to spontaneous behavior. The true social smile usually appears at 3 to 5 weeks of age. An infant who does not have a social smile by 8 to 12 weeks of age has a serious developmental problem.

It seems likely that babies differ in their tendencies to smile, and that larval smiles produced by premature infants have no substantial socializing implications. Bower (1977a) cites evidence that the social smile clearly elicited in a face-to-face relationship with another person appears at the same postconceptional age in all infants—about 46 weeks.

It has been said that the smile is first elicited by the sound of the other's voice in a face-to-face encounter, then (at 6 weeks) by the face itself of the other person, and finally by the smile on the face of the other. The discovery by the infant that he or she can produce a change in the environment—move a mobile, for example—becomes one of the most powerful eliciters of the smile, and it seems to be the responsive environment, rather than passive perception, which gives rise to the smile as a sign of enjoyment (Papousek, 1969).

In summary, then, during the first hours after the birth of a normal, unanesthetized, and unsedated infant, with the infant in a quiet, alert state, the opportunity may be particularly favorable for interactions that will facilitate bonding and attachment. Events at this time may have substantial influence upon the quality of the relationship established between mother and infant and, to a degree, between the infant and other persons sharing the experience, even if only as onlookers (say, as godparents). Whether *critical periods* comparable to those for imprinting in animals exist for bonding or attachment in humans is not known, and seems unlikely given the resilience with which many infants, parents, and families surmount neonatal experiences that might have had devastating effects. On the other hand, for some fragile infants or parents the loss of some opportunities for harmonious interaction may be irretrievable within a few days. These lost opportunities may be in some instances a first step in the development in later life of emotional disorders, child abuse and neglect, or failure to achieve potential levels of intellectual or social function. In any case, such effects are perhaps more likely to represent trauma to or changes in the relationship between parent and infant than to reflect any physiologic "now or never."

IMPLICATIONS

Growing appreciation of the importance of childbirth as a social event has led to substantial revision of traditional practices. The socialization of childbirth has been given much of its impetus in this country by young women who have sought through such organizations as the Childbirth Education Association and La Leche League to retrieve childbirth and the early care of the infant from the medical or (worse) from the surgical arena. Both mothers and fathers have become involved in prenatal programs oriented toward education for childbirth and for child-rearing. Such programs encourage family-centered activities for pregnancy and in preparation for childbirth, restraint in the use of analgesic and anesthetic medication in labor, adoption of breast-feeding, and provision of rooming-in arrangements in the neonatal period that will optimize the opportunities for newborn infants, their mothers, and their families to get to know each other within the first hours and days of life. Fathers are encouraged to share the experience of the delivery room, and sometimes godparents, too! For premature infants whose reception into the bosom of the family may have to be delayed, some investigators are putting pictures of parents and siblings in the incubators!

An important use of our growing understanding of the complexity and the abilities and equipment of the newborn infant may be to share this knowledge with parents and others for whom this understanding can make newborn infants more interesting. Enlightened observations and interactions can enrich parents' understanding of and involvement with their own infants. The nature and implications of these observations might also be made part of the curriculum of junior high schools, for both boys and girls as the parents of the future. Exposure to this knowledge and these issues can put their own lives in a new perspective, both retrospectively and in prospect.

ASSESSMENT OF THE NEWBORN INFANT

The assessment of the newborn infant begins with evaluation of *physiologic state, structural integrity, and maturity*. It begins most urgently with evaluation of respiratory and cardiac status. The evaluative instrument in widest use is the Apgar scale, which assesses respiration, heart rate, color, muscular tone, and response to the insertion of a catheter into the nostril (Table 3–1). The Apgar rating is usually made at 1 and at 5 min after delivery. The 1-min rating determines the need for immediate intervention in support of respiratory or cardiac function; the 5-min rating correlates more closely with the likelihood of death or of neurologic sequelae due to anoxia or to injury.

So far as evident anomalies are concerned, structural integrity can be established with a brief physical examination.

Developmental aspects of the physiologic state of the newborn infant will be related to maturity, structural integrity, and whatever metabolic or other features may reflect developmental processes. Developmental disorders (such as those due to inborn errors of metabolism, for example) will need to be differentiated from others (such as those due to trauma, drugs, or nutritional deficiencies). The clinical features of developmental disorders may not be at all distinctive, but be first reflected in the vital signs of the infant, or in respiratory or gastrointestinal or neurologic abnormalities that may have many possible causes. It is important that the possibility of a developmental abnormality not be overlooked in an infant who may have had other possible experiences (such as birth trauma) that might account for clinical difficulties.

Neurodevelopmental assessment of the newborn infant will draw upon classical neurologic findings, as described above, and upon such broader functional assessments as provided by the Dubowitz or Brazelton scales. The Gesell and Bayley scales begin to set standards for performances of infants who have reached the ages of 4 and 8 weeks, respectively.

The neurodevelopmental assessment of the normal newborn infant will be most effective when it can be carried out in the presence of the mother,

TABLE 3–1. Evaluation of the Newborn Infant (Apgar)*,†

SIGN	0	1	2
Heart rate	Absent	Below 100	Over 100
Respiratory effort	Absent	Slow, irregular	Good, crying
Muscle tone	Limp	Some flexion of extremities	Active motion
Response to catheter in nostril (tested after oropharynx is clear)	No response	Grimace	Cough or sneeze
Color	Blue, pale	Body pink, extremities blue	Completely pink

* Modified from Apgar V: Curr Res Anesth Analg 32:260, 1953.
† Sixty sec after the complete birth of the infant (disregarding the cord and placenta) the five objective signs above are evaluated, and each is given a score of 0, 1, or 2. A total score of 10 indicates an infant in the best possible condition.

and of the father also if possible. With the infant in the quiet and alert state, the opportunity given the parents to observe the behavior of their infant and to have it interpreted to them will be instructive and reassuring, and will help foster in them a sense of the personality and individuality of their child. This experience can give support to the processes of bonding and attachment, and make the decisions and actions of parents more informed, and parenthood more interesting. It will set the stage for that review of developmental status that should throughout childhood be a part of every health visit, not simply as a screening device but as an essential contribution to the enrichment of child-rearing and the prevention of misunderstandings that might otherwise lead to problems easily avoided.

The *psychosocial* assessment of the newborn infant ought to begin in the prenatal period with an interview with the parents-to-be that will explore their expectations of their infant, their previous experience of child-raring, their plans for delivery, and their wishes with respect to breast-feeding. It will be helpful to the clinician to know the composition of the family into which the infant is to be born, and what expectations the family members have of each other with regard to the care of the infant.

Observations made during labor and in the delivery room can add useful data to the clinician's estimate of the likelihood that the relationship between infant and parents will develop in a creative way. At the moment of birth clues may be gotten from the mother's reaction to the infant, her pleasure or displeasure at learning whether the baby is a boy or girl, her readiness to accept and hold the infant, and the like. During the next day or so it may be helpful to review with her her experience of pregnancy and delivery, along with findings made on examination of the infant in the nursery or at the mother's bedside.

The addition of a new member to a family, like the death of a family member, has a major impact upon the relationships between family members. The psychosocial assessment of the newborn infant should include an appraisal of this possible impact. There may be effects upon the relationships of family members to employment, to educational activities, and the like, as well as upon interactions among immediate family members, such as siblings, grandparents, and so on. It is appropriate that each of these areas be explored. As the infant emerges from the neonatal period, we will often need to assess the impact of day care or shared care (see pp. 208–212) upon the evolution of the processes set in motion by the remarkable machinery that the newborn infant brings to life.

Chapter 4

THE FIRST YEAR

GROWTH AND DEVELOPMENT DURING THE FIRST YEAR

The earliest days and weeks of life find the infant attaining control of reflex and homeostatic mechanisms, and entering into interactions with the personal and inanimate environment. Patterns or rhythms of feeding and sleeping evolve, along with the ability to control one's own state through self-quieting behavior, as through finger- or thumbsucking. The first month of life (the neonatal period) has been regarded as a time devoted primarily to the establishment of homeostatic stability and of some biologic rhythms, but we have seen that the newborn infant is endowed with complex reactivity, and with abilities that entrain caretakers in a growing social relationship. This relationship becomes increasingly personalized to the mother, if she is the principal caretaker, and to others who play significant roles in the infant's life.

Physical Growth in the First Year

During the first months of the first year, after the adjustment of weight that follows birth, the infant gains weight at a rate that represents a continuation of the rate of the last trimester of pregnancy. Most full-term infants regain their birth weights by the age of 10 days. The full-term infant will generally double the birth weight by 5 months (with an average gain of about 0.7 kg [1.5 lb] per month), and triple the birth weight by 1 year (gaining about 0.45 kg [1.0 lb] per month during the last 7 months of the first year). The length of the normal infant increases during the first year by 25 to 30 cm (10 to 12 in); about 65 per cent of this gain occurs during the first 6 months.

During the first year the premature infant is likely to gain about 6 to 7 kg (13 to 15 lb), which is close to the average gain attained by full-term infants.

The increase in subcutaneous tissue that typified the last trimester of pregnancy continues in the early months of life, and reaches its peak at about 9 months. Subcutaneous tissue is largely adipose tissue; adipose tissue is about two-thirds fat. The proportion of body weight that is adipose tissue varies from 15 to 30 per cent in normal persons.

Head circumference (normally 34 to 35 cm at birth) increases to an average of approximately 44 cm by 6 months and to 47 cm by 1 year (Table 1–1). The head circumference is slightly larger than that of the chest at birth, but the two become equal by the end of the first year. The anterior fontanel may increase in size after birth, but generally diminishes in size after 6 months and may become effectively closed between 9 and 18 months. The posterior fontanel is usually closed to palpation by 4 months.

The first deciduous *teeth* erupt in most children between 5 and 9 months. The first to appear are the lower central incisors, followed by the upper central and then the upper lateral incisors. The lower lateral incisors follow, then the first molars, cuspids (canines), and second molars in that order. By the age of 1 year most children have 6 to 8 teeth. Occasionally, an infant has as few as 2 teeth at 1 year without other evidence of any growth disturbance. Sometimes this represents a familial pattern.

THE FIRST THREE MONTHS

Physiology

As indicated earlier, in discussion of the newborn infant, the physiologic systems of the infant begin at birth to make the homeostatic adjustments that will ensure adequate temperature regulation, and respiratory, digestive, enzymatic, hepatic, and renal functions. Diurnal rhythms in feeding and sleeping begin to evolve.

Gastrointestinal

The infant nursed by his or her mother during the first months of life has the optimal nutritional intake. Breast milk has an ideal balance of nutrients for the full-term infant, with concentrations of protein and of solutes that present less burden to the kidney for their secretion than does cow milk, unless the latter is substantially modified.

The sucking, swallowing, and retention of milk by the very young infant are sometimes imperfect, and some regurgitation of milk is nearly universal. It may be minimized by "burping" the infant, which is to hold him or her upright, with gentle pressure or patting on the back, or by laying the infant prone on the lap, which has the effect of moving the bubble of air in the stomach to the cardia, where it can be most easily eructed.

Immunologic

As indicated earlier, during the first 3 months of life the infant's level of maternal immunoglobulin (Ig) G falls, at the same time that he or she is beginning to form endogenous antibody as a result of antigenic stimulation. For the nursing infant, on the other hand, there is a new source of antibody, with implications for protection. There are also immunologically active cells of maternal origin in breast milk; their role is uncertain.

Breast milk contains maternal antibodies not only against certain viral and bacterial pathogens, but also against some foods that have been in the maternal diet. When food proteins ingested by the mother reach the lymphoid immune system of her intestinal mucosa, specific lymphoid cells are stimulated to produce antibody. These cells migrate to the breast, where the antibody (virtually limited to IgA specificity) is secreted in breast milk. These antibodies offer protection for the infant against undue exposure to antigens of foods that have been in the maternal diet.

The protection offered by breast-feeding is not absolute. Infants sometimes form food antibodies in utero, including IgE. There is evidence that the infant who at birth already has a high titer of IgE will be at increased risk of development of food allergies.

Other mucosal defenses against absorption of intact food antigen consist of mucus, of the cells of the intestinal epithelium, and of the submucosal lymphoid, lymphatic, and vascular tissues. Plasma cells of the lamina propria form all classes of immunoglobulins, but particularly IgA and IgE, both of which act as secretory immunoglobulins.

The mucosal system of the newborn infant is more permeable to protein than that of the older infant, and that of the premature infant is even more so. As indicated above, the infant is protected passively by the IgA in breast milk against absorption intact of foods ingested by the nursing mother. Occasionally, however, there will be enough cow milk or egg protein in the mother's milk to produce symptoms in the infant; almost all such instances have been traced to IgE reactivity.

The above findings carry implications for the prophylaxis of food allergy in susceptible infants. Of prime importance is feeding the infant as exclusively as possible at his or her mother's breast.

A second implication is that the introduction of other foods into the diet of the infant ought to be postponed until the heightened permeability of the neonatal gut to food proteins has been effectively reduced. This appears to require at least 3 to 4 months, and may need 6 to 9 months or more in some infants.

A third possibility is that the first foods to be added to the infant's diet should be foods normally in the diet of the mother, and they should be added before breast-feeding is discontinued. In this way, the IgA in the mother's milk can modulate the exposure of the infant's mucosal immune system to those foods, while the infant develops his or her own specific IgA, IgE, or IgG.

A fourth prophylactic measure may be to avoid exposure of the injured gut of the infant recovering from gastroenteritis to food proteins likely to be sensitizing, with the substitution of relatively hypoallergenic food for cow milk. Enzymatic digests of casein may be effectively used until the integrity of mucosal epithelium has been fully restored.

These measures that might offer prophylaxis of allergy in infants are so simple that they might be effectively implemented for every child. For the infant at increased risk they may offer the best opportunity to forestall the development of clinical allergies in later life. The identification of infants at increased risk can be based on family history, upon the level of IgE in the serum of cord blood, and on the sex of the infant, boys being somewhat more likely to become sensitized than girls.

Neurodevelopment

Motor Activity

The newborn infant placed prone upon a firm surface is able to avoid suffocation by turning the face from side to side; by 4 weeks of age the head is extended and lifted above the surface as it is turned.

The newborn infant has a symmetric and somewhat stiff posture in semiflexion; by 4 weeks this has become relaxed, and he or she is likely to lie, when supine, in a tonic neck attitude (TNA; head turned to one side, with the extremities extended on that side, flexed contralaterally [a "fencing" posture]).

Many infants will be most comfortable in the prone position, in which the possibility of aspiration in the case of regurgitation or vomiting is minimal. In this position many infants in the first 3 months of life will move about their cribs by disorderly, scrabbling, crawling motions that bring them often into a corner of the crib, where progress stops. Safety measures include making sure that the infant cannot be trapped between mattress and side of the crib. The same scrabbling movements make it unsafe for the infant to be left unattended in the middle of a large bed by those who are under the illusion that an infant remains in one spot. Even premature infants move about their incubators.

Head Control

When the infant within the first 4 to 8 weeks of life is pulled from a supine to a sitting position, the flexors of the neck cannot bring the head up, and the head lags; with the infant in the upright position head control is poor or absent. By 12 weeks there is partial control of head lag as the infant is drawn to a sitting position. As the infant is held in the upright position, the head is tilted a little forward on the body; in this position irregular head control results in a bobbing motion.

Landau Response

When held in ventral suspension (Landau response—the infant is lifted from the prone position by a hand held under the trunk), the newborn infant will be in a posture of flexion of head and extremities around the supporting hand. By 1 month of age the infant will raise (extend) the head momentarily to the plane of the body, and by 2 months will be able to sustain the head in that plane. By 3 months the head will be raised above the plane of the body and the legs will be extended as well.

Visual Fixation

In the first days of life infants best fixate visually those objects that are placed close to or moved through their line of vision (see pp. 151–152).

Depending upon the characteristics of the stimulus, they may maintain fixation of an object placed before them in the midline and moved from side to side. If the object is sufficiently attractive, movement of the eyes and head may occur to nearly 90 degrees to either side of the midline. By 2 months of age an object presented to a supine infant at 90 degrees from the midline will be followed visually through an arc of 180 degrees.

Adaptive Behavior

Reflex grasp of an object placed in the hand persists until the age of about 8 weeks, after which, with growing eye and hand coordination, active, intentional grasp becomes more evident. Reaching and grasping evolve out of earlier coordinate but incomplete motions of the arms and hands in response to the sight of objects in motion nearby (Bower, 1974); by 12 weeks the infant attempts to make contact with an offered object and will hold it briefly if appropriate contact is made. The coordination of eye and hand implicit in this activity seems to have been facilitated by the tonic neck attitude (Gesell and Armatruda, 1941).

Temperament

From the point of view of temperament, about 10 per cent of newborn infants are not "cuddly." Such infants appear to have no need for and to find no pleasure in tactile stimulation; they cry a lot, are not easily consolable, have abrupt changes of state, and are irritable and fussy (see p. 87).

The cry of the newborn infant is an indicator of distress that most observers find undifferentiated as to meaning. Its intensity will vary with whether it represents an emergent or an urgent need to be fed, or some acute distress, such as pain. If the need expressed is not immediately or soon met, the cry may become "angry" in its intensity.

The cry of the newborn infant is a powerful motivator of his or her caretakers, and even serves as a distress signal to other newborn infants, who may be moved to cry on hearing one of their peers in distress. Caretakers are called by the cry to the infant's side to feed, to change a wet or soiled diaper, or to relieve distress in some other way.

It has been reported that by the fourth day of life most mothers will be able to differentiate the cries of their own babies from those of other infants. Mothers become increasingly skillful in differentiating between cries of hunger, of fatigue, or of distress. Those mothers who have had previous experience learn more rapidly than those who are caring for their first child.

Bell and Ainsworth (1972) found that a prompt response to the cry of hunger did not appear to act as a positive reinforcer of the crying, but that it may have opened other ways for the infant to communicate effectively. The mother who responds to the earlier restlessness of the infant, when the response is appropriate, may be spared the more energetic protest that evolves as unmet needs are prolonged.

Many infants have during the first weeks of life a fussy period at some time during each day, most often in the early evening. The fussy period may reach its peak at about 6 weeks, when the infant may cry for as much as 2½ hr per day. By the age of 3 months this fussy period, which sometimes takes the form of "colic," should be yielding to the infant's growing responsiveness and consolability.

It is noteworthy that there may be only two ways in which newborn or young infants can isolate themselves from sensory input or become relatively insensitive to it: one is by sleeping, the other by vigorous crying. Babies may at times use either of these strategies to shut out unwanted or distressing input.

Excessive crying is a common concern of parents, whose tolerance for it will vary, as will the reasons for it. "Colic" is a symptom that is based in some infants, if not in the majority, on temperamental factors, which may include those defining the "difficult" infant or child. The central problem is prolonged crying spells in the infant, during which the infant is inconsolable, over which the infant has no control through self-quieting behavior such as thumbsucking, and for which the parents can find no reliable solution.

Among the strategies that parents may find useful in support of the consolability or self-quieting behavior of crying infants are holding and talking to the infant, holding the infant's hands together across the midline, swaddling, or the use of a pacifier. Sometimes the infant is best left alone, in instances of fatigue or overstimulation. In some infants colic is rather difficult to manage for as much as the first 3 months of life, after which it disappears, while other aspects of temperament may persist.

Taubman (1984) found that colicky infants cried about 2.5 times as much (2.6 hr/day [SD 1.2]) as controls (1.0 hr/day [SD 0.5]). He investigated the efficacy of two procedures in the management of colic: 1) letting the infant cry, with minimal intervention; and 2) encouraging the parent to be persistent in efforts to find the cause of the baby's distress, with attention to be given to hunger, to need for nonnutritional sucking, to a possible wish to be held, to possible boredom, or to possible fatigue. Parents were encouraged to try to meet any need they thought might be unmet, in whatever sequence they thought might be most helpful, for periods of not more than 5 min per intervention, unless the intervention chosen was successful.

No success was achieved with letting the infant cry. The group of infants in whom intervention was encouraged had within 1 week an average of 70 per cent decrease in time spent crying, to the level in control infants.

Sleep

The infant at birth has no diurnal pattern of sleep and wakefulness, and may sleep about 15 to 17 hr/day during the first week (Ferber, 1987). The remainder of the day may be broken into 4 to 6 periods of an hour or more, in 3- to 4-hr sleep/wake cycles, with up to 6 to 8 hr for the longest sleep. The total amount of sleep and the longest uninterrupted period of sleep decrease and increase, respectively, until at about 2 months some infants will begin to sleep through the night, for a period of about 10 hr, with about three naps during the day. Sleep typically occupies about 15 hr of the day at 3 months. By 4 months the majority of infants will sleep through the night, and by 6 months nearly all. Breast-fed infants may be slower to arrive at sleeping through the night than bottle-fed infants, with an increase in sleep time (both of individual periods of sleep and of total sleep time) coming with weaning.

Communication

Within the infant's closest relationship develops an exchange of signals between infant and caretaker that enables each to recognize and respond to the other's needs. This signal system is integral to the sense of trust that develops in the infant that his or her needs will be met, both materially and emotionally.

Language

The infant begins at about 4 weeks to make small throaty noises; some vowel sounds will be produced at 8 weeks, and these will be uttered with smiles and evident pleasure on social contact by 12 weeks. Language at this age becomes an exchange of sounds between infant and mother, having more the characteristics of a musical duet than an exchange of ideas (Fernald, 1989).

Infants are particularly responsive to high-pitched voices in the first days and months of life, and mothers (and fathers) characteristically use such voices in vocal exchanges with their infants.

Maternal vocalization at this time, besides being high pitched, is typically "sing-song," slower in pace than in communications with older children, and with longer pauses and shorter utterances. This pattern has been called "motherese" (Fernald, 1985). Characteristic qualities of pitch and intonation appear to have imbedded in them syntax and structure that are the same in most languages and cultures. Certain of the patterns of intonation in motherese (high and rising) have the function of attention-getting or of alerting the infant, others (low and falling) the role of soothing.

Fernald questions whether the fact that some features of motherese seem to cross cultural barriers may not indicate an ethologic basis for this phenomenon, analogous to the observation that some patterns for the communication of affect in facial expressions tend to be universal (Hass [1970] and others). She suggests that the features of vocalization to which infants respond may correspond to similar features of visual stimuli, such as form, points of high contrast, or dynamic quality.

Fernald (1984) suggests that the purposes of certain biologically determined characteristics of the pattern of communication between mothers and infants may be: 1) to engage and maintain the attention of the infant, 2) to modulate the state of arousal of the infant, 3) to communicate affect, or 4) to facilitate in the preverbal child the ultimate actual comprehension of language. In the preverbal infant, in maternal utterances such purposes seem to be supported by a combination of affect and intent as these contribute to the tempo and melody. Attention-getting intent lends a rising inflection and pitch to words that are likely to be found at the end of sentences; praise starts with high pitch, rises a little, and then falls; protection or warning has a low pitch, high intensity, and falling pitch; and comforting utterances are of low frequency, prolonged, and of gradually falling pitch.

Psychosocial Development

The first year corresponds to the freudian period that is called *oral* and to the period in the eriksonian scheme during which the *basic trust* of the infant is developed.

With neonatal experiences fostering bonding and attachment, and with continuing social interaction, infants very soon show that they differentiate persons and objects in their environments, with evidence as early as 2 to 6 weeks of age that they are more comfortable with familiar persons than with strangers.

Newborn and even prematurely born infants often display fragmentary smiles, usually in response to internal stimuli of uncertain nature during rapid eye movement (REM) sleep or moments of drowsiness. A fully developed social smile becomes manifest usually between 3 and 5 weeks of age. There is evidence that the smile of the very young infant may be elicited primarily by the infant's discovery that he or she has control over some contingencies in the environment, such as securing care or attention from the mother or another caretaker, or from being able to control the behavior of inanimate objects. The infant who does not have a social smile by the age of 8 to 12 weeks (or by 48 weeks of gestational age, for prematurely born infants) should be regarded as possibly seriously deviant with respect either to developmental potential or to quality of environmental experience (see later in this chapter).

A major part of the interaction between mother and infant in the first weeks of life is initiated by the infant, not simply as changes of state indicating distress or immediate need, but as part of the growing and complex system of signals between infant and mother (and/or other caretakers) that was referred to above. Through these communicative exchanges emotional attachments are formed; the infant learns to sort out his or her own internal states for their meaning and to convey information regarding them. At the same time, the mother learns to read and to respond appropriately to the infant's signals, with activities that have the capacity to comfort, to reassure, or at times to make tolerable any appropriate or necessary frustration or postponement of gratification.

The first year has been treated in the past as a time for the early discipline of the infant ("let him cry" or "don't spoil her"). Current understanding of the needs of the infant in the first year indicates that the infant thrives best when his or her needs are met in a reasonably prompt and loving manner, without the prime caretakers becoming either over-protective or overindulgent. Neither should they feel that they have become so tyrannized by needs or demands of an infant that they are unable to find a comfortable pattern of family interaction within which each member's needs are adequately met.

In the responses of the caretakers to the behavior of the infant, both consistency and promptness seem important. In instances of defective mothering, the infant's normal or appropriate expression of need may not be consistently or reliably answered or rewarded by maternal nurturance that leads to reduction of tension; or an effective maternal response may come so late and after such prolonged tension or anxiety that the infant cannot reliably associate any specific action of his or her own (except perhaps crying) with relief of that tension. Such infants may come to feel that they have no way to affect their environments through their own actions. Long-term retreat, depression, anxiety, or hostility may be the consequences.

Conduct of Developmental Assessment

Developmental assessment in the first 3 months will focus upon the infant's physical progress, upon the degree to which he or she is achieving the goals of regularity of rhythms of feeding and sleeping, upon neuro-developmental progress, and upon the relationship between the infant's expressions of need and the understanding or skill with which the mother and/or other caretakers are meeting those needs. Inquiry should be made regarding vegetative functions, such as feeding and sleeping and elimination.

Useful information will be gained from observing the interaction of the mother and infant. How does the mother look (radiant, joyous, anxious, impassive, glum, fatigued, depressed)? How does she hold the infant? What, if anything, does she say to the baby? How much time does the mother spend in a face-to-face (en face) orientation with the infant? If the infant cries, how does she respond? (Some mothers cuddle the infant and seek to soothe with vocalizations; others jiggle the infant for long periods while the infant continues to cry or fret. [Such jiggling has not been shown to quiet such an infant.]) Does the mother smile? Does the baby smile? If the mother is accompanied to a health visit by the father or by a grandparent, what is the interaction between the mother and this other person?

Further information can be obtained from the interview with mother or father or other caretakers. Appropriate lines of inquiry include such questions as: How do you feel the baby has been doing? How do others (father, siblings, grandparents, etc.) feel about the baby? Have you had any surprises? Who helps you care for the baby? Are you able to get enough rest? Have you been able to find some time for yourself away from the baby? Have you gone out together and left the baby? Who looks after the baby when you are away? How do you manage? Have you thought about going back to work outside the home? Have you thought about day care? Any plans?

Such questions may discover nothing that is not reassuring, but they should be asked, in any case. They will help the mother (the parents) to put her (their) experience of motherhood (parenthood) into the larger perspective of the changes now under way in her (their) life and her (their) life-style. The same issues will need exploration at each age of infancy and early childhood.

Even in the first months of life the infant may give his or her own evidence that things are not going well. Failure of adequate weight gain, persistent spitting up, crying, or sleep disturbance may indicate trouble in the parent-infant relationship. Absence of a social smile by 8 weeks (or 44 weeks of gestational age) should be regarded as needing some explanation. The infant in difficulty may at 3 to 4 months lie relatively immobile and impassive at the approach of another person. If the infant averts his or her gaze from an approaching person, as if to shut out social contacts, some failure of socialization may be suspected, including the possibility of child abuse.

DEVELOPMENT FROM THREE TO SIX MONTHS OF AGE

Physiology

By the age of 3 months, physiologic homeostasis will have been achieved by most infants. No new developments of major significance take place between then and 6 months. By the age of 3 months many infants, and by 4 months most infants, will sleep through the night (for 10 hr), with two or three naps during the day. The breast-fed infant is likely to accomplish this later than the bottle-fed infant.

Neurodevelopment

By the age of 3 months infants placed prone upon a firm surface are generally able to raise head and chest from the surface, with their arms extended before them. By 4 months they are able in this position to raise the head to a vertical axis and to turn it easily from side to side. At 5 to 6 months of age the infant begins purposefully to roll over, at first from the prone to the supine position and then in the reverse direction.

When the supine infant of 4 months is pulled to a sitting position, the head is brought up without lag; in the upright position the head tilts a little forward, but is held steady without bobbing. The head will be maintained erect and steady by 5 months of age.

Between 3 and 4 months of age the infant gradually abandons the TNA as the predominant supine posture, and the head becomes generally maintained in the midline, with the arms and legs in more or less symmetric positions, and the hands often brought together in the midline or at the mouth *(symmetrotonic posture)*. In this position the 4- to 6-month-old infant often develops a bald spot over the occiput.

By 4 to 5 months the infant will enjoy being supported in an upright posture and becomes increasingly attracted to objects presented on a plane surface. By 6 months he or she will be able to change the orientation of the entire body to reach out toward the desired object, leaning forward when sitting, and by 7 months pivoting when prone.

At 5 to 6 months infants can often be pulled from a sitting to a standing position and will support their weight upon extended legs. At 6 to 6½ months in this same position they will often flex the knees momentarily and return to a standing posture. At 6 to 6½ months infants are often able to sit alone, leaning forward upon their hands, or with slight support of the pelvis; they will not yet have developed a lumbar lordosis, and the spine will have a gentle kyphotic curve from sacrum to cervical region.

Adaptive Behavior

By 4 months the infant becomes more adept in making contact with objects brought within reach and will often bring these to the midline and to the mouth for oral exploration. At 4 months of age the infant will be able to grasp readily an object of moderate size brought within reach, but he or she will have only limited interest in a small object (such as a pellet, pill, or raisin); these often receive only a glance with no sustained attention.

By 6 months the infant is usually able to *reach out* for a larger object not immediately within reach, by use of movements of the arms and trunk together.

By 6 to 6½ months most infants can grasp a large object, such as a rattle, and *transfer* it from hand to hand.

Communication

Like younger infants, the infant at 4 months attends preferentially to the higher pitch in the voice of the mother; and it has been shown that the response is to the cadence and melody of the utterance rather than to its qualities as speech conveying meaning. At this age, hearing a familiar attention-getting sound, which will generally consist of a rising inflection, will produce a reduction in heart rate, whether the sound is conveyed as words with explicit meaning or as the melody underlying such an utterance (Fernald, 1989). At the same age, maternal vocalization that consists of sustained and falling frequency will be experienced by the infant as soothing.

These features of the vocal interchanges between mothers and their infants have these qualities independent of the language or culture of the participants (Fernald et al., 1989). Moreover, such sounds as they relate to infants can be interpreted correctly by adults of other cultures, and even by adults who have had no recent or substantial past experience with infants or children.

Language

By 3 months 75 to 90 per cent of infants will utter cooing sounds, and most of them will engage in reciprocating sound production with their caretakers. By 4 months most infants will laugh out loud at pleasurable social interactions. By 6 months some infants will begin to babble spontaneously, at first in monosyllables and then in polysyllabic form. It is said that during this babbling period, which will last for several months, the infant will experiment with sound production, producing and repeating (in accordance with the piagetian stage of secondary circular reactions) most or all of the sounds heard on earth in human speech. These sounds will later be culled for those that belong to the speech of the infant's caretakers, and that the infant hears with increasing understanding of their meaning.

Psychosocial Development

As infants become more intricately related to objects and persons in the environment during the first 6 months, their smiles and vocal output continue to be catalysts of social exchange. By 4 months they begin to laugh aloud at pleasurable social contacts. They may also, on interruption of a pleasant social contact, show displeasure by changes of expression, fussing, or crying. Between 4 and 7 months of age infants become increasingly responsive to the emotional tone of social contacts, and by 7 months will respond to changes in the facial expressions of those having close rapport with them. For example, a maternal frown that interrupts an exchange of smiles may turn off the infant's smile.

By the end of the sixth month normal infants will have developed clear preferences for social contact with the persons giving them the most care, and will, particularly when in the mother's arms, begin to show anxiety at the approach of strangers. By contrast, in a setting where they are alone with a stranger, new social contacts may be accepted without protest. Development of separation anxieties and fear of strangers may depend in some measure on the depth to which infants have developed comfortable patterns of communication and emotional exchange with primary caretakers.

Conduct of the Assessment

During the first half of the first year, the procedure to be followed in the evaluation of the infant presents few developmental problems. The normal infant will generally readily acquiesce to physical examination. The concerns to be addressed in the assessment are substantially those indicated above for the infant in the first 3 months.

Relatively simple tools are required for informal neurodevelopmental evaluation. A simple kit is available for the Denver Developmental Screening Test; more elaborate kits accompany more formal examinations, such as the Bayley or Gesell scales. Gross and fine motor skills can be tested without much in the way of apparatus; adaptive skills should generally be evaluated with materials defined for each test.

By 4 months the infant can usually be supported by small pillows in a high chair, with tray or other flat surface before him or her upon which test materials can be presented (block or raisin, for example, or ring with string attached). Some infants will be more comfortable if a parent is at the side.

DEVELOPMENT FROM SIX TO TWELVE MONTHS OF AGE

Motor Development

By 7 months the infant is usually able in the prone position to *pivot* in pursuit of an object, but may be unable to attain it if it is not within reach. By 9 to 10 months most infants have learned to *creep* or to *crawl*.

Supine infants are able by 6 months or so to lift their heads with anterior flexion of the neck, and become increasingly interested in their legs and feet. By 8 to 9 months they are able to assume a sitting position without help and are soon able to maintain this with the back straight. They are often able at 8 months to stand steadily for a short while so long as the hands are held, and by 9 months may be able to take some steps with both hands held. The 10-month-old infant is generally able to pull him or herself to a standing position at the side of a chair, playpen, or crib and to *cruise* about, holding on. By the end of the first year an infant can be expected to be able to walk with one hand held. On the other hand, some infants may walk alone without support as early as 9 months of age or less.

The above standards for gross motor achievement are relatively useless as points of assessment of neurodevelopmental level, owing to the wide variability in the ages at which they are achieved. Fine motor and adaptive behavior are much more closely aligned with the true status of development.

Adaptive Behavior

By 6 to 7 months such small objects such as pellets, pills, or raisins are promptly seen and may be vigorously pursued by raking motions of the hand and fingers, but the infant is not likely to be able to pick such objects up.

After 6 months the functions of the hands are increasingly lodged in the structures on the radial side, the thumb first being used in conjunction with the side of the palm (radial palmar grasp).

Between 6 and 9 months the radial palmar grasp becomes clearly elaborated into movements involving thumb and forefinger. The index finger is used to poke at objects by 9 months, and at this time the thumb and forefinger can be brought into sufficiently accurate apposition to permit a raisin or pellet to be picked up with a *pincer* motion. This movement is apt to be made first with the ulnar surface of the hand supported on the same surface upon which the pellet lies. By 12 months the pincer will be executed without this ulnar support ("neat" pincer). Between 9 and 12 months one may see the evolution of the neat pincer pass through a stage during which the thumb and forefinger are steadied by the placement of only the tips of the other fingers on the surface on which the desired object lies.

Between 6 and 12 months the *imitative* aspects of the infant's behavior become more elaborate. At 6 months the infant may crudely imitate the tapping of a pencil upon a table. At 9 months the infant will wave bye-bye or bring the hands together imitatively (pat-a-cake). At 12 months a child may enter into a very simple game involving an intermediary object or toy, such as a ball (simply pushing it imitatively, for example).

At 9 months an infant may upon request release an object held in the hand if the object is grasped and given a gentle pull as the request is made. By 1 year most infants will on request extend the arm and hand holding the object and release it into an offered hand.

It is during the second half of the first year that the infant's earliest sense of *object permanence* can be shown to have developed. If an attractive object is placed before the infant, and covered with a cloth as the infant reaches for it, the 6- to 8-month-old infant will appear not to know where it has gone, and may appear perplexed, whereas the 9-month-old infant will usually promptly uncover and grasp the article. The same infant may not easily find an object that is hidden *behind* an obstruction, such as a screen; attention will be diverted to the screen. The 12-month-old, on the other hand, will peer around the screen to locate the object, and reach around to retrieve it.

By 12 months the infant will often be able to follow the movement of a hidden object (a toy under a cup, for example) as its position is moved (Bower, 1979).

Language

The infant begins to make repetitive *vowel* sounds by 6½ months and by 8 months is likely to produce repetitive *consonant* sounds, such as "ba-ba," "ma-ma," and "da-da," though not necessarily associating these sounds with objects.

Fernald (1989) finds that whereas the younger infant reacts to sound in accordance with its perceptual qualities and intrinsic affective quality, at around 6 months parental vocalizations begin to communicate affective content and meaning, as well as continue to gain and sustain attention.

Children of 8 to 9 months become attentive to the sounds of their own names spoken in their presence. By 12 months the parental vocalizations heard by the infant begin to highlight for him or her the phonetic structure and linguistic structures within the stream of sound, increasingly connecting sound and meaning.

By the age of 1 year infants will usually knowingly use one or more words besides "ma-ma" or "da-da," and may show by their behavior that they know the names of some objects.

Psychosocial Development

The preference for their mothers that was manifested at 6 months often evolves into separation anxiety between the ages of 6 and 8 months. About this same time a mother may experience difficulty in putting a baby to sleep who always went willingly before. Sometimes a mother whose child is fretful when she leaves the room can comfort him or her by maintaining vocal contact.

By 9 to 10 months infants begin to be less dependent upon the physical presence of their mothers, partly because they are increasingly able to follow her around. Moreover, it is at this time, as indicated above, that the infant's growing sense of object permanence permits him or her to know that the fact that an object or person is out of sight does not mean that it no longer exists or is not available. Peek-a-boo often becomes a pleasant game about this time, and gives the infant an opportunity to test and retest his or her ability to recreate the disappearing parent.

Sleep

About 25 per cent of infants who have slept through the night for some time will begin to awaken at night between 6 and 12 months, usually during periods of REM sleep. Lozoff and Zuckerman (1988) outline strategies that may be helpful to parents in dealing with nightwaking. These include reassuring the parents that infants may quite normally prefer being with their parents to going to sleep, and that this is a not-unexpected consequence of the infant's stage of recognition of dependency. A search needs to be made for those behaviors on the part of parents that give positive reinforcement to prolonged wakefulness or to protests at bed time.

Anders (1979) called attention to some of the features of nightwaking that call for further study, including that many infants who would be reported to have slept through the night actually are awake one or more times without requiring attention. Carey (1974) found a relationship between tendency to awaken during the night and low sensory threshold as a temperamental feature.

Assessment of the Infant

Like assessment at an earlier age, the developmental evaluation of the infant in the second half of the first year will be concerned with the physical, neurodevelopmental, and psychosocial status of both infant and family. Focus will be on age-appropriate developmental features, some of which may begin to complicate the evaluative process.

After the age of 6 months, with the infant's growing awareness of dependency upon his or her mother, protests at physical separation become common, and it will often be more useful to carry out *physical examination* of the infant as he or she clings to the mother or caretaker, or sits in a lap. The clinician's approach should be unhurried, but the examination should be carried out as expeditiously as possible.

At this age, the infant's anxiety can often be lessened by beginning physical examination with the extremities or abdomen, and postponing to last such invasive maneuvers as examination of the nose, throat, or ears. Some infants will gain reassurance from initial approaches to the ears that are little more than gestures, the otoscope being moved repeatedly from one ear to the other, each ear being examined more completely in turn. When restraint is necessary, it should be firm and gentle, and brought adequately to bear as soon as the need for it is recognized.

Investigation of *psychosocial* development can explore the ways in which the mother enjoys the infant, what games they play together, and the like, as well as how the infant spends his or her day, and what problems may have arisen, including discussion of those that have been referred to above.

During the first year, the need to make arrangements for day care may present problems for the mother who works outside the home. The issues involved are discussed later (pp. 208–212).

At the end of the first year, with a secure interactive system between infant and mother or other caretakers and with the development of locomotion, the infant is ready to move from a position of dependency toward more independent activities, and to explore a larger world.

Chapter 5

THE SECOND YEAR

GROWTH AND DEVELOPMENT IN THE SECOND YEAR

With the achievement of locomotion at the end of the first year, the infant gains a degree of autonomy that changes the relationship between infant and caretakers. He or she will need constant supervision and from time to time physical restraint in order to be protected from danger or from becoming a nuisance. The infant is called upon to yield aspects of developing autonomy to the need for safety or to meeting standards of behavior that will depend in some or great measure upon the goals of the parents or of the rest of the household or of the community, as all seek to find agreeable ways to live together.

Physical Growth

During the second year there is a further deceleration in the rate of growth, and at the end of this year, during which the child will gain about 2.3 kg (5 lb) in weight and 12 cm (5 in) in height, the child enters a 4- to 5-year period during which the increases in weight and height each year are nearly constant (about 2.5 kg [5 to 6 lb] and about 6 cm [2½ in] per year). After 10 months of age, owing to the diminishing rate of growth, there is often a decrease in appetite that extends well into the second year. The result is a loss during the second year of some of the subcutaneous tissue, which reached its maximal development at around 9 months; the plump infant begins to change gradually into the lean and muscular child. With the upright posture, the mild lordosis and protuberant abdomen appear that are characteristic of the second and third years of life.

The growth of the brain decelerates during the second year; head circumference, which increased approximately 12 cm during the first year, will increase only 2 cm during the second. By the end of the first year the brain has reached approximately two thirds, and at the end of the second year four fifths, of its adult size.

During the second year eight more teeth erupt, making a total of 14 to 16 by the end of the year. The first deciduous molars erupt, and the cuspids (canines). The order of eruption may be irregular; the cuspids commonly appear after the first molars.

Neurodevelopment

During the second year the infant moves from an awkward upright stance in which he or she could walk with support to a high degree of locomotor control. By 15 months infants are generally able to walk alone, and by 18 months may run stiffly. Between 18 and 24 months, running may become the preferred means of getting from place to place, as the child enters the age of the "runabout child." The child can now move quickly from a safe environment into danger and will need constant surveillance.

The 18-month-old infant can usually seat him or herself on a stool of appropriate height.

At 18 months the infant can climb stairs with one hand held, going up one step at a time; and by 20 months he or she is able to go downstairs, one hand held, and may be able to climb stairs by holding on to the stair railing.

The child who at 12 months was able to release a pellet into the hand of a person requesting it will at 15 months generally be able to put the pellet into a small bottle. He or she may attempt to remove the pellet from the bottle by inserting a finger, and by 18 months will be able to dump it from the bottle.

By 15 months the child is able to place a 1-in cube on top of another in response to a demonstration; by 18 months he or she is able to make a tower of three cubes and by 24 months a tower of six cubes.

Imitative and conceptual behaviors continue to evolve. By the age of 18 months, the child given a pencil or a crayon may make spontaneous scribbles on paper, and will imitate the production of vertical lines; by 24 months the child will imitate circular scribbles and horizontal lines.

Cognitive Development

Stages 5 and 6 of the piagetian scheme of cognitive development belong approximately to the second year. They consist of the development and exploitation of the *tertiary circular reactions* (12 to 18 months), through which the infant finds new ways to achieve familiar or novel effects, or (18 to 24 months) tries through experimentation to find more complex ways to achieve desired ends (see p. 66). Behavior typical of the age is absorption in the manipulation of objects such as pots and pans, blocks, books, or almost anything within reach that can be lifted by one hand.

During the first year infants are sensitive to events that deviate from previous experiences, reacting with surprise or with distress. During the second year these same responses occur to deviations from the expectations of the adults in their environments (see later in this section). During the 6 months before the second birthday, children behave as if they are acquiring a new set of functions that center on sensitivity to standards and the ability to meet them, as well as an awareness of the self's behavioral effectiveness.

Kagan (1981) has gathered together the evidence that it is during the second year that the infant becomes aware of him or herself as an entity different from others, particularly with reference to those processes through which one recognizes one's ability to act and to feel.

As features of this emerging self-awareness Kagan lists five classes of behavior that emerge during the second year: 1) intelligible speech; 2) attention to standards (a preoccupation with objects that are broken, incomplete, dirty, or out of place, or with toilet training); 3) enhanced quality of performance on tasks set by adults, avoidance of tasks that are too difficult, and the seeking of challenging activities; 4) social interaction (reciprocal interactions with another child or with an adult); and 5) the acceptance of the difference between pretense and reality (e.g., telephone play, or putting a doll to sleep).

A major change in intellectual function occurs at the end of the second year, according to Kagan. Its manifestation is a display of distress in some children when certain behaviors are carried out before the child that the child is not able to imitate, despite the implicit expectation that such imitation might be forthcoming. Kagan called this reaction *distress to the model*. An example would be the fretful behavior, pause in play, or appeal to the mother for help after another person had displayed certain well-defined actions involving toys, and the child had been told, "It's your turn to play." Kagan attributed the distress to the child's inability to carry out the proposed play, either because of uncertainty as to whether it was possible or because the sequence of play actions had been forgotten.

Distress to the model begins at 15 to 16 months in a few children, and reaches peak frequency at 24 to 26 months, when it involves about 50 per cent of children. Distress to the model is more likely when nonrealistic toys are modeled, and less likely when the mother models the behavior than with a stranger.

Communication and Language

The development of language has at last three principal elements: receptive language function, expressive language function, and articulation. Both receptive and expressive language functions are evident within the first months of life (Table 5–1), and upon these as a basis there evolve the *phonology* and *syntax* and *semantics* of language (Table 5–2), which give it meaning and usefulness as a means of communication.

Most infants will by the age of 12 months use with meaning at least one word besides "ma-ma" or "da-da." The imparting of meaning to utterances flows from the exchanges with parents and other persons, as sounds begin to convey meaning to the infant rather than continue to function simply as attention-getting or attention-directing sounds. Fernald and Mazzie (1983) has found that when mothers are instructed to try to teach new words to children of 12 to 24 months of age, they use the attention-getting quality of rising inflection. In English, the word to be taught is put at the end of a sentence, with rising pitch, just as in the speech of adults any new information is likely to be conveyed with stress and a higher pitch.

TABLE 5–1. Development of Speech and Language*

Age at Which Behavior Should Be Established (Months)	Receptive Language Behavior	Expressive Language Behavior
1	Random activity arrested by sound	Random vocalization; primarily vowel sounds
2	Appears to listen to speaker; may smile at speaker	Vocal signs of pleasure; social smile
3	Looks in direction of speaker	Cooing and gurgling; smile in response to speech
4	Responds differentially to angry vs. pleasant voice	Responds vocally to social stimuli
5	Responds to own name	Begins to mimic sounds
6	Recognizes words like "bye-bye," "Mamma," "Daddy"	Protests vocally; squeals with delight
7	Responds with gestures to words such as "up," "come," "bye-bye"	Begins to use wordlike sounds, some jargon
8	Stops activity when own name is called	Imitates sound sequences
9	Stops activity in response to "no"	Imitates intonation pattern of speech
10	Accurately imitates pitch variations	First words appear
11	Responds to simple questions ("Where is the dog?") by looking or pointing	Jargon well established
12	Responds with gestures to a variety of verbal requests	Announces awareness of familiar objects by name
15	Recognizes names of various parts of body	True words heard embedded in jargon, often with gestures
18	Identifies pictures of familiar objects when they are named	Uses words more than gestures to express desires
21	Follows two consecutive, related directions ("Pick up your hat and put it on the chair")	Begins combining words ("Daddy car," "Mamma up")
24	Understands more complex sentences ("After we get in the car we'll go to the store")	Refers to self by name

* From Behrman RE, Vaughan VC III (eds): *Nelson Textbook of Pediatrics*, 13th ed. Philadelphia, WB Saunders Company, 1987, p 101.

The normal child commonly has a vocabulary of 10 words by 18 months, but there is wide variation in the times at which words begin to flow readily. It is not unusual, for example, for an entirely normal child to have few or no sounds conveying definite meaning until 18 months or later. Some children with such delay in development of recognizable speech have a rich jargon before communicative sounds appear; this jargon often has many of the intonations and punctuations of speech, but otherwise conveys no meaning. In those normal children in whom speech is delayed to 18 to 20 months, there is often rapid acquisition of words and meanings after this time, with the result that most normal children by their second birthday are able to put three words together. These words are often in the subject-verb-object relationship ("me do it").

Growing self-awareness is illustrated in new uses of language that become apparent during the second year, including the use of the first person pronoun (first "me") that begins in some children at about 18 months. There may be confusion between "me" and "you" at first, with sometimes use of "you" to mean "me" (as "you want cookie"). By 24 to 26 months most children will use these pronouns correctly, and many will begin to use the nominative "I" correctly.

By 18 months most children will point to one or more body parts upon request, and between 19 and 26 months evaluative language reflective of concerns with standards generally emerges. The words likely first to be used are those such as "broken," "booboo," "dirty," "wash hands," "can't do," etc. By 20 months most children have used "bad," "good," "hard," "dirty," or "nice." Kagan reports that the same developmental course in evaluative language is found in other cultures.

Psychosocial Development

The second year appears to be the age in which the infant makes the greatest progress in self-awareness, and begins to exercise in a major way his or her own "will" in choosing activities or in making demands upon others. It is the time when the infant is first likely to become engaged in the effort to control such body functions as elimination or the choice of or amount of food.

Psychoanalytic theory proposed a change in investment of libido from predominantly oral to predominantly anal at this time, as the infant struggled for control of his or her own bodily functions, whether they be motor or eliminatory. Mahler et al. (1975) enriched the psychoanalytic view of the second year by their description of the *psychic* birth of the infant, which they saw as taking place over the first 2 years of life. This psychic birth freed the infant from an originally symbiotic relationship, chiefly with the mother. Mahler regarded upright locomotion and the emergence of symbolic representations as the keys to the growing individuation of the infant. Locomotion permits the infant to *choose* separation, for example; and for the period between 15 and 24 months of age the child vacillates between separation and rapprochement, ultimately achieving a balanced new relationship.

TABLE 5–2. Speech and Language Development*

Age	Phonology (Sound System)	Syntax (Grammar)/Semantics (Meaning)	Pragmatics(Use of Language)
6–12 months	Babbling—labial consonants dominant (p,b,m) Sound play Begins learning intonation patterns Imitates: First sounds that can be made spontaneously Later attempts to imitate new sounds not yet made spontaneously		Vocalizations have a range of functions/intentions: e.g., responding, greeting, protesting, attention getting Verbal and nonverbal turn-taking Shared eye contact (attends to object other looks at) Communication games
12–18 months	Consonant-vowel (e.g., ma) or consonant-vowel-consonant-vowel reduplicated (e.g., mama) Early consonants: nasals (m,n); front consonants (t, b, d); followed by back consonants (k) May not distinguish between voiced and voiceless consonants (t/d) Vowels—ah, ee, oo May use deferred imitation of words heard earlier	Begins using single words meaningfully Holophrastic words (one word = whole sentence) Uses a few function words (there, no, all gone); names (mama, pet); object labels (cup, doggie) Undergeneralizations—uses words more narrowly Overgeneralization of referrents Gesture and words About 50 words by 18 months	Intentions expressed: request for object or attention reject comment routine
18–24 months	18–48 months—simplification of adult syllable structures, e.g.: 1. Final consonants deleted 2. Delete unstressed syllables 3. Repeat syllable: byebye, mama, dada 4. Reduction of consonant clusters 5. Assimilation in which production of one sound is influenced by second sound in the word 6. Substitution of sounds, e.g.: front/back consonants (t/k), stop/fricative (d/s)	Sudden increase in vocabulary Onset of 2-word combinations Noun phrase, may include modifiers Verbs do not include inflectional ending except occasional -ing No or not used to negate entire phrase; Encode semantic relations such as: recurrence (more milk), cessation (no milk), disappearance (no doggie), possession (mommie juice)	Symbolic play emerges Onset of verbal dialogue Answers speech with speech

24–36 months	Develops voiced-voiceless distinction (e.g., t/d, p/b, k/g) Begins using consonants in final position of word	3–4 word "telegraphic" sentences Can name and tell use of common objects Noun phrases are elaborated to include modifiers, demonstratives, articles, and possessives Verb phrases used: -ing, regular past -ed, auxiliaries can, will, be emerge Yes/no questions marked by rising intonation Simple what and where questions asked: Why, who and how questions infrequent Negatives placed between noun and verb phrases; may include can't, don't and won't	Revises language secondary to listener's response Can put 2–3 sentences together to hold brief conversation Rapid topic change
36–48 months	By 3 years, all vowels acquired 3 years: p, m, h, n, w† Uses final consonants in words	Grammatically complete simple sentences Noun phrases elaborated to include adjectives Verbs: be-ing appears; begin use of modals: could, would, should, must, might Present tense contracted or uncontracted forms of can (e.g., can't, cannot), will, do, be Begins to move auxiliary for yes-no questions When questions emerge	Sustains topic Systematic changes in speech depending on listener
48 months and beyond	By 4 years: intelligible to strangers 4 years: b, k, g, d, f, y; early consonant clusters: sm, sn, sp, st, sk;† 6 years: t, ng, r, l;† 7 years: ch, sh, j, voiceless th;† 8 years: s, z, v, voiced th;† 8 years +; zh;† —Perfects consonant clusters —Develops accurate pronunciation of multi-syllabic, complex words (e.g., electrician, electricity, electrically) —Sophistication in use of stress, pitch changes and intonation patterns	Verb system completed Negation system completed Complex sentence structures, e.g.: Relative clauses (She sees the girl who's on the bike) Verb complements (Jaime thinks that John's stupid) Coordinates sentences by: Conjunctions (I went to the store and I bought some cookies) Embeddings (I went to the store to buy juice and cookies) Achieves full semantic contrast of word pairs such as more-less, before-after Continues to develop vocabulary and meaning of words into adulthood	Develops metalinguistic awareness (ability to think about language) Perfects social appropriateness of language use Develops ability to role-play and assume another perspective

* From Behrman RE, Vaughan VC III (eds): *Nelson Textbook of Pediatrics*, 13th ed. Philadelphia, WB Saunders Company, 1987, p 100.
† Customarily used by 90 per cent of children studied (Sander, 1972).

The psychosocial (eriksonian) view is that this age ushers in the period when the chief developmental feature of the psyche is the achievement of *autonomy*, and that failure in this leaves the child with senses of *doubt* or *shame*.

With the second year children enter a period when they will vigorously and imitatively exploit the objects in their environment. They can empty wastebaskets, drawers, and shelves and may try to examine everything within reach. Household poisons, drugs, and chemicals must be kept in places inaccessible to them.

During the second year imitative behavior extends to other persons, including siblings and playmates. Until the end of the second year, however, play is generally solitary and consists of active manipulation of available objects. During the third year of life, on the other hand, children move increasingly into play activities in which other children are involved. By the end of the fourth year the child is increasingly engaged in activity with other children in which the group begins to enact imaginative roles and activities. This tendency to role-playing will increase in the school years.

By 18 to 24 months most children are able to verbalize their toilet needs and can be helped at this time to begin to follow acceptable social patterns in meeting them. Where the young child has comfortable and adequate models, toilet training need not become the focus either of emotion-laden educational activity or of disciplinary concern.

It appears to be during the second year, with the growing sensitivity to adult standards, that the first experience of *shame* appears. Children know at an earlier age that their mothers may be angry or unhappy but not that it is because of them or their behavior. Scheff (1987) regards shame as a master emotion that has had too little study. It is a feeling that at any age is most difficult to admit or to discharge. It is not so clearly accompanied by any typical facial expression as are such other emotions as fear or guilt—there is simply a turning away of the eyes and face, as if not wanting to be seen. Shame emerges before guilt, with the child's discovery that the reactions of others are in response to his or her own behavior, and that others are directing emotional messages to him or her.

Laughter has been said to be the most effective management of shame—as manifestation of a sense of humor. Shame may be alleviated also when it can be admitted to one's self or to others and when one feels respected by others instead of being judged and adversely criticized by them. These principles may have limited applicability to the management of those events that produce feelings of shame in the lives of the very young, but do suggest that the deliberate creation of feelings of shame in children may be counterproductive as a means of instruction or management or in order to control behavior.

Pride appears at about the same time as shame, at about 16 to 18 months. Pride may be best indicated by a significant change in the meaning of the infant's or child's smile.

Kagan (1981) has identified six categories of smile:

    1. A social smile that is spontaneous or responsive, representing greeting or acknowledgment

2. A smile on recognition of a discrepancy—such as may occur to some unexpected event in the environment (a falling object, or a noise)
3. Smiles accompanying games
4. Smiles on hearing one's name
5. Smiles of mastery, that are produced by a discrepancy, by testing of limits, or when an adult conforms to some request or expectancy on the part of the child—in each case when the child is engaged in or completing a goal-directed activity
6. Ambiguous smiles

Smiles accompany action in children under 16 months, but before that age the event that provokes the smile is less likely than later to represent a response to achievement of a clearly goal-directed activity. The smile of mastery shows major enhancement during the second half of the year.

Discipline

The need for children at this time to submit growing control of their bodies and their environments to social and cultural pressures often produces frustration and anger in them. Temper tantrums, breath-holding spells, and less dramatic outbursts are common. These episodes respond best to management by firm and loving parents who are able to set the necessary limits for the child.

The manner in which limits are set for the young child may have both behavioral and intellectual implications. Maternal behaviors may be particularly important. Slaughter (1983) found that the children of mothers who are more affectionate, nurturant, accepting, and responsive fare better than children whose mothers are less so. The former mothers provide more positive reinforcement than negative. They are not highly punitive or restrictive. Children fare better whose mothers are more firm and insistent, but flexible, in controlling them; these mothers know their children's interests, see them as developing persons, and use these perspectives to motivate and engage them in activities. They feel, therefore, less need to be especially restrictive in response to the children's emergent and inevitable counterassertions.

Effective mothers provide play opportunities, and help to give structure to the children's ongoing play, in which the mothers themselves participate more often than do mothers whose children perform less well on measures of intellectual competence. The more effective mothers provide a more enriched verbal environment for their children, seeking and giving verbal responses. On the other hand, such mothers are not overly "intellectual." The type of speech they use is less important than the fact that they assist their children's early efforts to share and talk about their experiences. The results also of the study by Andrews et al (1975) clearly showed that it was not the maternal language per se but the socioaffective context of that language that was the crucial element in change (see also pp. 203–208).

ASSESSMENT OF THE CHILD

Measurements of height and weight and head circumference will generally reflect adequately the physical status of the child in the second year, particularly as these are related to earlier measurements. The metabolic status of the child will be reflected in findings on physical examination, including the state of dentition. Gross motor, postural and orthopedic findings typical of the age have been referred to earlier.

Conduct of the Assessment

During the second year, the conduct of the *physical examination* demands the same care to make the child comfortable that is required at the end of the first year. The child begins during this year to be ready to be brought into the social exchange that is part of history-taking. It is useful to know and to use the child's name (or nickname) and to explain quietly what is being done and what is proposed. The child's comprehension may be imperfect, but the procedure sets a desirable tone for the immediate and for future examinations.

When an anxious child resists examination or struggles, it is important to find and to exercise the needed restraint as soon as possible. Parents are often embarrassed by demonstrations of anxiety or of resistance on the part of the child, and may show their anger or frustration in words or actions, with teasing, scolding, shaming, or threats to leave or to punish. Both parents and child need to be reassured that such behavior is normal and acceptable; and whatever the circumstances, the child may be told that he or she has done as well as could be expected in dealing with a scary experience. The child may not fully understand the semantics of such efforts at comforting, but the emotional implications are likely to be felt, and may make future encounters more tolerable. Such management, additionally, provides a good model for parents.

There is rarely any reason to exclude a parent from the room while an examination is being conducted; such a decision should rest upon the comfort of the mother or father and their wish to leave rather than upon the degree of anxiety or struggling in the child.

Neurodevelopment

The neurodevelopmental and cognitive status of the child can be assessed informally by the administration of some items of the Gesell or Bayley scales, or through such screening instruments as the Denver Developmental Screening Test. Infants of this age, unless ill or fatigued or unusually anxious, will enter readily into play with blocks, pellets (such as vitamin tablets or raisins), small bottles, or other such paraphernalia, or will enjoy putting crayon to paper. The standards for performance have been given earlier and are summarized in Table 1–13.

Caution should be observed in the interpretation of any performance that seems to fall short of normal standards. The function of an informal evaluation is to identify those infants or children who need to have a formal assessment of their function by a physician, psychologist, or other technician who has had adequate training in the administration and interpretation of developmental tests.

Language

Assessment of the language of the child in the second year may be made using the Early Language Milestone Scale (Coplan, 1987) or the Clinical Linguistic and Auditory Milestone Scale (Capute and Accardo, 1978; Capute et al, 1987). Criteria for referral to a speech or language pathologist or therapist are given in Table 5–3.

Psychosocial Development

The evaluation of the psychosocial status of the infant in the second year will begin often with inquiry as to physiologic functions—appetite, sleeping, play, mood, temper tantrums, the occurrence of conflict over activities, the status of toilet training, and the like.

It will be helpful to have a description of the child's day (hours of sleep, meals, play, interests, etc.), and to know what opportunities there are for

TABLE 5–3. Signs of Problems in Language and Speech Development in Preschool Children*

1. At 6 mo of age does not turn eyes and head to sound coming from behind or to side
2. At 10 mo does not make some kind of response to his or her name
3. At 15 mo does not understand and respond to "no-no," "bye-bye," and "bottle"
4. At 18 mo is not saying up to 10 single words
5. At 21 mo does not respond to directions (e.g., "sit down," "come here," "stand up")
6. After 24 mo has excessive, inappropriate jargon or echoing
7. At 24 mo does not on request point to body parts (e.g., mouth, nose, eyes, ears)
8. At 24 mo has no 2-word phrases
9. At 30 mo has speech that is not intelligible to family members
10. At 36 mo uses no simple sentences
11. At 36 mo has not begun to ask simple questions
12. At 36 mo has speech that is not intelligible to strangers
13. At 3.5 yr of age consistently fails to produce the final consonant (e.g., "ca" for *cat*, "bo" for *bone*, etc.)
14. After 4 yr of age is noticeably dysfluent (stutters)
15. After 7 yr of age has any speech sound errors
16. At any age has noticeable hypernasality or hyponasality, or has a voice that is a monotone, of inappropriate pitch, unduly loud, inaudible, or consistently hoarse

* From Behrman RE, Vaughan VC III (eds): *Nelson Textbook of Pediatrics*, 13th ed. Philadelphia, WB Saunders Company, 1987, p 101.

interaction with other children or adults. Many children of this age begin to have experiences in day care. For those who do, it will be important to know what the arrangements are and the child's reaction to them. (Problems associated with day care are discussed in Chapter 6 [pp. 208–212].)

It will be useful to recognize that the mother of a child of this age may be easily exhausted by the demands of care and supervision, especially if she has no relief from others in her continuing responsibility for the child. An assessment of her support system is essential, particularly including the role of the father.

OTHER DEVELOPMENTAL ISSUES

Developmentally determined problems characteristic of the second year have been alluded to earlier. None are more characteristic or more likely to become the concerns of parents than the reduced appetite that comes with the diminished growth rate at the beginning of the year (10 to 16 months), or the later appearance of "negativism" (the ability to resist suggestion, to say "NO" with feeling, or to have a temper tantrum), or the first concerns with toilet training. These can generally be adequately handled with developmentally based interpretations, and with encouragement of parents to accept the normal (in the case of reduced appetite) or to learn techniques of positive reinforcement (in the case of temper tantrums or toilet training).

Parents have often been encouraged to "ignore" tantrums, unfortunately without this procedure being defined or its implications understood. The temper tantrum has been called the "normal psychosis" of infancy. The child in a tantrum is often inaccessible to reason or other persuasion, and may need nothing so much as to be moved to a neutral area where the outburst can run a natural course. When the parent trying to "ignore" the tantrum pays no attention to the unhappy child and, in effect, denies the existence of the child's misery, no useful message is conveyed. It is likely to be more helpful for the parent to remain accessible to the child, to indicate that the basis for the child's unhappiness is understood, and to indicate that when the child feels better, the matter can be discussed. When the tantrum subsides, the child can be congratulated for getting his or her feelings under control. When the child learns that tantrums have no power to change limits or restrictions, or to control the behavior of the parents, they will have a tendency to disappear.

Like tantrums, *toilet training* may become the focal point of a struggle between parent and child over control of the child's behavior. A traditional view once held that toilet training was to be achieved through the educational effort of parents or others, and that there might be no time too early for this education to begin. As a result, many parents invested frustrating effort in educational activities that often emphasized the disciplinary aspects of the goal-directed activity and that often led to child and parents being locked in a struggle for control of eliminatory behavior. Current views of toilet training, on the other hand, hold that if bladder and bowel controls are to be the achievement of the child, this result can be most effectively and comfortably obtained through the modeling of the desired behavior by parents or siblings, with encouragement of the appropriate steps, with forgiveness of failures, and with praise for behavior that moves the child step by step toward success. The first step in this process often occurs at about 18 months of age and consists of the child's complaint of being wet or soiled, which can be met with thanks and with encouragement to let one know beforehand next time.

By the end of the second year child and parents may often have entered upon a long process of adjustment and particular refinement of their relationship. The prominent and critical elements of this refinement will be acknowledgment by the parents of the child as a person, while they set appropriate limits upon the child's behavior, with flexibility and with a capacity for negotiation and compromise when these are appropriate.

Chapter 6

THE PRESCHOOL CHILD

GROWTH AND DEVELOPMENT

With the third, fourth, and fifth years of life the child generally moves increasingly into a larger sphere of activity than is represented by the nuclear family alone. With the child's discovery that he or she is a child and will become an older child and ultimately an adult, the child begins to seek and to find models for the future. Behavior must increasingly meet not only the standards of the home, but also those of the community, as experiences outside the home, such as day care and preschool arrangements, begin to play major roles in shaping development.

Physical Growth

During the third, fourth, and fifth year of life gains in weight and height are relatively steady at approximately 2.3 kg (5 to 6 lb)/year and about 6 cm (2.5 in)/year, respectively, as a continuation of the trend set in the second year. Most children become leaner than they have been earlier. The lordosis and protuberant abdomen of late infancy tend to disappear by the fourth year, along with the pads of fat that earlier underlie the normal arches of the feet.

By 30 months the 20 deciduous teeth have usually erupted. During the rest of the preschool period the face tends to grow proportionately more than the cranial cavity and the jaw to widen preparatory to the eruption of permanent teeth.

Neurodevelopment

Refinement of gross motor skills includes alternation of feet in ascending stairs by 3 year and alternation in descending stairs by 4 year. By 3 year most children can stand for a short period on one foot; by 5 year they are generally able to hop on one foot and soon to skip.

The child of 24 months builds a tower of six 1-in cubes; the tower reaches eight cubes by 30 months and nine cubes by 36 months. The increasing height of the tower is made possible by the improved precision with which the child places one cube on another. By 30 months the child is able to imitate construction of a "train" of four cubes and by 36 months to imitate construction of a "bridge" of three cubes. By 48 months the child is able to construct a bridge from a model and to imitate the construction of a "gate" of 5 cubes.

By 48 months the cross figure may be copied without prior demonstration, possibly as a four-element figure. By 48 months the child will generally be able to imitate the drawing of a square, and by 54 months to copy a square. By 4 to 5 years the child can make correctly proportionate copies of these figures and may at 5 years for the first time be able to handle figures with slanting lines, such as triangles. A diamond-shaped figure may not be accurately and proportionately copied until the sixth year.

By the age of 36 months the child becomes able to respond to the request to draw a person (Goodenough-Harris Draw-a-Person Test). Production of a circle establishes a basal developmental age of 36 months, with each additional feature adding 3 months ($1/4$ year) to the basal age (paired structures [eyes, ears, arms, legs, and so on] being counted only once). Other criteria exist for analysis of complex figures, including whether body parts or articles of clothing are shown in stick or two-dimensional form, as transparent or opaque, with or without emotional expression, and so on.

By the age of 36 months the child is able to count accurately three pennies, by the age of 48 months four pennies, and by the age of 60 months 10 pennies. (The child of 4 years may count seven pennies as 10, coming down on the seventh with "ten" at the end of a verbal sequence that has run correctly from "one" to "ten.")

Neurodevelopmental and Cognitive Growth as Reflected in Preschool Children's Art

Early in the second year the infant will make undirected scribblings in response to a demonstration of marks made on paper by a pencil or crayon. By 18 months he or she will imitate a vertical line, and by 24 months make a clearly horizontal line in response to a demonstration. A child shown at 30 months how to draw a cross may reproduce the vertical and horizontal lines without their intersection, whereas by 36 months a crude but adequate imitation of the cross will generally be made.

By 24 months the child will respond to the demonstration of a circle with a circular scribble, and by 30 months will be able to restrain the exuberant circular movement so that a single closed line representing a more or less circular figure is produced. Scribbling is otherwise non-directed so far as form is concerned. In the use of colors there is no sense of the natural relationships between their use and the colors of objects.

By the age of 36 months scribbling becomes directed. The Goodenough-Harris Draw-a-Person Test (Harris, 1975) draws upon the developing ability to translate what is felt into form, with scores achieved that bear a substantial relationship to other measures of the level of cognitive development.

By 48 months the scribbling of the child has communicative potential. The child can name what it is that he or she is drawing. By 5 years a figure of a person is likely to reflect a head-to-foot reality, with insertion of a torso in stick form between head and lower extremities. Color is still not used in a realistic relationship to the things colored.

This same progression of development of the ability to draw is said to be found in every community and culture.

Cognitive Development

The third year ushers in the *preoperational* period of cognitive development. As indicated earlier (see p. 66), this period (about 2 to 7 years) is marked by increasing sophistication in the use of language, in the appreciation of the consequences of manipulations, and in the way in which various aspect of objects are "conserved" in manipulation.

The preoperational period is marked also by the initial naiveté and the growing sophistication of the child in handling concepts of space, time, causation, and object permanence. This is the period that Piaget called *egocentric*, to indicate that the child's capacity to see phenomena from any perspective other than his or her own is still undeveloped.

Logical manipulations of concepts of space, time, size, speed, shape, and the like are still beyond the grasp of the child. For example: taller is older, but it might be possible to catch up; faster may be necessarily nearer without regard to the method of travel; to have a brother may not yet be to *be* one; or something that will happen "next Sunday" will be expected each day until the final day appears. Learning the sequences of the days of the week or the months of the year will not immediately resolve the child's confusion.

DeLoache (1987) has reported that a striking and significant change in the child's use of symbolism occurs between 30 and 36 months of age. She presented 2.5-year-old and 3-year-old children with a three-dimensional model of a nearby real room, showing where a toy was hidden in the model; she then examined their ability to find the toy in the corresponding place in the real room. The older children were able to make this translation, the younger ones not. The younger group, on the other hand, readily located the hidden objects from photographs of the real room that showed where the objects were to be found. DeLoache interpreted the findings as indicating an advance in cognitive flexibility, with the older children able to think of the three-dimensional model simultaneously in two ways, both as the model itself and as a symbol for the room. The photograph needed only to be regarded as a symbol.

By the age of 6 years the child begins to develop the ability to translate abstract conceptions into figures and structures (e.g., the sound of "T" into the letter T, the idea of "two" into the figure 2).

The resolution of the child's preoperational naiveté begins at the age of about 2 years, with the use of symbolizations, language, play, and growing experience. The process contributes to the developing personality of the child. It is not complete until the end of the preoperational period, at about 6 to 8 years, when the child enters the period of *concrete* operations.

Language

Language evolves rapidly during the preschool years, and, as indicated earlier, moves from a predominantly egocentric focus toward a more social one. The 18-month-old infant may have from zero to 50 single words, used mostly to label objects or persons. At 24 months three-word sentences are ordinarily formed in the subject-verb-object syntax. The rate at which the child develops receptive and expressive vocabularies will depend upon the richness of vocabulary in the home, and the degree of encouragement the child is given to use language as a means of communication of need or of pleasure.

During the third year the child learns to put two to three sentences together to hold a brief conversation, and to revise language in response to the listener's response. During the fourth year the child learns to sustain a conversation on a topic with grammatically complete sentences, and after 48 months uses language in socially appropriate ways, including role-playing.

During the third year the child begins to use *what* and *where* questions, with *why*, *who*, and *how* questions less frequent. *When* questions emerge during the fourth year, at about the same time that the child is able to accept for the first time the idea that something wanted immediately (e.g., dessert) can be postponed until something else (e.g., a clean plate) has been achieved.

Psychosocial Development

Psychoanalytic theory proposed that a central issue in psychic development during this period is the identification of the child with the parent of the same sex (oedipal complex). The eriksonian (psychosocial) view is that the period is marked by the growing *initiative* of the child in choice of activities, including the content of thought and of fantasy, with the possibility of feelings of *guilt* when these activities fail to meet the standards of parents, of the community, or of the self's growing superego.

By 3 years most children can state their ages and whether they are boys or girls. With increasing awareness that they are destined to become larger children and adults, children of 4, 5, and 6 years begin to exercise those habits of thought, feeling, and action that represent their growing perceptions or fantasies as to the future, and begin to seek adequate models from whom to learn. The most accessible models are, of course, the parents and other members of the immediate family, but other attractive models include others from the child's milieu or from television, such as Superman, airplane pilots, train engineers, and the like, in whom they may imagine their own futures. The child's imperfect perception of the realities of the future often engenders conflicting pressures and anxieties.

The *socialization* and *acculturation* of the child begin in the preschool years. Play is an important element in socialization (see pp. 104–108). For many preschool children, *siblings* may, whether older or younger, begin to make heavy impact upon cognitive and psychosocial development. In this period the child begins to identify the persons and groups in the environment outside the home with whom he or she will identify.

Gerard (1971) found evidence that as early as 5 years of age in a Southwestern community Anglo children have identified themselves as belonging to a social group that has a preferred status. He reports that black and Latino children learn that they belong to groups with less privileged status only after the age of 5 years.

Gerard's procedure was as follows: an ethnic pictures test was administered in which the subjects looked at six faces; two were identifiable as Anglo, two black, and two Latino. Children were asked to rank the faces along certain dimensions expressing favorable characteristics, such as kindness, happiness, strength, speed, best grades, and whom they would most like to have as a friend. With respect to best grades, for example, the black and Latino children at the age of 5 years do not appear to discriminate among the ethnic types portrayed, whereas the Anglo children already prefer the Anglo faces. By the time they reach the age of 12 years, the minority children prefer the Anglo faces even more than the Anglo children do. The results with respect to grades were not the result of experience in the classroom, since the children were in segregated schools.

Gerard believes that the Anglo children derive their views of their status from their observation of the structure of the community in which they live, and from television. The result is consistent with the hypothesis that the performances of children of differing ethnic groups during the school years on cognitive tests reflects a growing sense of "caste." One is reminded also of the observation that the performances of children can be significantly affected by the expectations of the teacher as to what the child may be capable of, without regard for the child's native ability or past history of achievement (see p. 73).

Sexuality

The normal interests, concerns, and fantasies of older preschool children about the world around them and about their future roles are likely to be expressed in dramatic play. The child's imagined future roles are likely to include playing the part of the parent of the same sex, and there will be increasing curiosity and concern as to what the realities of such a role may be.

The interest of children of this age in sex differences, which often appears as questions inside the home, may commonly appear in the form of sex play among children of both sexes, which is normal among 5- and 6-year-olds and up.

The growing senses of a time past and of a future, and often the pregnancy of the mother and the birth of a sibling, will generate in children of this age concerns with and questions about their own origins. The nature and timing of such questions will vary with the circumstances and experience of each child. The first question recognized by a parent as representing this concern is often heard first from the 3- or 4-year-old, and is likely to consist of "Where do babies come from?" or sometimes "Where was I before I was a baby?" Such questions are often anxiety-provoking to parents who are not ready to deal with the formal education of the child in matters of sexuality. As indicated earlier, however, the child's sexuality and the development of gender identity have had a long history before such questions come to the surface (see p. 97).

The order in which the child normally poses such questions will reflect the normal evolution of a purely conceptual concern rather than represent a concern having any emotional intensity. For example, if he or she is told that babies grow in their mothers' bodies ("stomachs" or "tummies"), the next concern is more likely to be "How do they get out?" than to be "How do they get in?"

These questions are given specificity when they are generated by the mother's pregnancy and birth of a sibling. Children generally respond well to simple and factual explanations of the growth and birth of the new baby that will help them understand the changes in the appearance of their mothers and the need for hospital or birth-home care when the baby is born. They may enjoy feeling the baby through the mother's abdomen, but this degree of participation is optional. Shutting the child out of consideration of the imminent birth of a sibling, on the other hand, or the attribution of the birth to storks or other magic, can only be confusing, and may breed a sense of isolation that will contribute to later sibling rivalry (see next section).

It will be helpful generally to use accurate anatomic descriptions and terminology in answering these questions of children regarding sexual physiology and childbirth. For example, the use of the word "stomach" or "tummie" (rather than "womb" or "a special place in the tummie") makes it easy for the child to develop the almost inevitable fantasy that babies exit the mother's body by the umbilicus or anus, or that they enter by the mouth, like food. Children handle simple, accurate, and matter-of-fact responses to these questions comfortably, as a rule, though the questions may be repeated from time to time, as the cognitive development of the child places them in a new perspective and the answers may need elaboration.

Sibling Relationships

Every child is born into a hierarchy of relationships within the family, and with the addition of any new member to the family the hierarchy is altered or upset. For the preschool child the birth of a sibling is a not uncommon event, with consequences that will differ with the circumstances of the child and family. For the first-born child in the family, in particular, the birth of a sibling may result in a sense of dislocation. He or she has been the unique focus of the childcare activities of the parents, and the needs of the new baby must inevitably change that. The transition will be easier when the child has been comfortably included in plans and discussions of the event beforehand, and has been given realistic expectations.

Children adapt better to the birth of a sibling when they are given a sense of sharing responsibility for the care of the young brother or sister. Such activities as helping with the bathing, feeding, dressing, or changing of the baby create a sense of participation. They will have consuming interest for the older child only for a short while, and should not become in any sense chores demanded of the child.

By the same token, if the new baby is the source of curtailments of normal activities or interests ("Don't make so much noise! You'll wake the baby," etc.), then anger, resentment, or regressive behavior is likely to follow. Some degree of such feelings is normal; they should be accepted with understanding, and when there appear to be simultaneous needs for parental attention from the new baby and from the older youngster, the needs of the latter should be given priority, if possible, at least during the first few weeks of this new relationship.

Among the regressive behaviors that should be regarded as normal are: to want to take a bottle again (once or twice), to wet again (a few times), or to cling to mother more than usual. If these lapses can be accepted without shaming, condescension, or scolding ("It's perfectly all right for you to want to be a pretend baby, to feel like it was when you were a baby"), then no ill effect should be expected.

Changing patterns of parent-child interaction and of other relationships in and out of the home often leave elements of anxiety, hostility, or aggression in the child's behavior, thoughts, or fantasies. Anxieties may be expressed as nightmares or as fears of separation, death, or bodily injury. Children with serious problems may display bedwetting or thumbsucking, speech or learning difficulties, inability to enter into a comfortable sharing relationship, temper tantrums, or other behavior appropriate to earlier developmental levels.

Ethologic

Ethologic studies have begun to examine the behaviors of preschool children. Blurton Jones (1967), for example, has studied the forms of greetings that take place when mothers come to retrieve their children from a nursery school setting, as well as the patterns of play characteristic of children in that setting. He noted the difficulty that a child new to the group has in being accepted into an already established pattern of relationships. Such studies underscore the need for attention to those actions that can facilitate the adjustment between groups of young children and newcomers to the group.

CONDUCT OF THE ASSESSMENT

Physical Assessment

With entry into the third year of life, the child begins to be able to take more responsibility for his or her participation in the clinical assessment. It is appropriate and often useful to ask the child why he or she is being brought to the office, clinic, or hospital. If this does not open a dialogue, then the child's permission may be asked to discuss the matter with the parents. This exchange affords an opportunity to assess the parents' tolerance for the child's being given initiative and to observe whether or how they will press the child to give some expected response. Intrusive parents (and the child as well) can be reassured that the child is not required to be responsive under such circumstances. It will often be possible and appropriate to include the child in the exchange of information that will follow during the visit by asking him or her from time to time for comment on his or her own experience of the matters being discussed.

The physical examination of the preschool child can often begin with the child standing on the floor, rather than sitting or reclining on an examination table. The child can be asked to stand in a particular spot while the clinician will "look you over from head to toe, and shine a light in your eyes, and ears, and throat." In this comfortable and nonthreatening position, and with the procedure described earlier for the examination of the younger child (p. 178), it is often possible to have the examination begin with the eyes or ears, rather than have these "anxiety-provoking" elements of the examination deferred to last.

A comprehensive examination on the floor can be followed by a request to the child to sit or lie on the examination table while "I have another feel of your tummy or another listen to your chest."

When a child is anxious, or when he or she is irritable or ill, examination may not go smoothly (owing in the latter instance to regression to a younger level of emotional or psychosocial function). It is important that the child be met at his or her functional level of the moment, and that when restraint is needed it be brought to bear with the same considerations that govern the management of anxiety or distress in the younger child (pp. 178 and 188).

It is inappropriate to regard the failure of a child to cooperate in the assessment as a disciplinary affair (e.g., "the patient was uncooperative" often has a pejorative ring to it). Whatever the circumstances, after some crisis is passed or the encounter is over, both child and parents can be told that he or she did the best possible under the scary or uncomfortable or painful circumstances experienced.

There is no place for teasing or rebuking or for trying to persuade children that what they have just experienced was trivial. They may discover that themselves, in which case they may let others know. Still less is there a place for shaming or for punishment. Rewards may be given, but they should come only after the fact and not be bargained for in advance, as part of a process of wheedling or cajoling; nor should they be contingent upon the child's meeting some arbitrary standard of performance. Children should emerge from every health care encounter with their self-esteem intact, insofar as it can be assured them.

Additional guidelines for the conduct of the clinical examination have been offered by Forman et al. (1987a). Among them (slightly revised) are:

1. Talk with children as with any patient, not in a condescending way.

2. Don't convey to the child that you consider his or her feelings, concerns, or ideas "childish."

3. Don't laugh at what a child says unless you are very sure that he or she means to be humorous.

4. Don't try always to be funny or amusing to children. Such efforts are best saved for few occasions only, and for children whom you know and who know you very well. Children know the difference between doctors and funny people.

5. Never *tease* a child unless you know him or her *very* well and the child knows that he or she has permission to tease you in return.

6. Try introducing initial or casual encounters with children by whispering to them. They may find this more personal, private, and reassuring than jollity; they commonly whisper in response.

7. When children are old enough (at 3 to 4 years), form the habit of discussing with them their symptoms, diagnoses, and treatments in terms they can understand. It may be particularly helpful to discuss with the child any measures to be taken that will involve his or her personal experience (e.g., modifications of diet, medications, hospitalization, and so on). Compliance with any prescribed regimen is more likely if the child even at the age of 2 or 3 years has been included in the discussion of it.

8. Never discuss in the child's presence the illness or treatment of a child who has receptive language function unless you mean to include the child in the discussion.

9. When a child fails to cooperate in his or her care, negativism or struggling is often perceived as immature, irritating, embarrassing, provocative, or frightening by parents or by other adults, but the clinician should assume first that the child is afraid and reacting to fear in a customary personal way.

10. One can always ultimately overpower a struggling child by words or force or both. This may be occasionally necessary, but there is always a cost to the child, to the physician, and to the relationship.

11. The task of controlling the child is often delegated by the physician to parents, nurses, students, or aides, or to drugs. This may give the physician a feeling of distance from the regrettable or unpleasant necessity, but he or she is ultimately responsible.

12. Calling upon naked power, whether it be verbal or physical, has at least three undesirable results: it increases the patient's sense of helplessness and powerlessness; it models the technique for students, residents, and other health care staff; and it narrows and restricts the clinician's own rapport, sometimes dulling sensibility to the feelings of others as well as to his or her own feelings.

Neurodevelopmental Assessment

Neurodevelopmental examination will take advantage of some of the features outlined above. Routine evaluation of the 2-year-old may employ blocks or paper and pencil, to see how high a tower or how complex a figure can be produced. By the age of 3 years the Goodenough-Harris Draw-a-Person Test will begin to elicit responses that can be scored. Care should be taken not to overinterpret results obtained under nonstandard conditions of testing.

Assessment of Cognitive Development

It is not before the third year that the cognitive status of the child begins to be an accurate predictor of future abilities or achievement. Language function may be the most valuable indicator, but it is susceptible to sociocultural pressures, especially in disadvantaged families. Cognitive status can be explored, along with neurodevelopmental status, with such instruments as the Denver Developmental Screening Test or the Revised Developmental Screening Inventory (based upon the Gesell scales, as modified by Knobloch and Pasamanick). More informal instruments include the Peabody Picture Vocabulary Test or the Raven Matrices. Such tests do not establish a definitive IQ, but may indicate those children for whom further testing will be appropriate.

When formal testing is indicated, such instruments as the Wechsler Preschool and Primary Scale of Intelligence or the Stanford-Binet Intelligence Scale may be used.

Whenever the cognitive function of the preschool child seems compromised in any way, it will be essential to explore the child's family and home environment for any factors or relationships that may interfere with learning or with emotional well-being. Whenever language function, exclusively or in particular, is impaired, examination of hearing has first priority.

Psychosocial Assessment

The psychosocial evaluation of the preschool child will usually be a matter of history-taking and observation of the behavior of the child in the clinical setting and in relationship with parents and others. Note can be made of the way in which the mother controls the child in the clinical setting, whether by suggestions, requests, or orders, for example; or whether the parent is able to give the child some initiative in the exchange between child and physician or other health personnel.

A variety of techniques may be used to elicit interaction between child and parent. Provence (1977) made the ingenious suggestion that much is to be learned when the suggestion is made to the toddler that he or she "give Mommie (or Daddy) a kiss." Observation of the responses of both child and parent will reflect the spontaneity, closeness, and warmth of their relationship.

When something is noted that might be further explored, the exploration can be initiated with an observation such as, "I notice you seem upset that Johnnie seems so active . . ." or "I notice that Johnnie seems pretty worried about what might happen here . . ." or "I notice (something else) . . ." Depending upon parental responses to such open-ended observations, the next ploy might be reassurance, or such requests for further information as "Tell me more about that" or "How do you feel about that?" or "What do you think is the reason for that?" It will be critical to know the parent's view of any problem or potential problem before any suggestion is made as to intervention or management.

OTHER DEVELOPMENTAL ISSUES

Fears

The growing experience and fantasy life of the preschool child may often produce fears or anxieties, sometimes with nightmares. For a discussion of their content and management, see "Fears" (pp. 116–118).

Discipline

As children enter the second and third years and the following preschool years, their growing thrust for independence in action inevitably creates recurrent conflicts with the needs of parents to protect, control, and instruct in the interest of the child's socialization and acculturation. In some areas (e.g., feeding) some parents may cling to rigid control of their children's activities long after a large measure of control could be safely left to the child.

At every age there are areas where responsibility for and control of childrens' actions and activities *must* reside with the parents, but an urgent duty of parents at every age of child is to prepare for the emancipation of the child through the appropriate transfer of responsibility and initiative and the slow relaxation of authority. The way is often difficult, and will be shaped by the experiences of the parents in their own childhoods, by the temperamental features of both parents and child, and by the unique experiences that they have shared and are sharing. Unbridled permissiveness has no place, nor does selfish love, which smothers with protection, nor selfish restraint, which stifles opportunities for learning through experience.

When parents and child become involved in a struggle for control of the child's behavior, health professionals will often be called upon for help or see opportunities to assist parents in handling feelings or symptoms aroused by the struggle. They will be adequately equipped to help only if they can understand the nature of the problem, and relate it to the rights and needs of the particular parents and children, and to the rights of the community as well.

There are at least five universal child-rearing practices: feeding, weaning, toileting, discipline, and control of sexual behavior. Conflicts may arise in the negotiation of any of them. Feeding is sometimes an area in which parents and children struggle for control of quality and quantity of input. Weaning (from breast or bottle) may be easy or difficult, and is accomplished suddenly in some cultures at appointed times, in others as a gradual accommodation of the needs of the infant to those of the mother. Control of elimination by the child has often been an area of struggle between parent and child, but need not necessarily become a disciplinary matter when the child has adequate models and appropriate encouragement for handling toileting needs in socially acceptable ways (see p. 190). The development of sexuality is discussed elsewhere (pp. 98–99).

By *discipline* we mean here the process through which children, adolescents, and adults learn to conform to the standards of the family or of the community in a variety of behaviors. To discipline in this sense is not to chastise or to punish but to develop self-control and obedience to standards, through instruction, models, and exercise. The salient behaviors that are modified by discipline vary with the age of the child or adolescent or adult, and include such aspects as manners, respect for the rights of others, truth-telling, sexual behavior, and moral or ethical issues.

Disciplinary issues first emerge in the second year of life, with the growing autonomy of the infant. As the disciplinary status of the preschool child is examined with his or her parents, it is useful to know what problems the parents perceive, if any, and how they are trying to resolve these problems. The parents must be encouraged to answer the following questions:

> What am I trying to teach?
> Why is this important to me?
> How am I trying to teach the child?
> What is my child learning?

The answer to the last question may be critical. For example, parents may need to be helped to examine such questions as whether through scolding they are helping their child to eat well or to dread feeding and mealtimes, or whether through shame or excessive punishment they are raising a child who is obedient or one who is resentful, devious, or fearful.

The roles of positive and negative reinforcement, extinction, punishment, and models in learning have been discussed earlier (pp. 70–71). For the preschool child the aim of discipline, using these modifiers of behavior, is the achievement of self-control (without [much] anxiety). Parents are likely to choose for the discipline of their children methods that will reflect the ways in which they were disciplined in their own childhoods. The choices will sometimes conform to family traditions, sometimes represent a welcome departure. Parents have a strong tendency to bring up their children as they *feel* themselves to have been raised. Some parents are happy with this; others deplore this tendency in themselves.

It is important that the clinician know whether the parents are in agreement or not as to the child-rearing practices to be adopted. Children may be greatly confused if they hear different messages from each parent, and may either become pawns in a primarily marital conflict or learn to exploit these differences in their own interests. In either case, discipline suffers. When parents are not in agreement, they must be helped to understand the needs of the child and each other's needs, and to negotiate their differences.

Parents may be regarded as having certain rights in the matter of discipline. Among these are: to expect a degree of conformity consistent with the child's understanding or safety; to be upset or angry from time to time at unacceptable behavior; and occasionally even to lose control (but not too often nor to a degree that endangers the child physically or emotionally). These rights are matched by responsibilities of parents to *understand the meaning of behavior,* whenever that is possible, and to let the child know that it is the *behavior* or the *act* that is disapproved of or punished, not the child. Whatever the disciplinary methods parents may choose, they will be most effective when the child learns that adults can be trusted to be consistent, fair, flexible, and loving.

In both individuals and families certain characteristic patterns or styles of parenting seem to evolve. These have been termed *authoritarian, permissive,* and *authoritative* by Baumrind (1966, 1968). These styles of parenting differ in the expectations they have of children, in the ways in which the values represented in these expectations are conveyed to the children, and in expectations about the behavior of children.

> The *authoritarian* style attempts to shape, control, and evaluate the behavior of children against absolute standards that emphasize obedience, work, tradition, and the preservation of order. Verbal give-and-take between parents and child is discouraged.

> The *permissive* style is tolerant and accepting toward the child's impulses, uses punishment as little as possible, makes few demands for mature behavior, and allows considerable self-regulation by the child.

> The *authoritative* style embraces clear setting of standards and an expectation of mature behavior from the child, with firm enforcement of rules and standards and encouragement of the child's independence and individuality. Communication is open between parents and children, with recognition of the rights of both.

The most salient disciplinary issue for preschool children is the *setting of limits.* The behavior of children must be regulated for their own safety, for the comfort of others, and to protect the environment. Obedience can be gained through persuasion, example, rewards, reminders, cautions, threats, punishment, or physical restraint. Each of these may be appropriate at some time or place. Forman et al. (1987b) discuss the role of these in the socialization and discipline of children, offering the following principles for parents:

> That they should help children to learn from the results of their behaviors, rewarding the acceptable and indicating disapproval of the unacceptable.

That they should understand the differences between hurting as retaliation, on the one hand, and teaching through discipline and punishment, on the other.

That they should resist using power or authority for its own sake.

That they should resist the tendency to demean or humiliate those who oppose their will.

That they should review their own childhood experiences with discipline to recognize those elements of their own attitudes or behaviors that are unreasonable residua.

Parents must be careful in selecting among suggestions, requests, warnings, and orders in attempting to control the behavior of their children. From time to time, at certain cognitive and emotional levels, suggestions or requests may in fact be intended to represent requests or orders, respectively; or simple cautions or warnings may actually represent threats. It is useful for parents not to issue suggestions or requests that they intend to have obeyed as if they were orders. Parents should be ready to have suggestions rejected or ignored from time to time, but to have appropriate requests or orders complied with, or negotiated. When an order is intended, it should be unambiguous.

The initiative and relative independence of the child can be nourished if orders can be phrased as the offering of alternatives, albeit representing limited choices: for example, not "Do this!", but "Would you prefer this or that way of doing this?" (presuming either "this" or "that" way to be equally acceptable). "Do you want red or gray pajamas?" or "Do you want your father (or mother) or me to tuck you in?" or "Do you want the hall light on or off?" may help resolve issues at bedtime, for example, the implicit instruction or order being "It is time for you to go to bed."

The *countdown* is a time-honored way of delivering control of the execution of an order to the young child: "You have until I count to ten to do that!" sets up a confrontation that the child can win, preserving his or her ego, and accomplishing the desired result. The count can be controlled as to pace to match the child's compliance, or the exercise can be aborted if it is likely to fail, with some other arrangement made (such as physical intervention or renegotiation). For the older child or for a more chronic problem, a *contract* may be useful, with duties and rewards to be agreed upon and lived up to to the letter by both sides (accepting, always, that some level of partial fulfillment of contract may be construed by the parent as sufficiently close to the letter to be acceptable and to warrant reward and congratulations).

In setting limits for young children, *physical restraint* is commonly necessary and sometimes urgently needed, for protection of the child or others. Such restraint may involve physical intervention to control the child's behavior or to remove the child from danger, or restriction of the child's mobility. The reaction of the child will vary with the circumstances; for example, if restraint is accompanied by expressions of fear or of anger on the part of the parent, it may be perceived as punishment by the child.

Punishment may be either psychologic or physical. In either case, it will be most effective if it is closely related in time to the behavior that is unacceptable, rather than postponed. Forman et al. (1987b) suggest that its intensity should be high enough to produce mild or moderate anxiety, but not so high as to produce fear in the young child (e.g., by excessive physical punishment) or anger in the older child (by either physical or excessively strong emotional punishment). The emotional context of punishment is important. It may be most successful when it clears the air, leaving intact the child's confidence in the love of his or her parents. It is important that parents understand that punishment and love are not incompatible in child-rearing.

Psychologic punishment may consist or reproof, shaming, scolding, deprivation of privileges, or demands for atonement or restitution. Its most salient feature for the young child may be the child's perception of loss of approval or loss of love. For the older child, punishment may be most instructive and useful if it is arranged in a way that clearly informs the child as to the normal consequences of unacceptable behavior. Loss of privileges can be tailored to the infraction; for example, restriction of bicycle riding might be appropriate for the child who repeatedly disobeys safe riding practices, such as the need to wear a helmet.

Time out is a useful form of control for unacceptable behavior that is not responding to appropriate reason or persuasion. It consists of removal of the child from the scene of conflict, usually to his or her bedroom, with instructions to return to the social setting when his or her emotions are under control and matters can be discussed more comfortably. A few minutes of isolation may clear the air.

Spanking, which we judge to be not more than one or two slaps on the buttocks, is likely the most common *physical punishment* meted out in our society. It is used most often in preschool children, with a peak use at around the age of 2.5 years, when the cognitive development of the child renders attempts at reasoning relatively futile, and when the child's response to frustration may often border on or consist of a tantrum. Some families are able to manage discipline of children with no physical punishment or with only rare recourse to a spank or two.

If spanking is to be effective, it is likely to be so mostly or only in an emotional atmosphere marked by basically loving and warm relationships and clear expectations as to the behavior of the child. It will often be the method of last resort and represent the exasperation of a parent pushed to the limit. Spanking gives evidence of loss of approval on the part of the parent and changes the nature of the interaction. When the reason for the spanking is made clear, with the expectation that no further punishment is anticipated, it may clear the air, restoring the earlier climate.

Spanking will lose effect when it is accompanied by rage, or followed by further reproofs, rebuffs, and other evidence of loss of the parent's acceptance and affection. It will be least or not at all effective when its use is impulsive, capricious, harsh, accompanied by scolding and shaming, and followed by a further period of rejection of the child as a beloved person.

Parents who use spanking must be careful not to let it become an outlet for pent up and smouldering resentment or explosive anger. Parents who find that this is the case should review their disciplinary procedures, with the aim of avoiding letting matters reach such a point. Children can be frightened by encounters with the naked anger of a parent, especially when this is associated with physical assault, and the disciplinary lesson may be lost. No physical punishment is acceptable that produces a significant injury to the child.

Television

Children may watch television as preschoolers, but it will at first be with limited appreciation of its meaning or content, so far as most programming is concerned. For example, the preschool child is at first unable to follow the time line as a story unfolds on television when the scene changes from one place to another or implicitly from one time to another. The 3- or 4-year-old child may not grasp that a change from one day to the next is presumed, or that two things shown serially are, in fact, intended to be understood as taking place substantially simultaneously, possibly at sites remote from each other. Cartoons and shows like *Sesame Street* must leave little to the imagination. Television is nonetheless riveting, however, and serves as the babysitter for millions of young children. The impact of television on children is discussed later (pp. 221–225).

Day Care

Within recent years, with the entry of greater numbers of women into employment outside the home, the growth and development of many infants and children has depended upon persons other than their parents for increasing periods of the day. The proportion of infants and children receiving part of their care from babysitters, housekeepers, neighbors, and day-care centers has risen steadily for two decades. Figures change constantly. It appears that now (1988) about 50 percent of infants under 1 year of age and about two thirds of children under 5 years of age have mothers in the workplace, including nearly half of *married* mothers whose youngest child is under 1 year of age. About two thirds of working mothers work full-time, including about two thirds of those who have children under the age of 3 years.

A second factor contributing to the need for day care has been the great increase in the number of single-parent families (usually involving the mother alone with her child or children). For the single parent who must work to support herself and child or children, problems are likely to be made more difficult by the fact that such heads of family are at increased risk of being poor and of having limited marketable skills. Within recent years the increasing numbers of families living below the poverty level has led to one in every four children under the age of 6 years living in such a family in the United States. For such children there is likely to be no easy access to day care of quality.

With the replacement of the extended family by the nuclear family, the arrangements for day care for children have grown, albeit not enough to meet the demand for care of high quality. And there has grown up a noisy debate as to the merits of mothers assigning the care of young infants to others for substantial portions of the day, and as to the need for either a national policy regarding day care or a commitment to day care of high quality. In provisions for day care, the United States has lagged behind most of the other industrialized nations, particularly in the West.

Types of day-care arrangements fall into three principal categories (Siegel-Gorelick, 1983): *home care,* given in the infant's or child's own home (by family members, such as siblings, grandparents, or father, or by a paid caregiver, such as a housekeeper or child care worker, who may live in as an *au pair* or governess); *family day care* (given by other mothers to small groups in their homes [shared care may rotate the homes involved]); and *day-care centers,* which care for larger groups of children with larger numbers of caregivers.

When day care is not given voluntarily, the costs are met by private nonprofit arrangements such as cooperatives, churches, industry, and the like; by public funds; by private for-profit organizations; or by the military for families of those on active duty.

The issues in day care that have the greatest implications for infant and child development include the appropriate age for entry, the qualifications of the persons to whom the responsibility for the care of infants and young children will be given, the standards to be met by an agency or center offering such care, the nature of the curriculum to be offered the children, and the numbers of children that it is appropriate to assign to any one or to any group of caretakers.

It seems likely that most infants and children adapt well to well-planned and sympathetic day care, but it is often difficult to know whether any given program of care meets the general needs of children, the specific needs of particular children, or any arbitrary standards. Most day care is probably given through informal arrangements made without any inspection or evaluation having been made by any professional accrediting body. When public funds are made available for day care, there is usually some local, state, or federal standard to be met. Federal standards were put in place in the 1970s, but these were aborted by deregulation set in motion by the Reagan administration, putting at risk the quality of staffing, free meals, and training for child care workers. The National Association for the Education of Young Children has begun to certify to quality in day-care centers, as a private effort to meet the need.

The possibility of deleterious effects of day care upon the development of infants or children or upon family integrity has been widely discussed, sometimes more emotionally than critically. We have seen that the first months of life have as one of their most important achievements for the normal infant the ripening of the relationship between mother and infant, with respect to both the bonding of the mother to the infant and the attachment of the infant to the mother. This involves the creation of a reliable signal system between the infant and mother or other caretakers that will ensure that the infant's needs are promptly recognized and met. Concern has been expressed that the entry of the very young infant into day care while his or her mother works may attenuate these processes, with injury to the infant's social development. There are conflicting opinions as to these effects, but no convincing evidence that secure attachment is threatened.

The Head Start program for preschool children of disadvantaged families has been shown to improve the social and academic performances of children when they enter school, though an earlier effect upon the results of intelligence tests has not been shown to be sustained for all of the participant children. Phillips et al. (1987) examine some of the data indicating such results, and report their own findings, which were that *in centers rated good* children seemed more intelligent, considerate, and achievement oriented. They appeared also to have a higher level of anxiety, for reasons needing further study.

Slaughter (1983) found that in a disadvantaged community the involvement in discussion groups of the parents of children in day care was helpful both to parents and to children. Such involvement holds the potential for redefining day care as a form of re-creation of the extended family.

Entry into Day Care

Siegel-Gorelick (1983) has suggested that only home care be considered for the infant in the first year of life, with family day care appropriate for the next 2 years, and with day-care centers being used only after the age of 30 to 36 months.

When parents are considering the timing of entry of an infant into child care outside the home, there are several nodal points in development to be considered: the first is at about 3 to 4 months, when the infant forms the first strong social bonds; a second is at 8 to 10 months, when the infant is dealing with separation anxiety and object permanence; and a third is at 16 to 20 months, when there may be a recrudescence of separation anxiety, possibly related to the emergence of concerns with standards and the sense of self-awareness.

Brazelton (1988) has urged that entry into day care be postponed until at least after 4 months. This may be as important for the mother's bonding and developing communication with the infant as for the infant him or herself. The mother should be encouraged, in any case, to find "quality time" with the infant, in which she can each day confirm their special relationship. In many developed countries it is expected that mothers will need at least 6 months for this early period of adjustment, and some countries have translated this conviction into programs of maternity and postnatal support that permit such an arrangement. When the use of day-care arrangements is delayed beyond 5 to 6 months, it may be preferable not to enter day care at 8 to 10 or at 16 to 20 months, which are other nodal points.

Assessment of Day Care Quality

Parents often bear alone the responsibility for assessing the adequacy of the day-care arrangement made for their infant or child. In home care arrangements they should be sure that the caretaker is experienced, warm, and affectionate with the infant or child, and that the responsibilities of the caretaker for other activities in the house (such as housekeeping chores) are well understood. There should not develop any competition between the parent and caretaker for care of the infant. The parents will get clues as to the adequacy of the arrangement from the behavior of the child and from any evidence of burnout in the caretaker.

In the evaluation of the day-care center, parents will examine the cleanliness of the site, the hygienic arrangements, and the behaviors of the caretakers. When they visit the center, they will want to observe whether the caretakers are involved with and talking with the children, or whether the children are watching television while the caretakers talk with each other. Here, too, the nature of the experience will become evident in the behavior of the child, or in the child's report.

The American Academy of Pediatrics (1987) has produced a manual for day care, in which standards are given, with a check-list for parents.

Concern has been expressed that the success of the Head Start program has led some communities to urge the admission of children to academic programs at an earlier age than usual, or the introduction of formal curriculum into kindergartens where they have not previously been the focus of attention. Elkind (1987) has urged that children not be forcefully accelerated by such efforts.

Effects upon Individual Children

Generalizations about the effects of day care may be irrelevant to the needs or experience of the individual infant or child, whose adjustment will depend upon his or her age, the duration of separation each day from parent or home, temperamental factors, cognitive style, the presence or absence of stress in the home (such as a recent move or conflict between parents), and the nature of the day-care program. Children of "easy" temperament may have the least trouble in adjustment, "difficult" children the most. For some of the latter, on the other hand, day care may be a blessing, in its provision of regularity in activities and models of behavior. As indicated above, infants and children may give their own reports as to the effects, verbally or nonverbally. For the infant, the nonverbal report may take the form of a psychophysiologic disturbance, such as vomiting, diarrhea, or failure to thrive.

When parents are planning for day care in the home, they should be urged to have the caretaker become familiar with the infant or young child for some hours or days prior to any separation, sharing with parents the care of the infant before the actual transfer of care is made. The same principle is served with the entry of children into care outside the home, when parents can spend time in the alternative home or center, with both child and parents becoming familiar with the caretakers, and the experience conveying to the child that he or she is among friends.

The question often arises as to how a child ought to be left at home in the hands of a babysitter or housekeeper, or in a day-care center. Seligman (1975) makes the important point that leave-taking should be discussed frankly and openly with the child, and the point of separation shared fully with the child, even when the child protests against the parent's departure. Attempts of the parents to leave unobtrusively when the child's attention is diverted, or when he or she is engrossed in some activity, run the serious risk of introducing into the child's life new and unexpected contingencies for which the child has had no preparation. The result may be that the child develops a generalized anxiety as to the whereabouts of parents, even when they are at home—with uncertainty as to whether they might be gone if they are out of sight, or that they may be suddenly gone even if they are plainly visible.

Chapter 7

THE SCHOOL-AGED CHILD

The school years prior to adolescence have been called the time of *middle childhood*. With the entry of the child into kindergarten or elementary school, a major change occurs in the origins of the motivations for behavior. These will now reside increasingly in relationships with teachers, with peers, and with the community. The central activity becomes education, and it will be more controlled and regimented than earlier activities. The child will increasingly be given responsibility for his or her own educational activity, and will be expected to meet certain standards of achievement.

Physical Growth

The early school years are a period of relatively steady growth. The average gain in weight during these years is about 3 to 3.5 kg (7 lb)/year, and in height about 6 cm (2.5 in)/year. Growth in head circumference is slower than earlier, the circumference increasing from about 51 cm (20 in) to 53 to 54 cm (21 in) between the ages of 5 and 12 years. At the end of this period the brain has reached virtually adult size.

The development of the facial bones is active during the school years, particularly with enlargement of the sinuses. The frontal sinus has usually made its appearance by the seventh year.

The first permanent teeth (the first molars) most often erupt during the seventh year of life. With these so-called 6-year molars in place, the shedding of deciduous teeth begins, following approximately the same sequence as in their acquisition. They are replaced at a rate of about four teeth/year over the next five years. The second permanent molars commonly erupt by the 14th year; the third molars may not appear until the early 20s.

The earliest changes setting the stage for the onset of adolescence come with the age of about 7 years in both boys and girls, and the steady growth of middle childhood ends in a preadolescent growth spurt by about the age of 10 years in girls and about 12 in boys. There will be an increase in subcutaneous fat in both sexes (''prepubertal fat spurt''); in boys the added fat will recede in adolescence, whereas that of girls will tend to remain. These developments are discussed further later (pp. 239–242).

213

The school years are a time of vigorous physical activity. The spine becomes straighter, but the child's body is supple, and postures may be assumed that are disturbing to parents and to teachers. Mild degrees of knock-knee or flat foot that may have been apparent in the late preschool years tend to correct themselves during the first year or two of the school years. The motor activities of the earlier years, such as running and climbing, become increasingly directed toward more specialized activities and games requiring particular motor and muscular skills.

Lymphatic tissues are at the peak of their development during these years and generally exceed the amount of such tissue in the normal adult. The abundance of lymphoid tissue during this time of life bears a relationship to the frequency with which tonsillectomy and adenoidectomy are recommended, often inappropriately. Respiratory infections are common during these years, and the response of the child to infection begins to be more like that of the adult than that of the infant or young child. The usual number of respiratory infections during the school years is high; as many as six to seven illnesses per year are not uncommon.

Neurodevelopment

By 5 to 6 years of age the normal child has developed a time sense that includes an orientation toward the future, and has conceptual, perceptual, and fine motor skills that make him or her ready to take on the work of learning to read and to write. Somewhat complex figures are reproduced with pencil on paper (see below). Self-care activities are reasonably advanced, and so it is usual and appropriate that formal education begin at this time.

The equipment that the child brings to this enterprise includes the ability to copy a square (by 54 months), to copy a triangle (by 60 months), to copy a rectangle with diagonals (by 66 months), and to copy a diamond-shaped figure (by 72 months). The building of a "gate" made of blocks is imitated at 48 months; the gate is copied from a model at 54 months.

The drawing of a person (Goodenough-Harris) will have four features by 48 months, a distinct body by 60 months, and neck, hands, and clothes by 72 months.

With entry into the school years the child continues a long period of refinement of gross and fine motor skills, with the disappearance of some of the clumsiness of an earlier age, and the acquisition of gross motor and manual dexterities that vary considerably from child to child.

The normal child may be expected (Levine, 1987): by the age of 5 to 6 years to skip or hop in place, to walk on heels, and to succeed in tandem (heel-to-toe) walk forward; by 6 to 7 years to manage a tandem gait backward and to stand on one foot with eyes open for 10 sec; by 7 to 9 years to crouch on tiptoes with eyes closed for 10 sec, to hop twice in place on each foot in succession for 3 cycles, and to stand in tandem position with eyes closed for 10 sec; by 9 to 10 years to accomplish tandem gait sideways, to catch a tennis ball in midair with one hand, and to throw a tennis ball at a target; and by 10 to 12 years to balance on tiptoes with eyes closed for 15 sec, to jump in the air and clap heels together, and to jump in the air and clap hands three times.

Fine motor features that are normal for preschool children but may persist into the school years include: mirror movements (synkinesis); awkward diadochokinesis; awkwardness in finger-to-thumb apposition; imperfect finger localization ("with your eyes closed, tell me which of your fingers I am touching"); imperfect finger differentiation ("with your eyes closed, tell me how many fingers I am touching"); imperfect detection of simultaneous stimulation of hand and face (likely to feel the face only [rostral dominance]); confused laterality (identification of own [or another's] right and left parts); execution of crossed lateral commands on self ("touch your right ear with your left hand, or touch my left knee with your right hand"); inconsistent hand preference; and unstable eye-hand preference (mixed laterality).

These responses tend to mature in the following order: diadochokinesis, finger discrimination, and consistent hand preference by 7 years; finger-thumb apposition by 8 years; identification of own right and left, and stable ipsilateral eye-hand laterality by 8 years; crossed lateral commands on self by 8 to 9 years (on others by 9 or later); synkinesis by 9 to 10 years; and finger localization by 11 to 12 years. When they do not mature at the usual times, they constitute the so-called soft neurodevelopmental signs commonly associated with learning disabilities (see later in this chapter).

As neurodevelopmental aspects of the child mature during the school years and adolescence, what one finds on examination of the child will increasingly reflect the individuality of the child and the child's unique experiences and opportunities. Moreover, the demands of scholastic achievement make increasing demands upon cognitive function rather than simply upon the maturation of innate neurophysiologic processes.

Cognitive Development

The school-aged child enters the period of concrete operations, according to the piagetian scheme. As indicated earlier (p. 67), this period (about 7 to 11 years) finds the child ready to deal with objects as perceived or imagined, but not to manipulate abstract concepts. By 9 or 10 the child has learned that weight is conserved against deformations of shape; by 11 or 12 the conservation of volume is also mastered.

The ability to monitor one's own mental processes increases during the school years, along with the ability to plan and organize behavior. The capacity for self-control and self-regulation increases, and impulsivity declines. By the third grade the academic achievement of the child will for the first time correlate highly with achievement measures at the 12th grade level.

The Art of School-aged Children

As indicated earlier, the child is able to copy and to produce a variety of forms with pencil and paper prior to entry into school. Besides the manner in which they draw a person, other aspects of the drawings of children reflect maturational and cognitive development. Five-year-olds exhibit a prime interest in drawing people. The 6-year-old will draw trees, and the 8-year-old houses (Lowenfeld, 1954).

By the age of 5 or 6 years the child begins to represent the body as a collection of two-dimensional masses (trunk, legs, arms, etc. being shown as open figures rather than sticks). "Scenes" begin to be drawn in the early school years, with houses and flowers, and usually a sun (occasionally two suns). The first trees are in "lollipop" form, likely to consist of a round top (sometimes green) and a straight trunk (perhaps brown). Naturalistic use of color is not to be expected before the age of 7 years. The sky is first drawn as a blue band across the top of the picture, and the ground as a green band across the bottom. The child's circle of awareness extends to the horizon by 9 years, when the sky and ground are depicted as meeting there, with figures beginning to be shown in perspective. Overlapping figures begin to be shown by the age of 11 years, by which age it begins to be possible to discriminate between the figures drawn by boys and by girls.

The way children *draw* reflects the way they *see,* which is often the way they *feel.* As children enter the school years and make more complex drawings, the content and quality of the drawings often reflects the child's perception of the quality of his or her life. Sunny scenes, with flowers and open doors and windows, and with smoke rising from the chimney, are likely to be produced by happy children, whereas sunless, stark scenes, with shut or darkened doorways may give a clue to depression. The sizes and placement of figures may reflect the child's sense of the power within the family, and the use of the available space on the paper may mirror the child's sense of confidence or power or self-esteem. Anger or fantasies of violence may be revealed in the expressions on faces or in the subject matter of drawings.

Psychosocial Development

Psychoanalytic theory once held that the demands of education were responsible for a suppression of the sexual aspects of the libido during this *latency* period. It is now understood that sexual interests and activities remain very much alive in the school-aged child. The psychosocial (eriksonian) view considers the principal challenge of this period to be the development of a sense of *industry* or of *duty and accomplishment.* When the child is unsuccessful in meeting this challenge, he or she may know for the first time a prevailing sense of *failure.*

With the removal of a large portion of the child's life from the home to the school environment, children begin increasingly to live independently and to look outside the home for goals and for standards of behavior. This shifting of interests is often anxiety-provoking for parents, and if earlier problems between parent and child have not been adequately resolved, adjustments to forces outside the home are apt to be difficult.

Peer-group activities become gradually less supervised by adults. They bring together children who can form relationships and share games in the early years of middle childhood, but the capacity for maintaining extended intimate relationships emerges only in late middle childhood.

The relationships between *siblings* cannot generally have the character of peer relationships except for twins or siblings born very close together. Preschool children may tease each other or younger siblings in a variety of ways (e.g., offer a toy and then refuse to give it over). Verbal teasing occurs at any age, and may seem to parents to be characteristic of the relationship between their children.

The verbal and material give-and-take between siblings is regarded as one of the ways in which children develop the social skills that will be useful to them in later life: the ability to ignore teasing or to develop repartee to a fine art, or to turn criticism into something constructive. Ultimately, they will learn through the development of empathy that teasing hurts, and will generally give it up as an instrument of social policy.

Parents should be encouraged to turn the encounters between siblings into models of empathic behavior. They should avoid taking sides whenever possible, and should deal with the *behavior* as unacceptable, not the character of the child. For the child who is sensitive to teasing and does not know how to avoid being hurt by it, McDermott (1988) suggests that the parents try role-playing with the child, teaching how to tease back or to ignore taunts or threats.

Vandell et al. (1987) found that during middle childhood the relationship between siblings tended to evolve toward more equal power and status, with less bickering and more cooperative activities than marked the relationships between preschool siblings. These changes took place, however, within the context of increasing conflict.

There is a possibility of great frustration for parents and children when the child's achievements in school do not measure up to parental hopes. The child unable to meet expected standards may learn for the first time the sense of failure and may react with anxiety, depression, or hostility. Antisocial behavior may develop through which the child attempts to gain recognition that he or she cannot attain otherwise.

CONDUCT OF THE ASSESSMENT

The developmental assessment of the school-aged child will give attention to physical status, to comfort with and achievement in school, to relationships with other family members and with playmates and peers, and to elements of the family's life-style (the places of television, or of a program of health fitness, or of things done together as a family, for example). The child will be increasingly able to participate in discussions of his or her health problems and health care, and may be given increasing degrees of responsibility for their management.

Physical Assessment

No major new developmental consideration enters into the conduct of the physical evaluation of the school-aged child. The examination should be complete, including evaluation of the optic fundus and the blood pressure. The evaluation should include screening tests for anemia, and for visual or auditory impairment.

In youngsters whose behavior in home or school suggests the possibility of attention deficit disorder or hyperactivity it will be useful to examine for the "soft" signs that indicate neurodevelopmental immaturity.

Assessment of Cognitive Development

The cognitive development of the child is now increasingly measured by academic achievement and by performance on standardized tests, such as the Stanford-Binet or the Wechsler Intelligence Scale for Children. When children are unsuccessful in their efforts at learning, the possibility of mental retardation or of specific learning disabilities will need consideration. Besides basic tests of intellectual function and of school achievement there will be a need for exploration of other aspects of the child's life, including the psychosocial and sociocultural aspects of his or her experience.

Levine (1987) has devised screening tests for various types of learning disability (Tables 7–1, 7–2, 7–3). There may be relatively discrete disabilities, for example, in visuomotor coordination, in memory, in the ability to give sustained attention to a task, in expressive or receptive language

TABLE 7–1. Tasks for the Assessment of Gross Motor Function*

AGE	GROSS MOTOR FUNCTION
5–6 years	Skip
	Walk on heels
	Tandem gait forward
	Hop in place
6–7 years	Tandem gait backward
	Stand on one foot, eyes open (10 sec)
7–8 years	Crouch on tiptoes, eyes closed (10 sec)
	Hop twice in place on each foot in succession (3 cycles)
	Stand in tandem gait position (heel-toe), eyes closed (10 sec)
9–10 years	Tandem gait sideways
	Catch tennis ball in air, one hand
	Throw tennis ball at target
10–12 years	Balance on tiptoes, eyes closed (15 sec)
	Jump in air, clap heels together
	Jump in air, clap hands three times

* From Levine MD: The elements of developmental function. In Behrman RE, Vaughan VC III (eds): *Nelson Textbook of Pediatrics,* 13th ed. Philadelphia, WB Saunders Company, 1987, p 89.

TABLE 7–2. Examples of Forms Standardized for Age*,†

	REVIEW	
AGE (YEARS)	FORMS FOR DIRECT COPYING	COPY FROM MEMORY (10-SEC EXPOSURE)
5		
6		
7		
8		
9–10		
11–12+		

* From Levine MD: The elements of developmental function. In Behrman RE, Vaughan VC III (eds): *Nelson Textbook of Pediatrics,* 13th ed. Philadelphia, WB Saunders Company, 1987, p 85.

† These forms can be utilized by pediatricians as screening devices for visual-perceptual-motor deficits. Impaired performance on such a task might also be due to other problems, such as inattention, inexperience, fine motor difficulties, or problems with conceptualization. These forms should never be used as the ultimate diagnostic indicator; instead, they might indicate the need for further evaluation of a visual-perceptual-motor problem.

function, in mathematical function, or in other skills. Learning disabilities are often associated with minor neurologic abnormalities, such as the "soft signs" that represent persistence of neurodevelopmental traits that normally disappear by or shortly after entry into school.

OTHER DEVELOPMENTAL ISSUES

Entry into School

Entry into systems of formal academic education has generally been deferred in the United States until about 5 years for kindergarten and about 6 years for first grade, when the average child is first ready to deal effectively with the symbols that are the heart of reading and writing. The beginning of formal education might be deferred until a later time, but the demands of an increasingly urbanized and mechanized society and the needs of industry and technology have become increasingly felt as demanding a more literate and skillful workforce, and soon. Recent years

TABLE 7–3. Tasks for the Assessment of Temporal-Sequential Organization

AGE (YR)	Digit Span Series of spoken numbers (1–9), given one per second, to be repeated by child	Object Span Series of objects tapped in random order; child imitates in same order	Block Tapping Series of squares tapped in random order; child then imitates in same order	Serial Commands Series of simple commands; child performs in correct order	Motor Sequence Child performs act after examiner
5–6	4 forward digits	4 objects	4 squares	3-step series	Simultaneously open and close both hands, arms extended
6–7	4–5 forward digits	4 objects	4 squares	4-step series	Imitative finger tapping (both hands, 3–4 steps)
7–8	5 forward digits	5 objects	5 squares	5-step series	Imitative mixed finger-foot tapping (4–5 steps)
9–10	6 forward digits 4 reverse digits	5 objects	5 squares	5-step series	Alternate left and right open and close fists, arms extended
11–12+	6 forward digits 5 reverse digits	6 objects	6 squares	6-step series	Imitate edge of hand on knee, then palm on knee, then clenched fist (4 cycles)

TASK DESCRIPTION

* From Levine MD: The elements of developmental function. In Behrman RE, Vaughan VC III (eds): *Nelson Textbook of Pediatrics*, 13th ed. Philadelphia, WB Saunders Company, 1987, p 86.

have seen increasing pressure from parents and others to have the "education" of children begin at earlier ages. Elkind (1987) has been a particularly articulate critic of this tendency.

It is clear that preschool experiences in school-like settings, such as the Head Start programs, can have beneficial effects upon the later adjustment in school of young children from disadvantaged communities (see pp. 209–210). The most consistent advantage seen in children who have had the Head Start experience appears to consist of greater social skills, better motivation, and greater confidence in later years. Elkind holds, on the other hand, that there is no convincing evidence that the introduction of *academic* instruction into the lives of preschool children conveys any advantage to them, even if it seems successful. He finds no evidence that early instruction will make more intelligent or gifted children, and emphasizes that young children will learn the things they need to know, at the times that they become relevant to the curriculum or to their life experiences.

Television

With the entry of children into school, a major portion of what they learn about the world in which they live begins to be learned through formal instruction. They have been exposed earlier to television (see p. 208), but now their exposure begins to reach its peak intensity, and there the child is exposed to a profoundly different curriculum.

Many studies have attested to the power of television to inform, misinform, and influence the perceptions and judgment of viewers. Concerns have been expressed about the amount of exposure there is of children to television, about the content of what the children see, and about the exploitation by the sponsors of childrens' programs of children as a market for the sponsors' goods. For example, the sales pitches delivered to children with programs for children have engendered conflicts between children and parents concerning priorities in family expenditures for food and other goods.

Palumbo (1985) reviewed the effects of television upon children. He reported that children between the ages of 2 and 11 years spend an average of 26 to 28 hr/week watching television; adolescents reduce the amount to about 23 hr/week. Acknowledging the potential of television for positive effects on education and on attitudes, Palumbo lists negative effects in five areas: violence, educational achievement, commercials, role models, and adolescent behavior and attitudes toward life-styles.

A Task Force on Children and Television of the American Academy of Pediatrics (1984) reviewed the literature on children and television and reported the following conclusions: that exposure to violence on television promoted a proclivity to violence in children and a passive response to its practice; that television viewing increased the consumption of snack foods and fostered the development of obesity; that television viewing as a passive activity detracted from time that might be given to learning through development of active learning skills; that unrealistic messages are conveyed regarding drugs, alcohol, and tobacco, with implicit encouragement of their use; that the portrayal of sexuality and sex roles on television is unrealistic and misleading (adolescence being portrayed, for example, as a constant state of sexual crisis, with rapid development of relationships, with little consideration of the possibility of pregnancy, and with the possibility of exposure to pornography on cable television); that television promotes ethnic and racial stereotypes; that television does little to promote understanding views of the handicapped; and that television conveys unrealistic views of problem-solving processes or of conflict resolution.

Gerbner (1984) has pointed out that children are now raised in homes in which the story-tellers intrude from outside, rather than coming from within the family, usually under corporate egis. Children learn less now from their parents, school, or church. Television sets their values in marked degree, taking value-setting out of the hands of parents or tradition.

He has found that television is used nonselectively by most viewers, much viewing amounting to a ritual, with watching providing information to people not seeking it, under the guise of "entertainment."

Children spend on the average more time before the television set than at school or at any other activity besides sleep. Television, then, is a major avenue through which children learn about life—how to live and how to behave, and particularly what behavior is expected at critical times.

During the growing years, Gerbner estimates, children see from 30,000 to 40,000 stories unfold before them, consisting of news, advertisements, fictions, and so forth. He has explored the nature of the world that television describes, and finds a distorted picture.

The depiction of women, of the aged, and of minorities on television has been disproportionately favorable to upper-middle-class white males, and has presented stereotypes that offer a distorted view of reality.

More roles and more opportunities are shown on television for men than for women, women's roles being stereotypical. Only one third as many persons under 18 years old and one fifth as many over the age of 65 years are given parts in television stories as are actually found in the population. A result may be that the more people watch television, the more they believe that old folks are less numerous, better off, and more powerful than a decade ago, whereas the reverse is true. Gerbner speculates upon the significance of this finding for the formation of public policy, as in social security legislation. Minorities are shown as equals of the majority in power, but are not proportionately represented in numbers.

During their time watching television, viewers see five violent acts per hour if they are watching adult programs and 18 per hour if they are watching children's television. There is now ample evidence that television programs depicting violent behavior are followed by escalation of such behavior in the viewing population.

Gerbner holds that television presents the message that violence is the medium through which social power is achieved, cultivating the notion that violence is an acceptable solution to problems. Television drama discloses who gets away with what against whom.

The exposure to violence fosters *fear* out of proportion to fact, and the notion that the world is "mean" (Gerbner et al., 1984). It fosters the notion that repression is justified in the name of security. The more that one watches television the more intense and diffuse this fear is. This seems true for both children and adults.

Violence involves more than 50 per cent of prime-time characters and more than 80 per cent of those on children's television. Violence needing medical attention is inflated on television, against about the 6 to 7 per cent need for medical attention in reality.

Singer (1989) summarizes the current status of the relationship between television and violence for children and adolescents.

Gerbner found the physician to be the most represented profession (12/week); in addition to physicians, the viewers see policemen (35/week), criminals (23/week), lawyers (6/week), and judges (6/week). Blue-collar workers, who are the most numerous group in the labor force, make up less than 10 per cent of television people.

The physician is represented as daring authority, omniscient, dominating and controlling the lives of others, risk-taking but winning, and accessible instantly.

Gerbner notes that *Healthy People: The Surgeon General's Report on Health Promotion and Disease Prevention* (1979) found that 50 per cent of deaths in the United States are contributed to by patterns of behavior associated with life-styles, such as drinking, overeating, faulty diets, and accidents on the highway. He has called these "manufactured diseases." Of other deaths, 20 per cent stem from environmental factors, 20 per cent from biologic factors, and 10 per cent from lack of access to health care. Gerbner has explored how television contributes to this pattern, and views television as central to a new battle for disease prevention.

Of about 25,000 advertisements monitored, Gerbner found that over 5000 were for foods; more than 50 per cent of these were for sweets, and 9 per cent made claims for nutritional excellence. There is a lot of eating and drinking on television, but obesity is rarely seen—only 6 per cent of men and only 2 per cent of women are obese. Only one or two leading characters are overweight. Most of the eating on television is snacking, like that shown in the advertisements.

Frustrations on television often call first for an alcoholic drink. Twice each hour someone is shown actually drinking, with drinking mentioned six times each hour. Less than 1 per cent of those drinking show any ill effect. If there is any effect of alcohol shown, it is likely to be portrayed as amusing or funny.

Gerbner (1984) has found that the views of heavy viewers of television about life, security, opportunity, education, physicians, safety, drinking, eating, and violence differ from the views held by those who view television less often. They expect too much from the physician and are more complacent about risk factors. (Neither the hero nor the villain of a television drama is likely to wear a seat belt while driving a car.)

For children television presents images that are not true, but that are taken by many to be the norms, and it cultivates dispositions that will govern future behavior. Moreover, television may then trigger such behavior. For example, the incidence of suicides has been reported (Gould and Shaffer, 1986) to rise by about 30 per cent in the days following the suicide of some prominent public person, and also after fictional deaths by suicide on television. They found the adolescent population to be particularly vulnerable, with increases in incidence of up to 100 per cent in females and 60 per cent in males.

Phillips and Carstensen (1986) reported similar findings, but a later study by Phillips and Paight (1987) cast doubt on the magnitude or existence of such an effect on television on suicide rates. Kessler et al (1988) also failed to find evidence supporting the earlier findings.

Educational achievement in children bears an inverse relationship to the amount of television viewing. Gerbner has found that the IQs of children tend to flatten in families of high socioeconomic status in which there is much television watching, whereas the IQs of children tend to rise in families of lower socioeconomic status in which television viewing is restricted. In the latter families the way seems more open for movement into the cultural mainstream.

Singer and Singer (1987) have suggested a guide for parents in support of constructive television viewing. The guide (here considerably abbreviated) includes the following:

1. Start early to develop the child's viewing habits. Limit television watching by setting some rules: no television before school, during meals, during daytime hours, before homework is done.

2. Encourage planned rather than random viewing.

3. Select children's programs featuring children in the child's peer group.

4. Keep a log of television hours.

5. Discuss sensitive television items with children. Share viewing. Discuss feelings. Analyze commercials. Examine differences between fantasy and reality.

6. Explain the function of advertising and that famous people say nice things about products for money.

7. Balance reading and television. Relate the two when feasible.

8. Balance the content for viewing. Designate a day a week for no television viewing and plan other family activities for that day.

9. Arrange for access to alternative programming (public television).

10. Point out that all ethnic groups make contributions to society.

11. Show examples of women performing competently at work and at home.

12. Write to the media and advertisers about programs that show excessive violence.

Gerbner suggests that for children television may be virtually unavoidable, only activities and actions organized within the community being powerful enough to control the impact of television, the actions of individuals not being sufficiently potent. Action for Children's Television (ACT) represents such a community effort.

Gerbner (1984) calls upon those professionals concerned with the care of children, without their becoming censors, to guard, propagate, and cultivate attitudes toward television; to instruct parents; and to demand that schools cultivate a sense of critical viewing of television, analogous to critical reading of literature, critical talking or discussion, and critical study. He calls upon citizens in general for political action, pointing out that the expenses of advertising as a deductible business expense are paid for by a levy on each household in this country that amounts to about $65 per year. He calls for a broader base of resources for television and for the story-telling that guides the growth and development of children in health-promoting ways.

Strasburger (1989) comments on the particular role that pediatricians may play in mediating the relationship between children, their families, and television.

Learning Disabilities

A learning disability (LD) is defined as a significant discrepancy between IQ and achievement in the absence of psychiatric disorder, of lack of schooling, or of sensory impairment. Learning disabilities take the forms of reading disorders, expressive writing disorders, arithmetic disorders, and language disorders.

Learning disabilities have a prevalence estimated by Rutter et al. (1976) to be about 3.8 per cent for children on the Isle of Wight, and about 6 per cent for children in London (in children of a different socioeconomic group). Estimates vary in the United States, according to definitions and population studied.

The causes of LDs are not fully understood. Neurophysiologic and neuropathologic studies indicate that some of the affected children have a decrease in the asymmetry of the brain that is ordinarily associated with differences in right and left hemispheric function (in right-handed persons, the right brain is predominantly concerned with form and relationships, and the left with speech and mathematical functions). Abnormal neural architecture has been reported in affected persons, especially in the parietotemporal areas. In some families the condition appears to be familial. In others it may be the result of prenatal or perinatal or other conditions, such as anoxia, drugs, or exposure to toxins such as lead.

The differential diagnosis of LD includes primary sensory deficit (of vision or hearing), mental retardation, primary emotional disorder (depression, autism, attention-deficit disorder), sociocultural deprivation, understimulation, low motivation, or poor self-esteem.

The child with a LD is often not recognized until entry into school, when he or she (the great majority of affected children are male) is found to forget material easily, to have difficulty in recognizing and writing letters or words, to be delayed in language development, or to have defective computational skills. Affected children often appear emotionally immature, dislike academic tasks, have a short attention span, and are hyperactive, distractible, and impulsive. They may also have a poor sense of time and difficulty in learning sequenced material (e.g., alphabet, days of week, or months of year). Delays in the development of gross and fine motor coordination are common (the evidence of these delays includes the so-called soft signs found on neurodevelopmental examination).

An assessment of the possibility of LD should be made for any child about to enter school. In addition to evaluation of vision and of hearing and a basic neurodevelopmental inventory, such an assessment should include inquiry of the parents as to the general behavior of the child and as to any problems that may exist, such as emotional lability or physical hyperactivity. The report of the parents may be more reliable than the observations of the physician in the office, where a hyperactive child may not display typical behavior. Assessment of developmental drawing ability, of language ability, and of parental reports of hyperactivity or distractability may be particularly helpful in identifying the preschool child with a LD.

Among the screening tests that have been found useful are the Peabody Picture Vocabulary Test, the Preschool Readiness Experimental Screening Scale (PRESS), and the Pediatric Examination of Educational Readiness (PEER). The PRESS focuses upon drawing and language abilities; the PEER is a complicated test better carried out by persons who have been specially trained to administer it. The Denver Developmental Screening Test may be helpful in identifying the child needing further evaluation for the possibility of developmental delay, but is relatively insensitive to LD in the child of normal IQ.

Management of the child with a LD generally requires close cooperation among physician, psychologist, teacher, and parents. Details of management will vary from child to child. For some, a special classroom arrangement may be required to protect the child from distractions, and for others individual tutorial efforts at compensating for specific deficits may be necessary. Such efforts may include reading to the child, or allowing the child to use oral dictation (rather than reading), tape recorder (to take aural rather than written notes), calculator (for mathematical computation), or word processor (to compensate for handwriting or spelling) (Wender, 1988).

For all affected children, a major need will be the fostering of supportive attitudes toward the child, correcting the misapprehension that he or she is "lazy" or "slow." There is a need to identify and build upon the child's strengths. For some children with attention-deficit disorder (with or without hyperactivity) the use of stimulant drugs may be effective in letting the child focus upon classwork with less distraction.

Prognosis for a LD varies with the nature of the condition in the particular child. When a predominantly visually based dyslexia is accompanied by good language skills, the prognosis is better than otherwise, reading and writing not being essential to education where language skills are intact. Poor language skills and attention-deficit disorder carry a particularly poor prognosis. Children with attention-deficit disorder are especially susceptible to emotional maladjustment. When the LD is of moderate to severe intensity, the disability is likely to persist and the academic discrepancy between the affected child and peers to widen with time.

A phenomenon as yet not fully explained is that the ranks of incarcerated antisocial adults contain a disproportionate number of persons who have had a LD in childhood. It is not known whether this is the result in some way of the primary process responsible for the LD or of the frustration, sense of failure, and anger felt by youngsters for whom achievement in school has always been denied.

Chapter 8

EARLY ADOLESCENCE

Early adolescence refers to that time in life when childhood has passed and puberty begins. It begins and is completed earlier for girls than for boys. The years that comprise early adolescence correspond roughly to the time between transition from sex maturity rating (SMR) 1 to SMR 2 and the time until, but not including, SMR 3.

Data from the U.S. Health Examination Survey (Harlan et al., 1979, 1980) indicate that by the mean age of 12 years 80 per cent of white girls have passed SMR 2, and by 14 years 98 per cent of girls will have done so. For boys the transition from SMR 2 to 3 is not reached by the majority until the average age of 15 years.

The wide range of normal pubertal development found at each chronologic age within the adolescent years is seen in Tables 8–1 through 8–4. There are also ethnic differences in the timing of sexual maturation: blacks are advanced, and Mexican-Americans delayed in comparison with whites.

A classification system based on biologic status, such as stage of puberty, has considerable merit, since most biologic and psychologic phenomena seem to correlate better during adolescence with pubertal stage than chronologic age. Such a system has limitations, however, inasmuch as in certain circumstances constraints imposed by chronologic age or grade in school may make age or grade level a better determinant of the attitudes or behaviors of young people, or may modify the effects of pubertal development. For example, among the age peers in a high-school class, late onset of puberty may present problems for males, whereas it may confer some advantage upon females.

It may be difficult for the physician to know how to treat a youngster whose physical development has been delayed (e.g., by chronic illness) but whose intellectual development has been unimpaired and who is attending school with age-matched peers. It is not clear whether this patient's reactions and needs will be governed predominantly by biologic or by social factors, and it is best to let the patient express his or her own readiness to be dealt with as a child or early adolescent. Open-ended questions such as: "What do you think may be wrong with you?" or "What did you think would happen when you came to the hospital this morning?" may provide insight into the adolescent's maturity level.

TABLE 8–1. Pubic Hair Stages in Females (%)[*]

STAGE AND ETHNIC BACKGROUND[†]

	1			2			3			4			5		
AGE	W	B	M-A	W	B	M-A	W	B	M-A	W	B	M-A	W	B	M-A
12	10.2	4.5	11.0	16.5	10.3	34.0	29.5	26.9	35.0	34.9	29.8	13.0	9.2	28.2	6.5
13	2.0	0.0	1.2	9.0	2.2	19.8	22.1	17.5	39.5	44.2	42.5	22.2	21.5	37.2	17.3
14	0.4	0.0	0.0	1.0	3.0	6.3	10.8	11.0	36.3	48.4	27.0	32.5	38.9	60.0	25.0
16	0.0	0.0	0.0	0.1	0.0	1.3	2.2	1.4	10.3	30.4	20.3	20.5	67.8	78.4	68.3

[*] Modified from Harlan et al. (1980) and Villarreal et al. (1989).
[†] W, white; B, black; M-A, Mexican-American.

TABLE 8–2. Breast Stages in Females (%)[*]

STAGE AND ETHNIC BACKGROUND[†]

	1			2			3			4			5		
AGE	W	B	M-A	W	B	M-A	W	B	M-A	W	B	M-A	W	B	M-A
12	5.3	5.7	7.4	20.4	6.8	32.4	32.8	23.5	37.0	27.4	33.2	13.0	14.2	30.5	10.2
13	0.8	0.0	4.9	9.2	4.4	17.3	23.4	19.7	33.3	35.3	34.3	25.9	30.0	41.0	18.5
14	0.4	0.0	0.0	1.4	3.0	2.5	13.8	8.0	35.0	41.0	38.0	25.0	42.9	52.0	37.5
16	0.0	0.0	0.0	0.3	0.0	2.6	5.1	3.7	10.6	33.1	23.2	15.6	62.2	73.2	72.8

[*] Modified from Harlan et al. (1980) and Villarreal et al. (1989).
[†] W, white; B, black; M-A, Mexican-American.

TABLE 8–3. Pubic Hair Stages in Males (%)*

	STAGE AND ETHNIC BACKGROUND[†]									
	1		2		3		4		5	
AGE	W	M-A	W	M-A	W	M-A	W	M-A	W	M-A
12	26.5	57.9	41.3	28.1	21.8	11.4	8.7	2.6	1.7	0
13	9.3	22.9	26.8	32.3	28.6	20.8	23.1	13.5	12.3	10.4
14	2.7	5.9	10.5	9.9	12.4	41.6	34.9	28.7	39.6	13.9
15	0.4	0	2.5	5.4	5.1	20.3	26.8	45.9	65.1	28.4
16	0.4	0	0.8	2.9	1.8	4.3	15.5	40.0	81.4	52.9
17	0	0	0	1.6	0.4	0	5.5	7.9	94.0	90.5

* Modified from Harlan et al. (1979) and Villarreal et al. (1989).
† W, white; M-A, Mexican-American.

NEUROENDOCRINOLOGY OF PUBERTY

Accidents of nature, such as the occurrence of tumors of the central nervous system, that result in precocious puberty have demonstrated that all of the structures and functional connections necessary for initiation and evolution of puberty exist from the time of birth. What triggers the pubertal process 10 or so years later remains a mystery, though considerable progress has been made in recent years in our understanding.

Even before birth, a feedback loop is established through which sex steroids (testosterone and estradiol) inhibit hypothalamic secretion of gonadotropin-releasing hormones (Gn-RH). In the absence of Gn-RH pituitary secretion of gonadotropins (luteinizing hormone [LH] and follicle-stimulating hormone [FSH]) is absent or negligible. The sensitivity of this feedback loop increases in early childhood (Grumbach, 1980).

A recently reported finding, not yet confirmed, is that the serum level of pineal melatonin remains elevated until approximately 7 years of age,

TABLE 8–4. Genitalia Stage in Males (%)*

	STAGE AND ETHNIC BACKGROUND[†]									
	1		2		3		4		5	
AGE	W	M-A	W	M-A	W	M-A	W	M-A	W	M-A
12	32.2	50.9	41.9	31.6	19.3	13.2	6.0	4.4	0.6	0
13	12.5	15.6	31.4	35.4	24.6	24.0	24.9	13.5	6.7	11.5
14	4.4	5.9	9.8	9.9	18.6	39.6	37.0	29.7	30.3	14.9
15	0.8	0	2.5	2.7	6.9	25.7	36.5	48.6	53.2	23.0
16	0	0	0.6	1.4	2.0	7.1	19.8	48.6	77.5	42.9
17	0	0	0	0	0	4.5	8.4	0	91.3	95.5

* Modified from Harlan et al. (1979) and Villarreal et al. (1989).
† W, white; M-A, Mexican-American.

after which it declines coincident with rising gonadotropin levels. This observation suggests that melatonin may be the source of suppression of Gn-RH secretion prior to puberty.

Endogenous opioids and dopamine also have been shown to exert a suppressive effect on Gn-RH production, whereas norepinephrine ap-

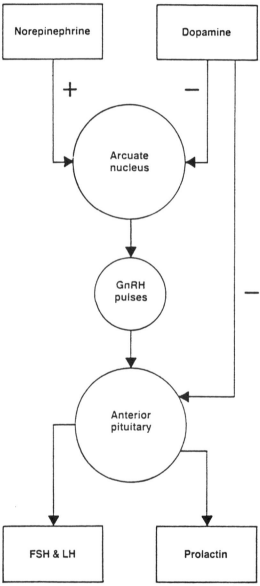

Figure 8–1. Neuroendocrine control of production of gonadotropins and prolactin. From Speroff L, Glass RH, Kase NG: *Clinical Gynecologic Endocrinology and Infertility,* 3rd ed. Baltimore, Williams & Wilkins, 1983.

pears to stimulate its secretion (Fig. 8–1) (Speroff et al., 1983). As puberty approaches, Gn-RH begins to be secreted by the arcuate neurons of the hypothalamus in a pulsatile fashion (Reiter, 1986).

Gonadotropins

The first sign defining the onset of puberty is increased secretion of LH by the pituitary in response to the pulsatile release of Gn-RH. The pulses occur in concert with sleep cycles, higher levels being found during sleep than in the daytime in early adolescence (Fig. 8–2), a phenomenon not observed at any other time of life (Boyar et al., 1972). The levels attained are higher in adolescents than in either children (SMR 1) or adults (SMR 5). The frequency and amplitude of LH pulses increase as puberty progresses until late puberty, when the adult pattern of approximately 12 pulses, evenly distributed over a 24-hr period, is achieved. This pattern must be considered in evaluating patients with pubertal delay so that blood specimens can be obtained at the appropriate times.

In early adolescence in boys LH levels increase dramatically (reaching a peak at SMR 2) and FSH levels rise gradually throughout puberty (Fig. 8–3). In girls, on the other hand, LH levels increase later in puberty and FSH levels manifest an early increase.

In addition to sex differences in absolute levels, another sex difference relates to patterns of gonadotropin secretion. The episodic or pulsatile pattern of release discussed above, and the tonic, or constant secretion (controlled by the negative feedback of circulating sex steroids acting on the hypothalamus) are equivalent in the two sexes but in the follicular stage of the menstrual cycle females manifest positive feedback of increasing levels of circulating estrogens, which causes a preovulatory surge of LH secretion (Fig. 8–4).

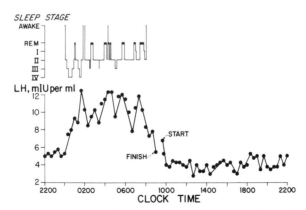

Figure 8–2. Plasma LH concentration in early puberty, expressed as mIU/mL. From Boyar R, Finkelstein J, Roffwarg H, et al: Synchronization of augmented luteinizing hormone secretion with sleep during puberty. N Engl J Med 287:582–586, 1972.

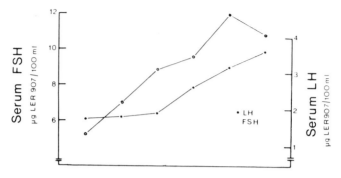

Figure 8-3. Blood levels of LH and FSH in 56 healthy boys studied semilongitudinally, plotted against stage of puberty.
From Marshall WA, Tanner JM: Puberty. In Davis TA, Dobbing J (eds): *Scientific Foundations of Paediatrics,* 2nd ed. Baltimore, University Park Press, 1974, pp 176–209.

Testosterone

LH and FSH stimulate the testes to produce testosterone. As a result, in the transition from SMR 1 to 2 in males there is, within less than a year's time, an increase in serum testosterone levels from around 10 ng/dL to around 200 ng/dL. A smaller and more gradual increase in plasma testosterone occurs in females between SMR 1 and 2, with levels typically ranging from 11 to 38 ng/dL.

Estrogen

In females, in response to FSH stimulation, the ovary produces estradiol in increasing amounts throughout puberty. Before breast development begins, serum estradiol levels are approximately 2 ng/dL. These levels rise to about 13 ng/dL at stage 3 of breast development and to around 30 ng/dL by stage 4.

Cyclical variations in estradiol production begin around the time of menarche. Some estradiol is converted peripherally to estrone, which is also derived from conversion of ovarian and adrenal androstenedione. Estrone levels are highest during SMR 2 and reach a plateau during SMR 3 and 4.

Boys have lower levels of estrone and estradiol (which result from conversion of testicular and adrenal testosterone and androstenedione) than girls, but in 30 to 50 per cent of boys the levels are sufficient to stimulate breast growth, with the occurrence of gynecomastia, primarily at SMR 2 and 3.

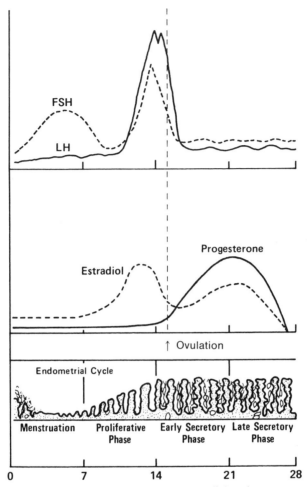

Figure 8–4. Patterns of secretion of gonadotropins, estradiol, and progesterone throughout the menstrual cycle.

Sex Hormone Binding Globulin

Another factor that contributes to the physiology of puberty is the level of sex hormone binding globulin (SHBG). Only unbound hormones are physiologically active. Puberty is associated with a fall in the level of SHBGs in males to a level approximately half that of females. A result is that plasma level of free testosterone in adult males is twice that of total testosterone in females.

Prolactin

Another sex difference is found in the secretion of pituitary prolactin during puberty. Prolactin levels increase in females but not in males, presumably owing to the fact that estrogen augments secretion of prolactin. The sex difference in basal prolactin levels reaches statistical significance at SMR 2 to 3. Responsiveness of prolactin secretion to thyrotropin releasing hormone (TRH) stimulation reaches a plateau, however, at SMR 4 to 5, with levels that persist for the first 2 years following menarche and decrease thereafter.

Plasma concentrations of prolactin up to 20 ng/mL may be found in adolescent females, compared to prepubertal levels in both sexes, and in adult males levels of approximately 5 to 7 ng/mL. Levels in excess of these should prompt consideration of the possibility of a prolactin-secreting pituitary adenoma. These tumors may be so small as to be undetected on conventional roentgenograms and may require computed tomography for detection.

It is thought that secretion of prolactin by the pituitary is controlled by hypothalamic production of an inhibiting factor (PIF). The pubertal rise seen in females may result from a decrease in PIF, from blockade of dopamine receptors on prolactin-secreting cells of the pituitary, or from blockade or suppression of dopamine production. The complex interactions between these hormones and neurotransmitters affect the timing of pubertal events and reproductive functioning in ways that remain to be elucidated and, as yet, have little clinical application.

Growth Hormone

Growth hormone, a polypeptide composed of 191 amino acids, is produced by the pituitary in response to hypothalamic secretion of growth hormone-releasing hormone (GH-RH). This hormone is secreted throughout childhood. In early puberty, however, production increases and the pattern of secretion changes such that it is enhanced by sleep and is produced in a pulsatile fashion.

Growth hormone affects somatic growth through its stimulation of production of somatomedin-C (insulin-like growth factor-1 [IGF-1]) by the liver. This effect is mediated by the state of nutrition of the individual (e.g., in anorexia nervosa or inflammatory bowel disease puberty is delayed and somatomedin-C production is low), as well as by other hormones such as thyroxin and testosterone. Somatomedin-C levels increase with increasing pubertal development (Luna et al., 1983). The range of normal somatomedin-C (IGF-1) levels at different stages of puberty are found in (Fig. 8–5).

It is rare that congenital growth hormone deficiency is first diagnosed during adolescence, as patients with this disorder manifest growth retardation from early infancy. Acquired growth hormone deficiency, resulting from a craniopharyngioma may, however, not become apparent until the youngster fails to manifest the normal pubertal growth spurt. The diagno-

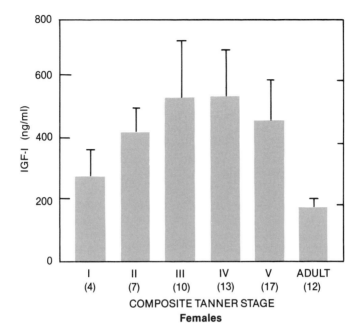

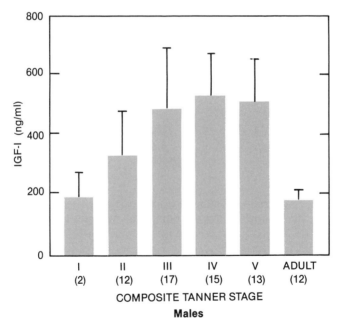

Figure 8–5. Mean somatomedin-C (SM-C)/insulin-like growth factor I (IGF-I) levels ± 1 SD for females (A) and males (B) for each composite Tanner stage. Numbers of subjects in each group in parentheses.
From Luna AM, Wilson DM, Wibbelsman CJ, et al: Somatomedins in adolescence: A cross-sectional study of the effect of puberty on plasma insulin-like growth factor I and II levels. J Clin Endocrinol Metab 57:268–271, 1983.

sis of growth hormone deficiency is made when there is failure to respond to at least two provocative stimuli, such as following administration of insulin, clonidine, or arginine, or with strenuous physical activity. In these studies, blood samples must be obtained every 20 min over the course of 24 hr in order to substantiate the diagnosis.

Patients with acquired growth hormone deficiency rarely have this as an isolated finding: accordingly, the possibility of other pituitary or hypothalamic lesions should be explored. For that reason, nuclear magnetic resonance or computed tomographic study of the head should be performed when growth hormone deficiency is diagnosed in the adolescent patient. Replacement therapy is now available through recombinant DNA technology and involves the daily intramuscular injection of 0.1 mg/kg/dose.

Adrenarche

Shortly before the beginning of puberty, there is an increase in adrenal androgen production in both sexes. Blood levels of dehydroepiandrosterone (DHEA) and dehydroepiandrosterone sulfate (DHEAS) double in males between the ages of 8 and 10 years and in females between 7 and 9 years. The only morphologic change that appears to correspond to these increased hormone levels is the prepubertal increase in fat (Tanner and Marshall, 1974). Plasma levels of androstenedione derive largely from the adrenal cortex and, to a lesser extent, the gonads in early adolescence. This hormone is converted peripherally to testosterone and contributes to the development of pubic and axillary hair.

GROWTH AND DEVELOPMENT

Physical

Height

Despite the fact that an increase in linear growth rate is one of the hallmarks of the pubertal growth spurt, this does not occur during early adolescence (at SMRs 1 and 2). The normal male or female growth rate is 6 to 8 cm/year, the same rate as during the childhood years. Early adolescence is a good time to begin to chart height velocity measurements, however, so that the imminent acceleration in height may be assessed and documented. This is accomplished by use of curves such as those in Figures 1-5A, B and 1-6A, B. Growth involves the cranium as well as the long bones and spine. The sequence and magnitude of skeletal growth is detailed in the section on middle adolescence (see pp. 294–295). The growth spurt of puberty is most pronounced for height of the mandibular ramus, at a rate of approximately 7 per cent yearly for males and 7.5 per cent yearly for females.

Weight

Upon entry into early adolescence, boys have achieved approximately 55 per cent of their adult weight, and girls 59 per cent. The weight gains during early adolescence are modest in comparison with those that follow and average 2.0 kg each year, not dissimilar from the rate of weight gain that characterized the later childhood years. There are major sex differences, however, in the tissues that predominantly contribute to the pubertal weight gain.

In females an increase in body fat content is associated with each successive stage of pubertal development, whereas in males the pubertal weight spurt is primarily due to increased muscularity (Fig. 8–6). Boys actually lose fat mass during puberty, despite their increase in weight, and this is reflected in the fact that the body density of boys increases more than that of girls. Girls have both larger and more numerous adipocytes throughout puberty.

Not only fat gain, but fat distribution as well, differs for boys and girls, with males accumulating fat particularly on the trunk and females on both the trunk and the extremities. Females accumulate more subcutaneous fat on the lower portion of the trunk, as compared to boys. In early adolescence, as during childhood, both sexes gain more subcutaneous fat on the lower than the upper body. Girls also accumulate proportionately more fat on the posterior thigh during early adolescence (Malina and Boucher, 1988).

Measurement of Weight Changes

Charting of weight velocity curves should be started during early adolescence. When incremental changes are so recorded, it is possible to

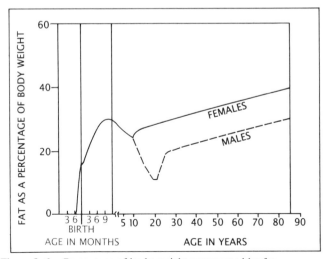

Figure 8–6. Percentage of body weight represented by fat. From Frisch RE: Fatness and fertility. Sci Am March, pp 88–95, 1988.

show that the acceleration in weight change has a peak approximately 3 to 6 months following the peak of the height velocity curve, which occurs generally at SMR 3 in girls and 4 in boys (see pp. 295–296).

During early adolescence, it is possible to show an actual deceleration in weight gain, particularly in males. Body fat content is assessed by a variety of methods, including measurements of body density and total body water, examination of x-ray studies, ultrasonography, and measurements of skinfold thickness (SFT), the last of which is the most practical for clinical management. The relationship between SFT and percentage of body fat is shown in Table 8–5 (Smith et al., 1978).

A number of sites have been used for the measurement of SFT, with varying results (the technique for measurement of skin fold thickness is illustrated in Figure 8–7 [Lohman et al., 1988]). Using the triceps and subscapular sites for SFT measurements, many investigators report a prepubertal gain of fat followed by a midpubertal fat loss in boys. These changes have not, however, been found at the subscapular site in girls.

Young et al. (1968) found a mean increase in SFT of 15 per cent between prepubertal and pubertal female adolescents, and an increase of 31 per cent between pubertal and postpubertal subjects. These increases were manifested in all skinfolds measured with the exception of the chin. The site of the largest increase with puberty was found to be the "pubic" fold on the abdomen, followed in decreasing order of magnitude by the umbilicus, the subscapular area, and the lower ribs.

In males the peak increase in muscle cell number occurs just as they enter early adolescence (approximately 10½ years) and its effect is to increase the number of cells by 14-fold over the number present at 5 years of age. The size of the muscle cell continues to grow throughout the third decade, in contrast to the situation with girls, whose ultimate muscle cell size is reached by the age of 10.5 years. The peak increase in muscle strength in males does not occur, however, until approximately SMR 4 at the peak of the height velocity curve. Muscle strength can be measured using a tenometer, which measures grip strength.

TABLE 8–5. Relationship of Skinfold Thickness to Percent Body Fat*

	PERCENT BODY FAT	
SKINFOLD THICKNESS (IN)	Boys	Girls
¼	5–9	8–13
½	9–13	13–18
¾	13–18	18–23
1	18–22	23–28
1¼	22–27	28–33

* Modified from Smith et al. (1978).

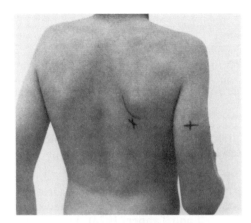

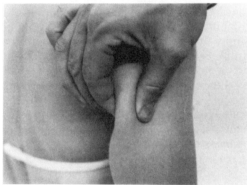

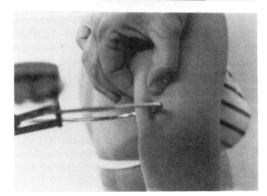

Figure 8–7. Technique for measuring skinfold thickness. *Top,* Landmarks for subscapular and triceps skinfolds. *Middle,* Position of thumb and index finger prior to grasping the fold. *Bottom,* Measurement of skinfold thickness with caliper. From Lohman TG, Roche AF, Martorell R: *Anthropometric Standardization Reference Manual.* Champaign, IL, Human Kinetics Books, 1987.

Reproductive Development

The *sine qua non* of maturity is the development of reproductive capability. The culmination of the process is the maturation of the gametes and of the system for their transportation, and for the fertilization and the secure development of the ovum. The first clinical indication that puberty has begun is enlargement of the testis or ovary, which occurs approximately 1 year prior to the first appearance of secondary sex characteristics. The latter, because of their conspicuousness and social significance, tend to receive much more attention than the primary sex characteristics in our society, and it is their appearance and progression that define puberty. Secondary sex characteristics are those that occur as a result of production of hormones produced by the testis or the ovary (testosterone and estrogen, respectively). As indicated above, these organs are capable of hormonal secretion from the time of birth but do not do so until stimulated by the pituitary gonadotropins LH and FSH.

"Primary" Sex Characteristics. In males, the first clinical sign of puberty, enlargement of the testes, results from the increased size of the seminiferous tubules and increased numbers of Leydig and Sertoli cells (Marshall and Tanner, 1974). During the course of pubertal development in Caucasians, the testes grow from the childhood volume of 6 ($\pm$2.6) mL to approximately 19 ($\pm$4.0) mL when puberty is complete. The relationship of testicular size to stage of pubertal development is provided in Table 8–6. (Testicular volume is conveniently measured using an orchiometer such as that developed by Prader, which consists of a graduated series of beads of known volume, which provide a reference standard for the visual or tactile assessment of the patient.) Enlargement of the epididymis, seminal vesicles, and prostate begins during early adolescence. Testosterone production is initiated and results in the secondary changes described below.

A major functional effect of these changes is the capacity for ejaculation, which occurs approximately 1 year after initiation of testicular growth and is coincident with the appearance of pubic hair (SMR 2). The first episode of ejaculation is typically in response to masturbation. Kinsey et al. (1948) found, contrary to popular belief, that ejaculation with nocturnal emission generally begins a year after masturbation-induced ejaculation. The same data showed that 90 per cent of males reported that first ejaculation occurred between 11 and 15 years of age. Within this age

TABLE 8–6. Testicular Volume (in mL) by Pubic Hair Stages in Males 12.5 to 20 Years of Age*

	PUBIC HAIR STAGES					
	1	2	3	4	5	6†
Mean	6.0	6.8	9.3	12.6	16.3	18.9
SD	2.6	3.6	3.8	4.2	4.6	4.0

* From Zachman M, Prader A, Kind HP, et al: Testicular volume during adolescence: cross-sectional and longitudinal studies. Helv Paediatr Acta 29:61–72, 1974.
† Represents further spreading of pubic hair in a masculine pattern.

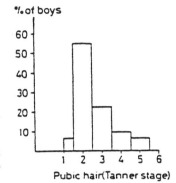

Figure 8–8. Estimated pubic hair stages at spermarche. Median 2.5, $n = 31$.
From Nielson CT, Skakkebaek NE, Richardson DW: Onset of the release of spermatozoa (spermarche) in boys in relation to age, testicular growth, pubic hair, and height. J Clin Endocrinol 62:534, 1986.

range, the first ejaculation was reported an average of 1 year later (14.6 years) in boys from lower socioeconomic strata.

Spermarche. Mature sperm appear in the ejaculate before the peak of the height velocity curve, but this may occur at any stage of pubertal development, from SMR 2 to 5 (Fig. 8–8) (Nielsen et al., 1986). Various studies have found the median age for appearance of sperm in the first morning urine sample to be between 13.5 and 14.5 years (see also Fig. 8-9). Complete fertility in males is not reached until Stage 5 of pubertal development, but it is apparent that impregnation is possible much earlier. Anticipatory guidance in the area of pregnancy prevention must therefore be initiated during early to middle adolescence.

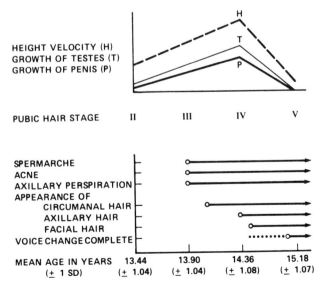

Figure 8–9. Sequence of maturational events in males. Adapted from Marshall and Tanner (1969).
From Litt IF: Adolescent development. In Behrman RE, Vaughan VC III (eds): *Nelson Textbook of Pediatrics,* 13th ed. Philadelphia, WB Saunders Company, 1987.

Ovulation. The ovary contains its full complement of ova at the time of birth. With the onset of pituitary gonadotropin stimulation at puberty, these ova begin to mature and estrogen is produced. The uterus at this stage of development is equally divided between the corpus and the cervix, as it is in the child. The secretion of estrogen results in endometrial thickening and differentiation, as well as increase in cellular content of actinomysin, creatine phosphokinase, and ATP of the myometrium, presumably in preparation for menses and childbirth. The ratio of size of the corpus uteri to the cervix increases.

Menarche. The onset of menstrual periods (menarche) now occurs in the United States at an average age of 12.5 years, with a normal range of 10 to 16 years. This was not always the case. A change toward an earlier average age of menarche of 3 to 4 months per decade has occurred over the past 100 years. This trend appears to have recently leveled off. Amundsen and Diers (1973) have reported that during the Classical period (4th century BC to the 7th century AD) and in Medieval times, menarchal age was not very different from that of today (approximately 13 years of age). Why it was as high as 17 years in the late 18th and early 19th centuries is not understood.

The timing of menarche is closely related to other pubertal events (Fig. 8–10) (Litt, 1987). For example, 10 per cent of girls have their menarche at SMR 2, another 20 per cent at SMR 3, another 60 per cent at SMR 4, and the remaining 10 per cent at SMR 5. As seen in Figure 8–11, there is a close association between the timing of the weight spurt and the onset of menstruation: the latter is coincident with the peak of the weight velocity curve, which occurs approximately 6 months after the peak of the height velocity curve. The relationship between skeletal development and menarche is so close that failure of menses to begin by the time that bone age has reached 14.5 years is generally considered a signal for medical evaluation for primary amenorrhea.

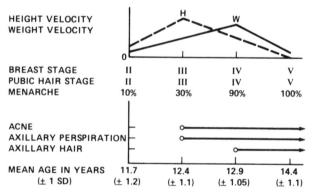

Figure 8–10. Sequence of maturational events in females. Adapted from Marshall and Tanner (1969).
From Litt IF: Adolescent development. In Behrman RE, Vaughan VC III (eds): *Nelson Textbook of Pediatrics,* 13th ed. Philadelphia, WB Saunders Company, 1987.

With menarche typically occurring at the peak of the weight velocity curve, the relationship between weight (fat tissue) and menarche has received much attention. A hypothesis (Frisch, 1976) that body fat must reach 17 per cent in order for menarche to be reached has not been substantiated (Trussell, 1980), but it is apparent that girls with more fat tissue have earlier menarche than those who are lean. In addition, weight loss of as little as 10 per cent of body weight may cause cessation of menses, as well as loss of pulsatile secretion of Gn-RH, LH, and FSH (Schweiger et al., 1987). Weight loss of even 5 per cent may result in shortened luteal phase. The profound weight loss associated with anorexia nervosa results in amenorrhea (primary or secondary, depending on the age at onset), as well as pubertal delay in the young patient of either sex (Palla and Litt, 1988).

Vigorous athletic training is also associated with delay in menarche and/or interruption of normal menstrual function (Shangold, 1985). A number of possible explanations for this phenomenon have been suggested. Some have attributed the menstrual dysfunction to the often-associated weight loss, others to the physical and/or emotional stress of competition. Malina (1983) observes that the body habitus characteristically found in amenorrheic ballet dancers and runners (that is, a lean, tall body with a relatively low ratio of upper to lower body segments) is also typical of late maturers. He suggests the possibility that girls with the desired body type may self-select into these activities, rather than that the body type and menstrual dysfunction are the result of such activities.

The timing of menarche is also determined largely by familial patterns, with close concordance ($r = .4$) between the menarcheal ages of mothers and daughters. Siblings' menarcheal ages are more closely related even than those of mothers and daughters. One study found the average difference in age at menarche between nonidentical twins to be 8 months, whereas the difference between identical twins was only 2 months.

There are ethnic differences in age at menarche: for example, in the United States it is earliest in Hispanics, later in blacks, and latest in Caucasians (Litt and Cohen, 1973). Menarche occurs later in rural than in urban areas, and earlier at lower altitudes. Birth order also appears to affect mean age at menarche, which is 0.19 years earlier with each subsequent birth.

Other factors, such as chronic illnesses, particularly those that interfere with nutrition or tissue oxygenation, will delay menarche (Table 8–7) (Litt, 1983a). For reasons that are not understood, blindness is associated with earlier onset of menarche. Medications may also cause amenorrhea (Table 8–8) (Litt, 1983a).

The commonly held view that menarche signals the onset of reproductive capacity is somewhat misleading, since most girls do not ovulate regularly with menstrual periods until the second year after menarche. On the other hand, although it is rare, pregnancy has been reported to have occurred before the first menstrual period.

TABLE 8–7. Chronic Illness Associated with Delayed Pubertal Development and Amenorrhea[*]

Endocrine
 Hypothalamic tumor
 Pituitary
 Insufficiency Tumor
Thyroid
 Hypersecretion
 (Rarely hyposecretion)
Adrenal
 Insufficiency
 Hypersecretion
Diabetes mellitus (poorly controlled)
Hematologic
 Sickle cell anemia
 Thalassemia major
Gastrointestinal
 Inflammatory bowel disease
 Cystic fibrosis
Cardiac
 Congenital cyanotic heart disease

[*] From Litt IF: Menstrual problems during adolescence. Pediatr Rev 4:203–212, 1983.

TABLE 8–8. Drugs That May Cause Amenorrhea[*]

Hormones
 Estrogens
 Progestogens
 Testosterone
Antihypertensives
 Methyldopa
Antidepressants
 Phenothiazines
Chemotherapeutic agents
 Cyclophosphamide
 Chlorambucil
 Vincaleukoblastine
 Methylhydrazine
Radioisotopes
 ^{32}P
 ^{131}I
 ^{198}Au
Vitamins
 A (in toxic doses)
Illicit drugs
 Heroin

[*] From Litt IF: Menstrual problems during adolescence. Pediatr Rev 4:203–212, 1983.

"Secondary" Sex Characteristics. Bodily changes that occur at the onset of puberty as the result of the influence of testicular or adrenal androgens or of ovarian estrogens are called secondary sex characteristics. These include changes in genitalia and breasts and the appearance of sexual hair, which is rather variable in timing of onset, except in the pubic region. In both sexes, the first sexual hair is nearly always pubic.

The progression of development of sexual hair in males is outlined in Figure 8–11. Axillary hair appears approximately 1.3 years after the first pubic hair, followed about 1 year later by facial hair. The latter typically begins at the corners of the upper lip and spreads medially to create a moustache. This is followed by appearance of hair on the upper cheek, under the lower lip, and on the chin. Circumanal hair appears at approximately SMR 3. Tanner and Marshall (1974) suggest that growth of hair on the chin signals completion of puberty. Growth of chest hair in males is a later, postpubertal event. The first appearance of body hair is coincident with that of axillary hair. Recession of the hairline (male pattern baldness) begins during late puberty in one third of males.

In females, axillary hair appears approximately 1 year after pubic hair. Around the time of appearance of pubic hair, apocrine glands of the vulva and axilla become functional. Other secondary sex characteristics that appear in both boys and girls include acne and the apocrine gland secretions (the origin of dreaded "body odor"). In males, change of voice

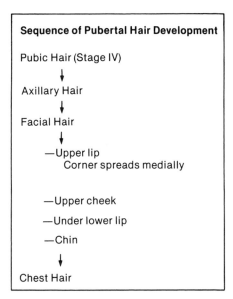

Figure 8–11. Sequence of pubertal hair development.

occurs, typically at SMR 3 to 4, as well as marked growth of external genitalia.

Those pubertal changes that are most consistent in the order of their occurrence and in their progression involve breast development in females, the appearance and evolution of pubic hair in both sexes, and the development of external genitalia in males. These characteristics are, therefore, used to establish the sex maturity ratings (SMRs 1 to 5) that Tanner proposed to describe the successive stages of puberty (Figs. 8–12 through 8–14). The SMRs are often referred to as "Tanner stages," though others had made similar observations earlier (Greulich et al., 1942).

SMR 1 corresponds to the childlike stage, before signs of development of secondary sex characteristics appear. SMR 5 describes the final stage of pubertal development, which corresponds to fully adult bodily habitus and reproductive maturity. Between these extremes, an amazing transformation occurs within a relatively short period of 3 to 4 years.

SMR 2 in Males. The interrelationships in development of secondary sex characteristics for males are outlined in Fig. 8–9.

The early signs of increased production of testosterone are found in changes in the external genitalia and pubic hair. The scrotal skin begins to redden and thin as it becomes more vascular. The scrotum itself assumes the adult configuration of a narrower proximal portion with the left testis lower than the right. Enlargement of the penis begins shortly thereafter; it remains relatively thin in proportion to its length until later in puberty (SMR 3 to 4), when acceleration of the growth of the corpora cavernosa eventuates in adult penile width.

The evolution of the consistency and distribution of pubic hair follows a predictable pattern in both sexes, and consequently is a reliable index of

Pubertal development of female pubic hair.

Stage 1. There is no pubic hair.

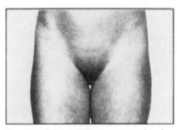 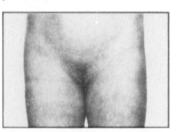

Stage 2. There is sparse growth of long, slightly pigmented, downy hair, straight or only slightly curled, primarily along the labia.

Stage 3. The hair is considerably darker, coarser, and more curled. The hair spreads sparsely over the junction of the pubes.

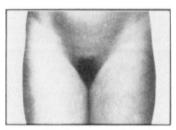 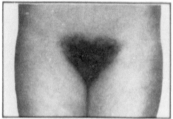

Stage 4. The hair, now adult in type, covers a smaller area than in the adult and does not extend onto the thighs.

Stage 5. The hair is adult in quantity and type, with extension onto the thighs.

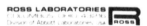

ROSS LABORATORIES
Division of Abbott Laboratories, USA

Figure 8-12. Pubertal development of female pubic hair. From Tanner JM: *Growth at Adolescence,* 2nd ed. London, Blackwell Scientific Publications, 1962.

Pubertal development in size of female breasts.

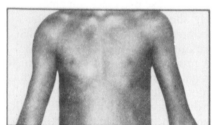 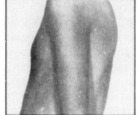

Stage 1. The breasts are preadolescent. There is elevation of the papilla only.

Figure 8-13. Typical progression of pubertal development in size of female breasts. From Tanner JM: *Growth at Adolescence,* 2nd ed. London, Blackwell Scientific Publications, 1962.

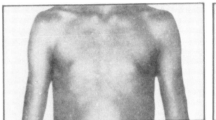 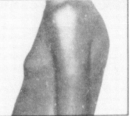

Stage 2. Breast bud stage. A small mound is formed by the elevation of the breast and papilla. The areolar diameter enlarges.

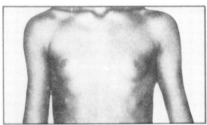 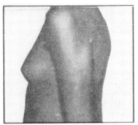

Stage 3. There is further enlargement of breasts and areola with no separation of their contours.

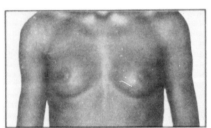 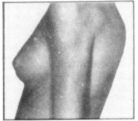

Stage 4. There is a projection of the areola and papilla to form a secondary mound above the level of the breast.

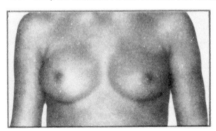 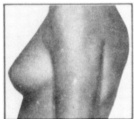

Stage 5. The breasts resemble those of a mature female as the areola has recessed to the general contour of the breast.

Figure 8-13. (*continued*).

Pubertal development in size of male genitalia.

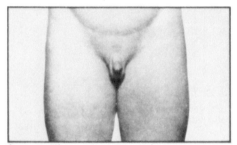

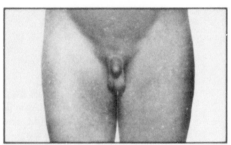

Stage 1. The penis, testes, and scrotum are of childhood size.

Stage 2. There is enlargement of the scrotum and testes, but the penis usually does not enlarge. The scrotal skin reddens.

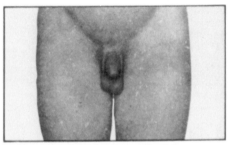

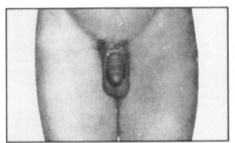

Stage 3. There is further growth of the testes and scotum and enlargement of the penis, mainly in length.

Stage 4. There is still further growth of the testes and scrotum and increased size of the penis, especially in breadth.

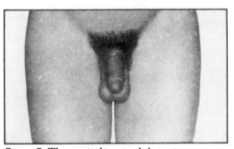

Stage 5. The genitalia are adult in size and shape.

Figure 8–14. Typical progression of pubertal development in size of male genitalia. From Tanner JM: *Growth at Adolescence,* 2nd ed. London, Blackwell Scientific Publications, 1962.

pubertal progression. At SMR 2 pubic hair is fine, long, silky, and lightly pigmented, and appears mainly in the midline, surrounding the base of the phallus. The mean age for attaining SMR 2 in males is 11.64 years (± 1.07) for genitalia, and 13.44 years (± 1.09) for pubic hair.

The areola of the nipple increases in diameter in males with the onset of puberty, and approximately one third of males experience breast tissue enlargement (gynecomastia) as well, at an average age of 14 years (usually at SMR 2 to 3). The enlargement usually consists of a dime to quarter-sized mass directly beneath the nipple. The mass may be tender, and the nipple as well.

Gynecomastia is unilateral in 40 per cent of cases and occurs more often on the left side. Areolar enlargement persists for life, whereas that of the breast tissue mass itself is usually transient, typically regressing within 18 months of onset and only very rarely requiring surgical intervention (Nydick et al., 1961).

Gynecomastia has been attributed to a pubertal rise in serum estradiol levels (to about 25 pg/mL) that approximates the rise that occurs in females at the time of breast budding. Were this the only factor, however, the regression of breast tissue enlargement in males would be difficult to explain. The rare pathologic causes of gynecomastia are listed in Table 8–9.

TABLE 8–9. Causes of Gynecomastia in the Adolescent

Physiologic
Nutritional (refeeding)
Genetic/Congenital
    Klinefelter syndrome
    Hermaphroditism
    Testicular feminization
Endocrine
    Adrenal hyperplasia
    Thyrotoxicosis
    Testicular failure
Neoplastic
    Testicular
    Prolactin-secreting
Pharmacologic
    Amphetamines
    Cimetidine
    Cyclophosphamide
    Isoniazid
    Ketoconazole
    Marijuana
    Phenothiazine
    Reserpine

TABLE 8–10. Hematologic Values for Adolescent Males

	SMR AND HEMATOCRIT (%)				
	1	2	3	4	5
Whites					
Mean	39.5	39.8	40.9	42.3	43.8
Range	37.1–41.8	36.7–42.8	38.2–43.5	39.7–44.8	41.1–46.4
Blacks					
Mean	37.7	38.4	39.7	41.1	42.7
Range	35.2–40.2	36.0–40.9	37.3–42.0	38.3–43.8	39.6–45.9

* From Copeland K, Brookman RR, Rauh JL: Assessment of Pubertal Development. Columbus, Ohio, Ross Laboratories, 1986.

The hematocrit rises above childhood values in males at SMR 2, owing largely to the stimulatory effect of androgens on erythropoietin production. This rise must be taken into account in evaluating the hematologic status of males in adolescence (Table 8–10). Serum alkaline phosphatase activity rises at SMR 2, reaching an average of 90 IU/L in males at this stage.

SMR 2 in Females. Breast development is the most salient secondary sex characteristic for the female. SMR 2 begins with the appearance of a breast bud and with an increase in the diameter of the areola. Less apparent effects of estrogen stimulation involve the external genitalia: thickening and softening of the vaginal mucosa; increased pigmentation, vascularization, and eroticization of the labia majora; and slight enlargement of the clitoris. The hymen thickens and the diameter of its orifice increases to a maximum of approximately 15 mm.

Increased deposition of glycogen within the cells of the vaginal mucosa, another estrogen effect, favors the growth of Döderlein (lactic acid–forming) bacteria. This results in a change of vaginal pH to acid, as well as increased susceptibility to yeast infections.

Bartholin glands begin secretion, and the upper portion of the vagina becomes more distensible. Cervical secretion of mucoid material begins, giving rise to a milky, nonmalodorous discharge. Cervical enlargement is followed by growth of the uterine corpus, with the lengths of the two segments of the uterus becoming equal just prior to menarche.

In females at SMR 2, as in males, pubic hair first appears as fine, long, silky strands, usually first in the midline of the labia, or rarely first on the mons pubis. In addition to their effect on hair growth, androgens produce in both sexes increases in the size and secretions of sebaceous follicles; these changes are forerunners of acne.

The mean age for achieving SMR 2 for breast development in girls is 11.15 years (±1.10) and for pubic hair is 11.69 years (±1.21).

In contrast with males, in whom advancing stages of puberty are associated with increasing hematocrit levels, in females there is a decrement related to pubertal stage. The possible diagnosis of anemia is again related to these levels (Table 8–11).

Height and Weight. According to Tanner and Marshall (1974), in approximately 30 to 40 per cent of girls the peak of height velocity curve is

TABLE 8-11. Hematologic Values for Adolescent Females

	SMR AND HEMATOCRIT (%)				
	1	2	3	4	5
Whites					
Mean	39.1	39.2	39.6	39.2	39.2
Range	36.1–42.1	37.1–41.3	37.0–42.2	36.9–41.6	36.2–42.2
Blacks					
Mean	37.3	38.9	39.0	38.4	38.7
Range	34.6–39.9	35.7–42.1	35.2–42.6	34.9–42.8	35.9–41.5

* From Copeland K, Brookman RR, Rauh JL: Assessment of Pubertal Development. Columbus, Ohio, Ross Laboratories, 1986.

reached at SMR 2 (breast). This corresponds to an average age of 12.14 years (± 0.14). The average increase in height for girls from the beginning to the end of the pubertal growth spurt is 25 cm. For boys, it is 28 cm. Although the lower extremity experiences its growth spurt earlier, most of the increase in stature that takes place at this time is in the trunk.

The peak of the weight velocity curve is reached approximately 0.5 year after that of the height velocity curve for girls and 0.2 year later for boys. Those boys who experience their growth spurt during early adolescence are both taller and stronger than their later maturing peers at this time; these findings are associated with athletic and social advantage in our society. The early maturing female, on the other hand, appears to be at a disadvantage in some respects (see p. 300).

Dentition

The cuspids (canines) and first molars of the primary dentition are shed by early adolescence. The permanent cuspids, first and second premolars, and second molars erupt during this period and assume the positions of their predecessors (see Table 1–7). Eruption of permanent teeth occurs slightly earlier in girls than boys. There is close correlation between the timing of eruption of the second permanent molar and of menarche ($r = .62$). Hyperthyroidism and precocious puberty are associated with accelerated eruption of teeth, as are certain anomalies such as hemifacial hypertrophy.

Adolescence is the time of the second peak in incidence of caries. A study by the National Institute of Dental Research (National Caries Program, 1981) found that by the age of 12 years, children in the United States had an average of four decayed, missing, or filled permanent teeth, and that by the age of 17 years, this number has risen to 11. Excessive ingestion of refined carbohydrates, particularly of sucrose, by adolescents is thought to be responsible for this increase. A specific microorganism (*Streptococcus mutans*) is thought also to play a role. Prevention of caries may be promoted by substitution of snacks that do not stick to the teeth, as well as by use of dental floss and by brushing teeth with a fluoride dentifrice.

Late childhood and early adolescence are the preferred times for most orthodontic therapy, but maintainance of results may require continuation of certain devices until growth has ceased. The form of malocclusion that is associated with tonsillar and adenoidal hypertrophy tends to occur primarily during early adolescence and involves constricted upper dental arches. Treatment requires coordination between pediatrician, orthodontist, otolaryngologist, and, often, an allergist. The posterior surfaces of the teeth should be examined, as enamel erosion in that location may provide a clue as to the possibility of bulimia (binge eating with self-induced purging) (see later in this chapter).

Skeletal Development

For a discussion of skeletal development, see pp. 294–295.

Neurodevelopment

By the age of 10 years the brain has achieved 95 per cent of its adult weight. There are no further gross changes in brain morphology during adolescence. Epstein (1974) has proposed that there is a spurt in brain circumference between the ages of 10 and 12 years, and another around the age of 15 years, with slow growth at the ages of 13 to 14 years. Epstein's data are controversial, however, and inconsistent with other growth data in the finding of sex differences in the timing of various growth phenomena. It is of concern that he may have failed to consider the differences between early and late maturers.

The electroencephalogram gives evidence of continuing neurodevelopmental maturation, with an increase in alpha-2 wave activity paralleling a decrease in theta activity. This phenomenon is most dramatic in girls during early adolescence. Organization of sleep also undergoes change during pubertal development; there is increased daytime sleepiness and decreased sleep latency during middle adolescence (SMRs 3 to 4) (Anders et al., 1980).

By this stage of development, the adolescent should manifest a "mature" response on all items of a standardized neurodevelopmental assessment, such as the PEEX (Levine, 1983). The last items to mature do so by the age of 12 years. The last items include the abilities: 1) to identify correctly stimulated fingers in a finger localization task; 2) to distinguish left and right starting from new bases, such as those in marching commands; and 3) the ability to separate the third and fourth fingers without "overflow" movement to other fingers.

Cognitive Development

Cognitive development has in the past generally been assessed largely in relation to chronologic age. As a result, the relationship between stages of pubertal development and cognition has been unclear and remains so. The few recent studies that have attempted to account for the effects of puberty on cognitive function have given inconsistent results. Carey et al.

(1980), for example, using face recognition as the assessment tool, concluded that the onset of puberty has a disruptive effect on cognition in girls. Peterson (1983), on the other hand, using different measures of cognition, failed to find any such disruption.

Piaget classified his subjects on the basis of chronologic age, rather than in relationship to stage of pubertal development (Table 8–12). At 12 or 13 years of age, therefore, there is considerable overlap of youngsters who would be considered to be still at the piagetian stage of concrete operations with those who have advanced to formal operations.

At the piagetian stage of formal operational thinking, the individual is

TABLE 8–12. Piaget's Eras and Stages of Logical and Cognitive Development[*]

Era I (age 0–2) The era of sensorimotor intelligence
Stage 1. Reflex action.
Stage 2. Coordination of reflexes and sensorimotor repetition (primary circular reaction).
Stage 3. Activities to make interesting events in the environment reappear (secondary circular reaction).
Stage 4. Means/ends behavior and search for absent objects.
Stage 5. Experimental search for new means (tertiary circular reaction).
Stage 6. Use of imagery in insightful invention of new means and in recall of absent objects and events.

Era II (age 2–5) Symbolic, intuitive, or prelogical thought
Inference is carried on through images and symbols which do not maintain logical relations or invariances with one another. "Magical thinking" in the sense of (a) confusion of apparent or imagined events with real events and objects and (b) confusion of perceptual appearances of qualitative and quantitative change with actual change.

Era III (age 6–10) Concrete operational thought
Inferences carried on through system of classes, relations, and quantities maintaining logically invariant properties and which *refer to concrete objects*. These include such logical processes as (a) inclusion of lower-order classes in higher order classes; (b) transitive seriation (recognition that if a > b and b > c, then a > c); (c) logical addition and multiplication of classes and quantities; (d) conservation of number, class membership, length, and mass under apparent change.
Substage 1. Formation of stable categorical classes.
Substage 2. Formation of quantitative and numerical relations of invariance.

Era IV (age 11 to adulthood) Formal-operational thought
Inferences through logical operations upon propositions or "operations upon operations." Reasoning about reasoning. Construction of systems of all possible relations or implications. Hypothetico-deductive isolation of variables and testing of hypotheses.
Substage 1. Formation of the inverse of the reciprocal. Capacity to form negative classes (for example, the class of all not-crows) and to see relations as simultaneously reciprocal (for example, to understand that liquid in a U-shaped tube holds an equal level because of counterbalanced pressures).
Substage 2. Capacity to order triads of propositions or relations (for example, to understand that if Bob is taller than Joe and Joe is shorter than Dick, then Joe is the shortest of the three).
Substage 3. True formal thought. Construction of all possible combinations of relations, systematic isolation of variables, and deductive hypothesis-testing.

[*] From Kagan J, Coles R: New York, WW Norton & Co, 1972.

presumed to be capable of generating hypotheses to be tested before action is initiated, of thinking abstractly, of entertaining multiple contingencies simultaneously, of generalizing, and of considering possible consequences of behavior in a logical manner without actually having experienced them. This notion is currently being reexamined (see below). If it is accurate, it poses interesting questions for physicians and others as to when the relationship with the teenage patient should be changed from that which existed during childhood to the confidential patient-physician arrangement appropriate for adult patients.

Health behaviors are influenced by the patient's ability to understand the consequences of proposed therapy. Is it necessary for the teenager to have reached the stage of formal operations in order to be capable of engaging in such a relationship? If so, how can one judge when this has happened? Attainment of this stage is often associated with the young person's development of interests in the occult, the mystic, and the religious, which may have their own implications for his or her health status. Vegetarianism or adherence to a spiritually prescribed dietary regimen may occur at this time, challenging the health care provider to offer nutritional counsel appropriate to the young patient's belief system (see pp. 277–280).

A recent challenge to piagetian theory has been primarily directed at his emphasis on clear-cut, discrete stages. A revised view, as articulated by Flavell (1985), emphasizes "developmental trends" that are thought to evolve during childhood and adolescence and that involve more overlap and variation than previously thought. These trends include:

1. *Information-processing capacity.* Adolescents appear superior to younger children in their capacities for information-processing functions, but it is not yet known whether this is associated with any increase in their structural capacity with age.

2. *Domain-specific knowledge.* As a child ages, he or she accumulates more and more organized knowledge in different, specific domains, allowing for problem-solving by memory processes unavailable to the younger child.

3. *Concrete and formal operations.* The piagetian notions are viewed as trends, rather than specific stages, such that the younger child's approach is viewed as more "empirico-deductive," whereas that of the adolescent is more "hypothetico-deductive."

4. *Quantitative thinking.* Adolescents tend to approach problems with a "more quantitative, measurement-oriented set" than younger children as a result of acquisition of "the concept of a unit measure."

5. *A "sense of the game."* With increasing age, children become increasingly interested in thinking as a game and are challenged by it.

6. *Metacognition.* This concept refers to thinking about thinking and is divided by Flavell into metacognitive knowledge and metacognitive experiences. The first "refers to your accumulated declarative and procedural knowledge concerning cognitive matters," and the second to affective experiences of the "Eureka!" or, conversely, the "This doesn't make sense to me" variety. Metacognition develops considerably between childhood and the end of adolescence.

7. *Improving existing competencies.* The maturation of competencies once acquired is a continuing process during development. Sex differ-

ences appear to emerge during early adolescence, boys performing better in areas of spatial ability and mathematics and girls excelling in verbal ability (Jacklin and Maccoby, 1983). (It is not clear to what degree these sex differences reflect cultural expectations, rather than biologic imperatives.)

Closely related to cognitive development is that of **moral thought.** As earlier indicated, Kohlberg and Gilligan (1971) proposed a developmental theory about moral reasoning that they believed evolved in six stages. The first two stages are included in the *preconventional level*, which includes most children who view rules and social expectations to be external to the self and is rather egocentric in terms of comprehension of fairness. In Stage 1, authority is unquestioned and obedience is valued in order to avoid punishment. In Stage 2, right is defined in terms of fulfillment of one's own needs and interests.

At the *conventional level*, which includes late adolescents and adults, the rules and expectations of the society have been internalized. At stage 3 the concept of fairness is rooted in societal consensus, with right defined in terms of shared needs and interpersonal relationships leading to conformity. Stage 4 focuses on maintenance of the social order.

The highest, *postconventional* level is reached by a minority of adults, who attain Stage 5. (Stage 6 has been discarded from the original schema because of lack of validation in Kohlberg's longitudinal study). Stage 5 is the stage in which what is right is conceptualized on the basis of reciprocity of standards that have been agreed upon by the whole society and freestanding logic. This highest level is characterized by the ability to use deductive reasoning when faced with moral dilemmas, to see flaws in the law, and to be able to see differences between law and morality. As such the "major thrust [is] toward autonomous moral principles which have validity and application apart from authority of the groups or persons who hold them and apart from the individual's identification with those persons or groups" (Flavell, 1985).

The rate of attainment of these progressive stages of development, the order of which Kohlberg believed to be invariant, is based on cognitive developmental attainment and experiential prerequisites. At the time of entry into formal operations in the piagetian schema, for example, an adolescent is considered to have reached the postconventional level of moral development.

Just as piagetian theory is currently being reexamined, so, too, is that of Kohlberg. There is concern that the basis for his scheme of moral development, rooted as it is in progression toward autonomy and power, may be more applicable to the experience of males in our society than of females, for whom relationships and feelings are more relevant to the ontogeny of moral decision-making. Gilligan's examples (1982) of differing responses of male and female early adolescents illustrate this point.

The moral dilemma that Gilligan posed to male and female adolescents involved a man who is considering whether or not he should steal from a druggist the medication that he cannot afford in order to save his wife's life. The 11-year-old male is clear that the only recourse is to steal the drug, conceptualizing the conflict as being one between property and life; in so doing he acknowledges limitations of the law. The 11-year-old female, on the other hand, responds that the husband should not steal the drug because he would go to jail, and then his wife would lose him; in this the subject is highlighting the importance of relationships. "Instead, seeing a world comprised of relationships rather than of people standing alone, a world that coheres through human connection rather than through systems of rules, she finds the puzzle in the dilemma to lie in the failure of the druggist to respond to the wife. . . . Thus she considers the solution to the dilemma to lie in making the wife's condition more salient to the druggist or, that failing, in appealing to others who are in a position to help."

From Kohlberg's perspective, the girl's response to the above dilemma would be considered less mature than that of the boy for it suggests powerlessness, an inability to think systematically about issues of morality and law, and a reluctance to challenge authority. As Gilligan points out, however, the young girl's world is one of "relationships and psychologic truths where an awareness of the connection between people gives rise to a recognition of responsibility for one another, a perception of the need for response." Gilligan's criticism notwithstanding, the weight of Walker's review (1984) of the literature on possible sex differences in development of moral reasoning found that there have been few, if any, sex differences reported.

The way a young person behaves when faced with pressure to smoke, drink, use drugs, or have premature sexual experiences will be determined by a number of factors, one of which is his or her stage of development of moral thought. Accordingly, it is less important for the physician who is providing anticipatory guidance to judge the level of development than it is to be able to provide the necessary factual information for the young person to process at whatever his or her developmental level may be.

Psychosocial Developmental Tasks

Some of the literature on adolescence suggests that the development of self-image and of independence are tasks exclusively of this age group. Such a view is misleading, as both are significant factors throughout the earlier years of life. Separation-individuation is a salient issue to be negotiated by 2-year-olds, for example (see pp. 88–94, 183), and self-image has its origins in experiences that occur soon after birth and continue throughout life, shaped by ongoing interactions with the environment and with significant people and events.

Burns (1984) describes the process by which self-concept develops as: "never really ends; it is actively proceeding from birth to death as the individual continually discovers new potentials in the process of 'becoming'. . . . To have a self-concept, the child must come to view himself as a distinct object and be able to see himself as both subject and object, distinguishing himself from other objects. He must then become aware of other perspectives, for only in that way can he become aware of the evaluations of others about him."

Burns further identifies five major sources of self-conception, the importance of each of which varies over the life span: body image, language, interpretation of relative standing in relation to societal norms, sex role identification, and child-rearing practices. What is unique to the adolescent years is the advent of puberty, which may upset the homeostasis established during childhood and requires integration of one's new physical self and the social definition of such maturational changes into one's self-concept (see pp. 94, 300).

Autonomy

The early adolescent must function in three arenas: family, peer group, and school. In each there exists a complex interplay of determinants of successful functioning.

A popular view is that adolescence is a time of separation from parental influence and that such separation is achieved through deviance and rebellion in the context of peer group influences. This is not necessarily the case. When populations of normal adolescents are studied, rather than those drawn from psychiatric cases or delinquent groups, it appears that the emotional ties between teenager and parent undergo transformation during adolescence in continuity with relationships established during earlier childhood. Studies by Brittain (1967) show, for example, that peer influences dominate decisions that relate to style of dress, but that parents still hold sway over moral decisions and those that determine employment.

Baumrind (1988) sees parents as being most influential in the context of long-range educational aspirations and occupational plans, whereas adolescents "comply with peer standards up to a point to achieve status and identity within the peer group." Baumrind writes that a competent adolescent will be one from a family system that "avoids both enmeshment, in which family members are expected to act and think alike, as well as disengagement, in which family members are so separate that they have little effect on each other. Family processes that balance expressions of individuality (both self-assertion and differentiation of self from others) with expressions of connectedness (permeability to and respect for the views of others) are most effective in generating competence."

Offer (1973), on the basis of a comprehensive study of middle-class, Midwestern suburban teen-aged males, states: "The transitional period of adolescence does present the adolescent with a special burden, a challenge, and an opportunity. He has to individualize, build up confidence in himself and his abilities, make important decisions concerning his future, and free himself of his earlier attachments to his parents. Our observations have led us to conclude that the majority of the teen-agers in our sample cope with these tasks successfully. They lack the turmoil of the disturbed adolescent precisely because their ego is strong enough to withstand the pressures. In their task they are greatly helped by the parents."

Offer reported that turmoil did occur, however, during early adolescence (ages 12 to 14 years), according to both the teenagers and parents. Offer believes that this turmoil or rebellion is in the service of emancipation from parents and "is characterized by chronic infighting (lasting one to two years) with parents and school teachers in the pre-high-school years. This infighting is over issues that seem small or undramatic. The rebellion does not involve serious or repeated delinquencies, nor does it involve the plunging and rising of great emotional states. "Bickering" is the word most characteristic of these disturbances."

Offer continues: "The adolescent is in conflict over his desires to be emancipated, and the rebellious behavior is a compromise formation that supports his efforts to give up the parent and at the same time gratifies his dependent longings for them. That the adolescent is not confident of his emancipation—has not completed the process of emancipation—might imply an underlying persistance of unacceptable dependency wishes." The majority of teenagers in Offer's sample described their parents as supportive and were proud of their close relationships with them. Accordingly, it is not surprising that most researchers find that adolescents choose peer groups with values not very dissimilar from those of their parents.

Mussen et al. (1969) hold that when conflict between parent and teenager occurs, it tends to fall into one of two categories. The first involves "issues involving greater adolescent demands for independence than the parents are willing to grant," and the second, "issues involving more dependent, or childish, behavior on the part of the adolescent than the parents feel able to tolerate." Assumed under the first would be such topics as bed time and choice of friends, whereas the second would include parental criticism of behaviors such as sloppiness, teasing of younger siblings, or failure to perform assigned household chores.

The Relationship of Parenting Styles to Development of Autonomy. Kandell and Lesser (1972) compared family and peer relations of secondary school students from Denmark and the United States. With autonomy subjectively defined as teenagers' perception as to whether they are given sufficient freedom, Danish teenagers were found to feel that they are given more freedom than American youngsters. Those who described themselves as autonomous, regardless of country, lived in families with few rules. "The families were more often democratic in decision-making than authoritarian or permissive and they were families in which, whatever the authority structure, parental rules and judgments were more often explained than not. . . . The feeling of being granted independence was associated with positive interactions with parents. There was not estrangement but avowed closeness and positive feeling: The number of young people who brought their problems to their parents to talk over *increased* over the years from 14 through 19 from 9% to 48%." Those who perceived themselves as being independent were also those who enjoyed their parents company, felt closer to them, and aspired to be like them.

Elder (1968) broadened the definition of autonomy to include the cognitive dimension of confidence of judgment and a behavioral dimension of help-seeking. His findings agreed with those of Kandell and Lesser to the extent that subjective independence was associated with democratic decision-making, but differed in that he found adolescents from permissive families to be more autonomous.

The effect of parenting styles on the development of autonomy has been extensively studied by Baumrind (1968) in a longitudinal study of middle-class youngsters. She distinguished four patterns of nonlenient parenting: traditional, authoritarian-restrictive, punitive, and authoritative.

In *traditional* families, those who value conformity and continuity, teenagers "may circumvent altogether the adolescent individuation crisis. . . . However, there is a price to be paid for bypassing . . . [as] these young people are likely to show deficits in the areas of autonomy and creativity."

In *"authoritarian-restrictive"* families, teenagers are kept in subordinate roles without a voice in family discussions and responsibilities. "When coercive authority is not relinquished during the adolescent transition, children are less likely to attribute responsibility to themselves as moral agents and therefore not to feel obliged to abide by the explicit or implicit contracts they have with their parents or with society. Authoritarian parents, unlike traditional parents, are likely therefore to incite reactive rebellion in some adolescents as well as to reduce the moral maturity of most."

Harsh and *punitive* parents raise teenagers who believe that "morality is inevitably arbitrary and self-serving, thus providing a rationale in experience for immoral behavior" often leading to little experience of guilt and antisocial aggression.

Authoritative parents are firm, consistent, and responsive to their children. During adolescence, they encourage democratic participation and share power with their youngsters. Baumrind found that their daughters, as young adolescents, were most socially assertive, and their sons most socially responsible.

Family Interaction

The major developmental task of early adolescence is to initiate the process of establishing independence from the family. The negotiation of this task is typically gradual and often symbolic, although, as indicated above, some of the less common features involving outward rebellion have tended to be widely accepted as the norm and have given adolescence "a bad name."

Hill and Holmbeck (1986) have written: "There is considerable evidence that . . . emotional attachments of adolescents to their parents are strong and this is unlikely to change. Parents, by and large, continue to be a major force in socialization in their functions both as models of adult behaviour and as sources of sanctions for behaviour of which they approve or disapprove. Occupational and educational aspirations are, for example, more strongly influenced by parental than by peer standards. Conflict between parent and peer pressures most often occurs in matters related to adolescent behaviour in the peer group and less often in relation to socialization for achievement."

Adolescence does have an impact on the family, often upsetting earlier homeostasis. The adolescent's unspoken wish for limit-setting is often in conflict with his or her need for autonomy, and unresolved parental needs are often reawakened by these stresses.

The prime stimulus for shifts in family balance during adolescence in our society is typically the onset of pubertal development, which is a potent signal to adults that their youngster is becoming capable of reproduction. The previously affectionate parent of the opposite sex may suddenly become uncomfortable with physical closeness and the adolescent may suddenly demand privacy, both reactions resulting in increased distance and decreased opportunities for interaction. The need for privacy extends to the examining room, as well. Gowning and draping, as well as care and sensitivity in the wording of the medical history and maintaining confidentiality, show respect for this often unspoken need.

Steinberg (1988) found that from the onset of puberty to its apex, male adolescents and their mothers interrupt each other with increasing frequency. Male adolescents defer to their fathers more and their mothers less; mothers and sons explain themselves less frequently; and there is increasing rigidity in patterns of familial interaction. In late adolescence, mothers' interruptions of their sons decrease and there is some lessening of rigidity. Throughout pubertal development, there is increased paternal assertiveness. The temporal relationship of events suggested that the conflict is initiated by the adolescent, rather than by his mother, and that the increase in her assertiveness was in response to his, not vice versa.

The shift toward more deferential treatment of fathers during early puberty is in marked contrast with the mother-son pattern and warrants exploration in a population of daughters. This change in family homeostasis results in a shift of the male to a higher position in the hierarchy, above that of the mother in family decision-making.

In both sexes, pubertal maturation is associated with distancing between the adolescent and the family. For example, among girls and their mothers pubertal maturation increases the number of arguments and decreases the number of calm discussions they have with their fathers. Steinberg found that the midpoint of the pubertal growth spurt was associated with dimunition of father-daughter cohesion. Interestingly, data from nonhuman primates and more recently from studies by Steinberg and others, support the hypothesis that family relations may impact on the timing of puberty, at least in girls. It was found that there was an acceleration of puberty by increased distancing in the mother-daughter relationship.

According to Baumrind (1988), "increased symmetry of power typically characterizes family structure following puberty. . . . Power cannot be used by parents to legitimate or enforce their authority once the young person acquires formal operational thought. While head-on confrontation may serve to strengthen parental authority in the authority inception period, negotiation and intellectual exchange are most effective during adolescence. A renegotiation of entitlements and obligations among family members following puberty is appropriate and should enable adolescents to accept reasonable parental control."

Many of the negative behaviors of adolescents that are assumed to be related to adolescent rebelliousness, such as use of alcohol and drugs and sexual promiscuity, may have their origins in experiences and observations from early childhood. The modeling by parents of specific behaviors, such as drinking, or of general traits such as distrust or exploitation, may have a greater impact on the development of risk-taking behaviors than peer group or other influences. Baumrind has written, "adolescent negation of convention usually expresses simultaneous emulation and rejection of parental standards. For example, in emulation of their elders, adolescents use drugs to assuage immediate or anticipated discomfort, and in rejection of their elders, they seize on certain drugs of which their elders disapprove. The use of illicit substances offers young adolescents an opportunity to rebel against the rules their elders set down while simultaneously conforming with underlying parental attitudes.''

Jessor and Jessor (1975b) found that such family characteristics as religiosity also affect subsequent adolescent behaviors. Their longitudinal study found that parents' reactions to events that occurred during childhood (such as the child's accidental viewing of the "primal scene" or being caught in the act of "playing doctor") may have more powerful effects than the experience itself on the youngster and on sexual attitudes and behavior during adolescence.

The implications of these findings for relationships between physicians and their adolescent patients are just beginning to be examined. Friedman et al. (1986), for example, found an inverse relationship between the degree of intrafamilial conflict and adolescents' satisfaction with the physician and compliance with medication, suggesting that there is carryover of conflict from the home to the health care delivery system.

Not only may the young adolescent unconsciously transfer feelings from the parent to the physician, as a parent figure, but the reverse often occurs. The physician who has cared for a patient since early childhood may continue to be parental (paternalistic) in his or her interaction with the teenager. Such an orientation may create barriers to obtaining a proper medical history in areas of sexuality and drugs, or taint counseling with an aura of judgmental advice.

Peers

According to Erikson (1968), strong peer group interaction is a normal and healthy component of adolescent development. Even in a family characterized by comfort and cohesiveness, the adolescent is likely to turn to the peer group in matters of sexuality and aggression. As discussed above, teenagers will comply with the standards of the peer group so far as is necessary to achieve status and identity within that group. Some have argued that it is parental relegation of authority and withdrawal from their children's lives (increased permissiveness) or, at the other extreme, parental authoritarianism, which pushes adolescents toward increased peer group involvement.

During early adolescence, the peer group tends to be composed of same-sex members, and friendships that form at this time center largely on a particular shared activity rather than on personal interactions per se. Douvan and Adelson (1966) found that friendships during early adolescence were relatively devoid of depth or mutuality and that they emphasized conformity in both sexes (see discussion of friendships, pp. 108–109).

The peer group, but especially a best friend, is particularly influential in determining initiation into use of drugs and alcohol, as well as smoking. There are also data, however, that show that the influence of the peer group can also be mobilized to prevent the onset of abuse of harmful substances during the early adolescent years, as well as to enhance normal adolescent development. These data have derived from a variety of peer programs, including those modeled on positive peer influence, peer teaching, peer counseling, facilitating, helping, and peer participation.

DELIVERY OF HEALTH CARE

Assessment

Providing appropriate health care to the early adolescent (SMR 2) requires that the special concerns of this period of development be considered, taking into account the accompanying physical changes of puberty. The routine medical assessment of the early adolescent should include the items listed in Table 8–13.

Physical Examination

In addition to addressing the items included in examinations of the younger child, the physical examination of the early adolescent should be directed at those organs and systems likely to be affected by puberty and/ or to have special psychosocial implications at this time. The importance of obtaining blood pressure determinations has been stressed. Males are at greater risk than females of developing hypertension in adolescence. Height and weight should be plotted on velocity curves rather than on the traditional growth charts used during earlier years. Grip strength should be assessed as a measure of muscle development. The frequency with which musculoskeletal problems occur during puberty requires that the back and extremities be carefully examined, and the gait observed.

Skinfold thickness should be measured (the technique for performance of skinfold determination is found on p. 241). The stage of development of secondary sex characteristics (SMR) should be ascertained, using standardized pictures and descriptive material. Testicular size should be measured using a standardized reference, such as the orchiometer (Prader, 1966), and the testes should be palpated for the presence of a discrete mass or varicocele.

There should be an examination of the skeletal system, including the vertebral column (both in the upright and bent-forward positions to rule out scoliosis [pp. 269–270]), of the gait for the possibility of slipped capital femoral epiphysis, and of the tibial tubercle for signs of Osgood-Schlatter syndrome. The thyroid gland should be examined for enlargement and for masses. The presence and extent of acne should be evaluated using a system such as that devised by Pillsbury et al. (Table 8–14).

There is no need to perform a pelvic examination unless:

1. The patient is sexually active and therefore at risk for pregnancy and for sexually-transmitted disease.

TABLE 8–13. Package of Care for the Well Adolescent, Visit I: Early Adolescence (Tanner 1 and 2)*

	FEMALES	MALES
Screening		
Physical	Hematocrit	—
	Urine culture screen	—
	Rubella titer (once)	—
	Tuberculin	
Psychosocial	Self-image	Self-image
	Depression	Depression
	Peer interaction (including sexuality)	Peer interaction (including sexuality)
	School performance	School performance
	Substance abuse	Substance abuse
Health Promotion	Self-examination of breasts	Self-examination of scrotum
	Nutrition counseling	Nutrition counseling
Prevention	Smoking	Smoking
	Cycle safety	Cycle safety
	Automotive passenger safety	Automotive passenger safety
	Immunization update	Immunization update
Anticipatory Guidance	Developing independence	Developing independence
	Dealing with peer pressure	Dealing with peer pressure
	Confidentiality	Confidentiality
	Variations in growth and development	Variations in growth and development
	Dating	Dating
	Preparation for menarche	—
Physical Examination	Blood pressure	Blood pressure
Special attention to:	Height, weight	Height, weight
	Skinfold thickness	Skinfold thickness
	—	Grip strength
	Stage of sexual development	Stage of sexual development
	Scoliosis	—
	Goiter	
	Acne	Acne
	—	Gynecomastia
	Tibial tubercle	Tibial tubercle
	Gait	Gait
Symptomatic Treatment	Acne	Acne
(anything revealed by	Dysmenorrhea	—
the above +)		

* From Litt IF: Adolescent health care. In Green M, Haggerty RJ (eds): *Ambulatory Pediatrics III.* Philadelphia, WB Saunders Company, 1984, pp. 80–103.

2. The patient's mother took diethylstilbestrol (DES) during pregnancy, thereby predisposing to the development of adenocarcinoma of the vagina following the onset of puberty, in which case plans for periodic colposcopy by an experienced gynecologist should be made.

3. The patient has symptoms that may be gynecologic in origin (e.g., vaginal discharge, abnormal or no vaginal bleeding, abdominal pain, etc.).

4. The patient is interested in having such an examination to satisfy her own curiosity about her normality.

TABLE 8–14. Classification of Acne*

Grade 1—Comedones.
Grade 2—Comedones and superficial pustular and inflammatory lesions, confined to the face.
Grade 3—Comedones, small pustules, deeper inflammed lesions of the face, neck, tops of the shoulders, and presternal region.
Grade 4—Extensive cystic acne.

* From Pillsbury DM, Shelley WB, Kligman AM: *A Manual of Cutaneous Medicine.* Philadelphia, WB Saunders Company, 1961.

The technique for performance of a pelvic examination in the adolescent is outlined in Appendix A.

Throughout the performance of the physical examination, the patient's modesty should be respected through the use of appropriate drapes (males should be offered disposable trunks as an alternative to a gown!). The presence of a female chaperone will be appropriate for the examination of young adolescent female patients by male physicians. Should an erection occur in the male patient during the course of the examination, he should be reassured that this is not unusual or worrisome.

In addition, it is very reassuring to the teenager to have constant feedback about the normality of the physician's findings as the examination progresses.

Screening

As at other ages, screening tests should be done if they are cost-effective, either in dollars or in discomfort; that is, if the condition under investigation occurs with sufficient frequency or is so serious that the test is warranted. Normative data relating to the condition (as to its incidence, cost of screening and of therapy, etc.) should be available for the age and sex group of the patient. These data are often not available for adolescents, owing to the infrequency at which youngsters at this age are seen by physicians. Moreover, in considering the timing of performance of a screening test, particularly one of dubious importance or for a condition for which no effective intervention exists, the physician should consider whether detection of a condition of potential future clinical relevance is warranted at this time in the adolescent's development.

It may, perhaps, be prudent to delay performance of some tests, such as those for the carrier states of genetic diseases, until such time as the youngster can deal with a positive result without feeling inadequate or flawed. With any such form of genetic screening, counseling must be built into the program. Naturally, decisions as to timing must also take into account the need to have such information before it becomes imperative, such as before making plans to become a parent.

Routine Laboratory Tests/Procedures

Hematocrit. The frequency with which iron-deficiency anemia may be detected during adolescence suggests that the hematocrit be obtained during early adolescence as a baseline value. With the pubertal growth spurt in females, with the advent of menses, or with participation in strenuous athletic activity, the risk of anemia increases; the hematocrit should be evaluated at least yearly. The criteria for the diagnosis of anemia depend upon the stage of pubertal development (see Tables 8–10 and 8–11). For adolescents at high risk of anemia (such as athletes), a serum ferritin level may be measured, in addition to the hematocrit, in order to detect iron deficiency before it has caused anemia and/or to monitor the athlete's iron status at frequent intervals during a season of strenuous activity (Rowland et al., 1988).

Urinalysis. A screening urinalysis or urine culture is another worthwhile laboratory test in females during early adolescence since asymptomatic urinary tract infections are relatively common at this time. The finding of white blood cells in the urine sediment may also be a clue to vaginitis or cervicitis if the urine culture is negative for usual urinary pathogens. A pelvic examination should be performed under such circumstances.

Rubella Titer. Unless it is decided to immunize the young adolescent female regardless of immunization history or clinical history of infection, a rubella titer should be obtained (see p. 289). Recent data indicate no risk to the developing fetus from inadvertent immunization during pregnancy, but if immunization is undertaken, the physician should establish that the patient is not pregnant and be sure she understands the importance of preventing pregnancy for 3 months after immunization.

Gynecologic Screening. Adolescents who have had or are having sexual intercourse should be screened at yearly intervals for sexually transmitted disease and cervical neoplasia, without regard to chronologic age or to stage of pubertal development. Accordingly, a Papanicolaou (Pap) smear is performed. The Pap smear should include a second cervical scraping, in addition to the standard cervical and vaginal pool samples. The second sample will increase the detection rate of carcinoma-in-situ of the cervix (Davis et al., 1981). Cervical culture for *Neisseria gonorrhoeae* and *Chlamydia trachomatis* should be obtained.

Human Immunodeficiency Virus (HIV). At the time of this writing no recommendation has been made regarding routine screening for HIV. Those in high-risk groups (such as prostitutes, male homosexuals, and intravenous drug abusers or their sexual partners) should, however, be screened.

Tuberculosis Testing. A yearly tuberculin test is indicated in adolescence, as in earlier years. Because of the risk of activation of latent tuberculosis with the pubertal growth spurt, the finding of a positive test, even in the absence of information about previous tests, is an indication for prophylaxis with isoniazid, 300 mg daily, unless the patient has been so treated previously.

Screening for Genetic Disease. Screening tests for genetic diseases (such as sickle cell trait or other hemoglobinopathies, or Tay-Sachs disease) should be performed sufficiently early to be useful in future reproductive planning, yet late enough for the youngster to be able to cope with the emotional pressure that may result from a positive result. Whenever this screening is performed, age-appropriate counseling should be provided to prevent any untoward sequelae.

Physical

The following procedures are often performed by health personnel other than physicians, as part of the physical assessment.

Hearing. An audiogram is indicated during the initial evaluation of the young adolescent even if this procedure has previously been performed during childhood and found to be normal. Elevations in audiometric threshold may result from exposure to highly amplified music, fireworks, or gunfire at any time during adolescence. Conductive hearing loss may result from chronic middle ear infection.

Vision. Vision screening should be performed routinely during adolescence. The adolescent growth spurt is shared by the optic globe as well as by other organs. Myopia may occur in genetically predisposed individuals.

Blood Pressure. Blood pressure normally rises during puberty. Those adolescents who have an earlier growth spurt reach adult levels of systolic blood pressure sooner than the later maturing ones. By the age of 17 years these differences disappear in males.

Hypertension. Age-appropriate references standards are necessary for diagnosis of hypertension in adolescents (Table 8–15). The currently used standards based on chronologic age fail to take into account the effects of different stages of maturation (SMRs). Current standards consider a patient to be hypertensive if his or her blood pressure exceeds by 2 SD the mean for chronologic age.

Most of the teenagers who are found to have elevations of blood pressure at one time or another will have normal readings at other times and will, therefore, be considered to have labile hypertension. Extensive evaluations of such individuals typically fail to reveal any basis for hypertension and are not cost-effective. On the other hand, biannual reevaluation of blood pressure is indicated in adolescents with labile hypertension since 50 per cent of them will progress to essential hypertension during adulthood.

Whenever an adolescent is found to have *sustained* hypertension, further evaluation is indicated. If a cause can be found, it is most often renal or endocrinologic.

TABLE 8–15. Correlation between Blood Pressure and Stage of Pubertal Maturation[*]

		MALES Stage of Pubic Hair Development		Stage of Pubic Hair Development
Age	Systolic BP		Diastolic BP	
10	110 ± 9.0	0.26	59 ± 9.6	0.17
11	109 ± 9.5	0.24	59 ± 10.1	0.14
12	114 ± 10.1	0.25	58 ± 11.2	0.16
13	113 ± 10.3	$0.42^{\dagger}$	55 ± 10.9	0.13
14	116 ± 10.6	0.24	58 ± 9.0	0.25

		FEMALES Stage of Breast Development			Stage of Breast Development	
Age	Systolic BP		Menarche	Diastolic BP		Menarche
10	108 ± 9.3	0.00	—	63 ± 7.8	-0.2	—
11	110 ± 9.8	0.19	$-0.45^{\ddagger}$	59 ± 7.4	-0.24	-0.14
12	113 ± 9.4	0.08	-0.14	58 ± 11.8	0.01	0.1
13	112 ± 10.0	0.19	0.11	59 ± 9.6	0.18	0.1
14	115 ± 7.2	-0.09	$-0.41^{\ddagger}$	66 ± 9.8	-0.24	-0.06

[*] Modified from Londe S, Johanson J, Kronemer NS, et al: Blood pressure and puberty. J Pediatr 87:896–900, 1975.
[†] $p = <.01$.
[‡] $p = <.05$.

This discussion presumes that the blood pressure determination has been accurate. Reliable sphygmomanometric readings depend upon:

1. Selection of the proper cuff size (i.e., the largest cuff that will fit snugly with the bladder completely encircling the arm without overlapping).
2. Proper positioning of the patient (in a comfortable sitting posture with his or her right arm fully exposed and extended, and supported at the level of the heart.
3. Applying the cuff with its lower edge above the antecubital fossa and placing the diaphragm over the brachial artery.
4. Inflating the cuff rapidly to approximately 30 torr (30 mm Hg) above the point of disappearance of the radial pulse, followed by deflation at a rate of about 3 torr/sec, the point at which a clear tapping sound begins being taken as the systolic blood pressure, and its change to a low-pitched, muffled, softer sound as the diastolic blood pressure.

Scoliosis. Screening should be done for scoliosis, which has its onset most commonly at the peak of the height velocity curve. Idiopathic scoliosis has an incidence of 5 to 6 per cent in boys and 10 to 14 per cent in girls. The finding of a structural curve or any curve greater than 10 degrees in an early adolescent is an indication for periodic close follow-up until growth is complete.

Here, too, the technique for evaluation is important. For proper examination for scoliosis, the disrobed patient should turn his or her back to the examiner. The heights of the iliac crests should be noted. If they are not equal, the patient may have a leg length discrepancy as the cause of scoliosis. The patient should next be asked to bend forward 90 degrees with his or her hands clasped in the midline. The rib cage should be symmetrical. If there is asymmetry (that is, a "hump" is seen on one side), a rotation of the vertebral bodies with a lateral curvature is likely. Whether a curvature is present or not should also be noted. Curvature in excess of 30 degrees will be apparent upon inspection.

Scoliosis is diagnosed upon the finding of a lateral curvature with rotation of the vertebrae. The most common type of idiopathic scoliosis has the apex of the convexity in the left thorax ("left thoracic scoliosis"). A "right lumber scoliosis" would have the apex of the convexity of the curve to the right in the lumbar region.

Psychosocial Screening (Interviewing the Adolescent)

Self-Image

Early adolescence is a time of heightened self-consciousness, which results both in the increased empathy that comes from understanding the perspective of another person and in increasing self-centeredness. The enhanced cognitive competencies of this age may be used to construct a personal fable as a way of "reaffirming their specialness and separateness" (Baumrind, 1988).

Between the ages of 8 and 13 years, there appears to be a decrease in the individual's sense of self-worth, particularly among high-achieving, middle-class adolescents. A poor self-image appears to be a risk factor for a number of problematic behaviors during early adolescence, including depression, premature sexual intercourse and pregnancy, and noncompliance with medication. Accordingly, it is useful to identify the youngster with problems in self-image. Standardized tests are available for this purpose, including the Piers-Harris Self-Concept Scale (1964), the Offer Test of Self-Image (1973), and the Rosenberg test (1972). We have had considerable experience with the first and find it to be easily administered and comprehensible to anyone with more than a third-grade reading level. A shortened, 40-item revision is now available that takes no more than 10 min for self-administration.

If the health care provider can, in the course of obtaining a medical history, include a few open-ended questions aimed at assessing self-image, this may be felt to be more natural than such tests as the above. For example, this purpose can often be served by asking the young teenager what he or she might like to change about him or herself or considers to be his or her best and worst features.

Depression

The frequency with which depression occurs during adolescence mandates that we attempt to identify and alleviate it. Depression is not only the forerunner of suicide, the second leading cause of death during adolescence, but also appears to be a contributing factor to the high incidence of automotive accidents and drug and alcohol abuse.

Prior to adolescence it is uncommon to see the affective symptoms typically associated with adult depression, and the child is more likely to express distress "through anti-social behavior, restlessness, lack of attention and 'psychosomatic complaints'" (Mechanic, 1983). In Mechanic's words, "only as children approach adolescence is there an internalization of some of the cognitive conditions for depression." Epidemiologic studies show that most adults with bipolar and unipolar depression experienced onset of symptoms during adolescence. As children, most of those with the latter form of depression were described as being "shy, conscientious, sensitive, and having good judgement." Accordingly, Mechanic (1983) believes that a learned disposition toward self-attention or introspection develops during adolescence and that this is central to understanding the timing of onset of depression. It is at this time that a person first learns to monitor his or her private experience.

Since wide mood swings are common during early adolescence, it is not always easy to ascertain which youngster is seriously depressed and needs help. Persistence of a depressed mood without intervening periods of elation warrants concern. Puig-Antich and Rabinovich (1983) feel that depression should be considered to be persistent if it lasts more than three consecutive hours for three or more periods each week. In addition, withdrawal from friends and social activities, decrement in school grades, increase in the number of days absent from school or frank truancy, use of drugs or alcohol, and sexual promiscuity are all signs of possible depression in the adolescent.

The "vegetative" signs more typical of depression in adults, such as sleep disturbance and diminished appetite, may not be present in adolescents. When sleep problems occur, they tend to be characterized by initial insomnia, often with the result of sleeping all day and remaining awake all night, without ever feeling rested. Concern is heightened when the youngster expresses hopelessness and helplessness about the future. A family history of depression, particularly if it includes suicide or an attempt at suicide, is an additional risk factor in the assessment.

To evaluate the adolescent with signs of depression, it may be helpful to inquire about plans for the future. A response along the lines of "I won't be here much longer" obviously belongs to severe depression and requires immediate psychiatric intervention. Another useful probe is a question as to what the adolescent would like to change in his or her life. When a desire for change is expressed, it may be useful to follow-up with questions about possible steps taken to effect such change in order to open a dialogue. If depression is revealed, the physician should not hesitate to inquire if the patient has ever felt so sad that death was considered a preferable alternative to living. If the patient admits this to be the case, further questioning about the existence of a plan for self-destruction should follow. The existance of such a plan is an indication for immediate psychiatric evaluation. The sudden appearance of a cheerful demeanor in a previously depressed adolescent is not always a cause for optimism:

such a change may also signal the resolution of ambivalence with a decision to commit suicide.

Standardized instruments for assessment of depression in adolescents include those devised by Zung (1967) and by Beck et al. (1974).

Problems of Sexuality

For the early adolescent, problems of sexuality typically involve insecurities about what they perceive to be abnormalities in development of secondary sex characteristics or about sexual preference. Occasionally, they include dilemmas about whether or not to engage in sexual intercourse.

Ascertainment of these concerns will facilitate counseling and anticipatory guidance. Knowing that the teenager has been sexually active will assist in identifying contraindications for medications and indications for diagnostic tests. Obtaining a sexual history should not be undertaken solely in response to the physicians' subjective impression as to whether or not the adolescent is "sexually active." It should not be embarrassing for either physician or patient.

Taking the Sexual History. A mutually productive interaction is facilitated by discussing sexuality with the patient alone, rather than in the parents' presence. This arrangement gives an implicit statement of respect for the teenager's desire to protect his or her parents from concerns or information that might be upsetting to them, as well as respect for what he or she wishes to have kept altogether confidential.

Just as teenagers often feel protective toward their parents, so may they also toward their physicians. By the same token, if the physician harbors "parental" feelings toward the youngster, whom he or she may have had as a patient since birth, there may be difficulty in initiating a discussion about sex.

The choice of an approach that seems comfortable is the best approach. The alternatives may fall into one of the following models: the "physical development" approach; the "preventive" approach; the "social development" approach; or the "medical" approach (Table 8–16).

The "physical development" approach rests on the observation that when there is any deviation from the peer group norm in development of secondary sex characteristics, or when gynecomastia is present in boys, anxiety is often created. It is therefore useful for the physician to mention these normal variants before the physical examination is undertaken. By simply mentioning that concerns about pubertal development are common among people of the patient's age, the physician may relieve some anxiety and facilitate a dialogue.

As he or she obtains a history of the chronology and pattern of development of the patient's secondary sex characteristics, the clinician may wish to comment that these physical changes are commonly accompanied by new and often overwhelming sensations or emotions, which may be sexual in nature. This may be amplified by a discussion of the variety of ways in which "other" teenagers have dealt with such feelings (e.g.,

TABLE 8–16. Identifying the Sexually Active Adolescent

Medical model
1. "These laboratory tests (medications) may be affected by use of contraceptives . . ."
2. "This medication may be harmful in pregnancy. Is there *any* chance that you are pregnant?"

Previsit questionnaire
1. "Have you ever been concerned that you will become pregnant (make someone pregnant) before you're ready?"
2. "Have you ever worried that you may not be able to have children when you are ready?"

General
1. "Is there anything you would like to change in your relationship with your boyfriend (girlfriend)?"
2. "We can check for V.D. and provide birth control here. Let us know if we can help with these matters."

masturbation, petting, or intercourse), in order to ease the transition to discussing how these issues affect the patient.

The "preventive" approach uses the physician's accepted role in disease prevention to raise comfortably the issues of prevention of sexually transmitted disease (STD) and pregnancy. Without the need for any confrontation as to whether or not these risks are relevant to the patient, the physician may simply state that information about prevention and testing for STDs and pregnancy is available in his or her office to any teenager who might benefit from it and that such requests will be kept confidential.

The "social development" approach may use inquiry into typical weekend activities to help place the teenager in the hierarchy of social relationships (see Table 8–17), and in that way lead to identification of the one who is now dating (a same- or opposite-sex partner). Follow-up with an open-ended question, such as: "Is there anything about your relationship with (the date's name) that you would wish to change?", is often answered in terms of sexual pressures and conflicts.

The "medical" approach may provide a straightforward entree to taking a sexual history by exploring drug interactions with oral contracep-

TABLE 8–17.
Hierarchy of Social
Relationships among
Adolescents*

Same sex groups
Both sex groups
Dating
Desire for steady dating
Steady dating
Sexual intercourse

* Modified from Chess et al. (1976).

TABLE 8–18. Interactions of Oral Contraceptives with Other Drugs*

INTERACTING DRUGS	ADVERSE EFFECTS (PROBABLE MECHANISM)
Acetaminophen (Tylenol and others)	Possible decreased pain-relieving effect (increased metabolism)
Alcohol	Possible increased effect of alcohol
Antidepressants (Elavil, Norpramin, Tofranil, and others)	Possible increased antidepressant effect
Barbiturates (phenobarbital and others)	Decreased contraceptive effect
Benzodiazepine tranquilizers (Ativan, Librium, Serax, Tranxene, Valium, Xanax, and others)	Possible increased or decreased tranquilizer effects, including psychomotor impairment
β-blockers (Corgard, Inderal, Lopressor, Tenormin)	Possible increased blocker effect
Carbamazepine (Tegretol)	Possible decreased contraceptive effect
Corticosteroids (cortisone)	Possible increased corticosteroid toxicity
Griseofulvin (Fulvicin, Grifulvin V, and others)	Decreased contraceptive effect
Isoniazid	Possible decreased contraceptive effect
Penicillin	Decreased contraceptive effect with ampicillin
Phenytoin (Dilantin)	Decreased contraceptive effect, possible increased phenytoin effect
Primidone (Mysoline)	Decreased contraceptive effect
Rifampin	Decreased contraceptive effect
Tetracycline	Decreased contraceptive effect
Theophylline (Bronkotabs, Marax, Primatene, Quibron, Tedral, Theo-Dur, and others)	Increased theophylline effect
Troleandomycin (TAO)	Jaundice (additive)
Vitamin C	Increased serum concentration and possible increased adverse effects of estrogens with 1 g or more per day of vitamin C

* Modified from Hatcher et al. (1988).

tives (Table 8–18), or contraindications to prescription of certain other drugs or to immunizations with live viruses or diagnostic techniques during pregnancy. These interactions require information about use of oral contraceptives or the possibility of pregnancy.

Inclusion of Parents. The need for privacy and confidentiality in taking a sexual history from the adolescent has been stressed, but the physician must also make provision for a separate interview with parents. This allows for discovery of their concerns, as well as an opportunity to provide them with anticipatory guidance without breaching the confidentiality extended to the teenager.

Parents vary widely in their reactions to their youngsters' adolescence and its implications for emerging sexuality. They often feel and act in accordance with their own experiences as adolescents, their experiences with older children, their perception of this child's vulnerabilities, and possibly, their own midlife sexual adjustments. Encouraging them to express concerns and ask questions will often remove barriers to communication between parents and teenagers themselves. Discussions of sexuality with parents also provide the physician with information about the adolescent's concerns that the latter might have been reluctant to raise.

Because of the implication that physical maturity indicates readiness for adult sexual activity in our society, parents may react to pubertal development in their daughters with fear that it will signal their readiness for sexual intercourse. Without an opportunity to articulate these fears, parents may impose stringent curfews, make arrangements for chaperones, and exhibit other behaviors likely to be misinterpreted by the teenager as expressions of mistrust. The teenager may, in turn, react by rebellion, which often includes sexual acting-out, often more as a way of testing the injunctions aimed at control than necessarily out of desire for the sexual experience itself.

Despite widespread concern among adults that the child's entry into puberty marks imminent transition from the virginal, fewer than 20 per cent of early adolescents experience intercourse. Among those who date, heterosexual activities are typically limited to petting. Most early adolescents do not date at all and the majority of their time spent in social activity is in the context of same-sex friendships (see Table 8–17). Accordingly, it is useful to inquire if the youngster has at least one very good friend with whom he or she can share the most intimate thoughts. Absence of such a confidant, particularly for a girl, may be an indication that the youngster is "at risk" for social isolation and for depression.

Mention was made earlier of the frequent occurrence during early adolescence of mutual masturbation among males. Discovery of such behavior by parents often causes anxiety that it may be a manifestation of homosexuality: in fact, the available evidence suggests that it provides a means of experimentation, self-exploration, comparison, and reassurance in the service of later heterosexual relationships. The homosexual male will have displayed in early childhood such behaviors as cross-dressing and a preference for female playmates, roles, and toys (Green, 1979). Mutual masturbation as a normal occurrence in early adolescence among heterosexual males never involves an adult male.

School Performance

Since early adolescents spend a great deal of their time in school, it is useful to assess performance in this setting as an indicator of general psychosocial functioning. Asking the youngster how he or she is doing in school is usually not very productive since this closed-ended question will typically be answered with a disyllabic "OK." More productive is an open-ended question such as: "How do your grades in school this year compare with last years'?" or "How has your attendance in school this year compare with last?" As indicated above, evidence of a decrement in school performance or increased absenteeism may be signs of depression.

Substance Abuse

Despite the importance of identifying the adolescent involved in substance abuse, physicians often have difficulty taking an appropriate history. It is not easy to find an approach that will obtain the necessary information without offending the adolescent, whether abstinent or user. The nonuser may misinterpret such questioning with resentment at unjustified stereotyping of adolescents as "drug users." The user, on the other hand, will resist intrusion into his or her private life, particularly if the use of drugs has been rationalized as harmless.

Despite these potential barriers, a nonjudgmental, patient approach can open a discussion that can be rewarding both to the physician, who may learn a good deal about the physical and psychologic status of the patient, and to the adolescent, who may gain valued information about certain drugs, as well as about him or herself. In taking a "drug history," the following steps may be useful:

1. Inquire if there is any habit the youngster might like to break. This question may be answered by expression of a wish to stop smoking, for example.

2. Indicate that a lot of misinformation has been promulgated about drugs, and that the physician is a resource for obtaining factual information about them. This may prompt an "I have a friend who . . ." response that will lead profitably to a discussion about the pharmacologic effects of various substances. Such an approach will be less emotional than one that came only in the context of the patient's own drug use having been established.

3. Ask if there is pressure at school to try drugs. If answered in the affirmative, one might then ask what the patient has done to resist this pressure, indicating that it is not always easy to do so even when you know it may be harmful.

4. Remember that teenagers make fine distinctions about abused substances, such that inquiry about "drugs" may not be construed to include marijuana, inhalants, or alcohol. It is useful and sometimes necessary to be specific.

5. Remember that teenagers are generally bored by being lectured to about the dangers of using drugs. Techniques aimed at arousal of fear have been shown, in fact, to be counterproductive. Establishing a dialogue is a preferable approach.

6. Assure confidentiality. This is the only way to get accurate information. Most states have laws permitting treatment of adolescents for alcohol and drug abuse without parental consent or knowledge; on the other hand, it may not always be possible to guarantee confidentiality. If, for example, the physician discovers that the teenager is engaged in extensive illicit or otherwise self-destructive behavior and is unwilling or unable to get help for it by him or herself, it may become necessary to involve parents. In addition, if the patient has been referred to the physician by the school or another agency for assessment of possible drug abuse, a promise of confidentiality cannot be extended to the patient without having a prior commitment from the referring agency to honor such confidentiality.

7. Explain the importance of the physician's knowing about any use of drugs (including oral contraceptives) that might interact with prescribed drugs (Table 8–18). Examples of potentiation or dimunition of effect may be offered (e.g., the potentiation of the effect of anticonvulsants or antihistamines by alcohol, or the prolongation of an elevated level of alcohol in the blood with the use of oral contraceptives.)

HEALTH PROMOTION

Breast Self-Examination

Teaching young women to examine their breasts for masses or nipple discharge is offered with the hope that they will early develop a habit that will be sustained throughout years of high-risk for development of breast cancer. There are as yet, however, no data that show that teaching this technique during early adolescence leads to its lifelong practice. We teach it nonetheless, partly with the hope that it will accomplish its goal, but also because emphasizing the participatory aspects of the procedure often diminishes the embarrassment that might otherwise occur when an early adolescent undergoes examination of her breasts by a male physician. We have also found that the patient often reminds her mother of the need and/ or teaches her mother the examination.

The proper technique for breast self-examination is shown in Figure 8–15.

Scrotum Self-Examination

Teaching self-examination of the testes serves a similar function for the male adolescent, who may be less embarrassed by a female physician's examination when he is asked to focus on the procedure itself in order to be able to perform it himself in the future. The procedures serves as an important screening device because the peak incidence of testicular malignancies, in contrast with those of the female breast, occurs in late adolescence and early adulthood. (See Appendix B.)

Nutritional Counseling

Not only are early adolescents particularly opinionated and selective about food preferences, but they often, as a result of newly espoused religious or spiritual beliefs, adopt diets that are nutritionally deficient. In addition, many young adolescent females view their pubertally altered shape with displeasure and diet for weight reduction. For these reasons the primary care physician should screen for the possibility of dietary inadequacies and provide counseling.

In the extreme, concern with diet may eventuate in anorexia nervosa or bulimia. These also may be discovered by sensitive questioning of the young adolescent patient. Administration of a standardized test for detection of eating disorders (such as the Eating Disorders Inventory) is advisable if this is suspected.

Nutritional counseling should respect the adolescent's belief system (e.g., "vegetarianism is compatible with good nutrition if the following principles are incorporated into the diet") and should acknowledge that

HOW TO EXAMINE YOUR BREASTS

Examining your breasts once a month is an excellent health habit to begin during your teens. One out of 11 women will develop breast cancer one day (usually after age 40). Breast cancer has an excellent chance of cure if found early. Fortunately, most breast lumps in young women are *not* cancer.

There are three good reasons for doing monthly self-exams when you're young:
- It's easier to develop the regular habit
- You'll become comfortable with the normal variations in your breast tissue
- You'll be taking responsibility for your own health care.

When to do the exam

It is best to do the examination at the same time each month, immediately *after* your period is over. Your breasts will be the least tender or swollen then. If you are taking birth control pills, the day you start your new pack each month is usually a good time for the exam.

How to do the exam

1. You can do the exam either in the bath or shower or while lying down on your back.
2. First, lift one hand and place it behind your head.

3. Hold the first three fingers of your left hand firmly together.
4. Press the outermost part of your right breast (near the armpit) firmly in a little circular motion with

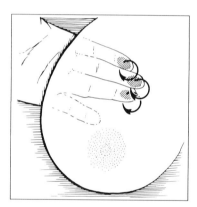 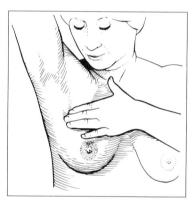

Figure 8–15. Self breast examination technique. From Beach RK: Routine breast exams: a chance to reassure, guide and protect. Contemp Pediatr Oct:70–100, 1987.

during the pubertal growth spurt one needs between 2000 and 3000 kcal for sustenance. Failure to consume this amount may restrict linear growth, as well as potentially that of muscle.

The adolescent's diet is often deficient in iron-containing food and, for girls, in food containing adequate amounts of calcium. Iron is important for males during the pubertal growth spurt, since the growth of muscle requires 18 mg/day, the same amount required for a menstruating adolescent female. Athletes of both sexes are at risk for losses of iron, which occur through the gastrointestinal tract (either spontaneously or second-

HOW TO EXAMINE YOUR BREASTS

the pads of your fingers. Then continue in a large circle all around your breast.

5. Move your fingers an inch closer to the nipple and feel another circle around the breast. Continue circling until you have felt every part of the breast, including the nipple.

6. Squeeze the nipple gently to see if any fluid comes out.

7. Now change hands and repeat the procedure for the other breast.

The drawings that accompany this instruction sheet will help you learn the self-examination technique.

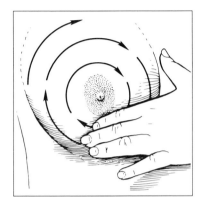

What you might feel

Your breasts are made up of fat, glands, and fibrous tissue, with muscle tissue underneath. Occasionally tender cysts will develop before your period and shrink afterward. As you do your exam each month, you will become very familiar with the normal tissue in your breasts.

When to see your doctor

If you find any lump or thickening that lasts over a month, or if you find fluid when you squeeze your nipples, or anytime you feel something that worries you, see your physician. Most findings will be harmless and do not mean breast cancer, but let your physician make the diagnosis.

As you get older

After age 30, you will be taught a more detailed examination that can detect even smaller lumps. Also, after age 35 or 40, your doctor may recommend regular mammograms (breast X-rays that detect cancer). Until then, practice this simple self-exam every month.

Figure 8–15. (*continued*).

ary to the common practice of use of nonsteroidal antiinflammatory drugs for musculoskeletal injuries), through the kidney, through the skin in perspiration, or secondary to hemolysis. These needs notwithstanding, most teenagers refuse to eat spinach and females tend to shun red meat, fearing its high fat content. Motivation to increase iron intake may be increased by pointing out that when iron stores are adequate oxygen-carrying capacity is improved and performance also, as a result.

Fear of fat also often causes female adolescents to avoid dairy products and not to consume sufficient calcium (the recommended level is 1.5 to 2 g/day). This does not become clinically significant unless other risk factors are present, such as prolonged amenorrhea (in which case osteoporosis may result) or pregnancy. In counseling a weight-conscious adolescent about her need for calcium, it is useful to point out that nonfat yogurt (with no cholesterol) is high in needed protein (typically 10 g/pint) and in calcium (35 to 45 per cent of the Recommended Daily Allowance [RDA]). Tables 8–19, 8–20, and 8–21 list the RDAs for adolescents.

TABLE 8–19. Mineral RDA Values for Healthy American Adolescents Aged 11–18 Years*

NUTRIENT	11–14 YEARS	15–18 YEARS
Males		
Calcium (mg)	1200	1200
Phosphorus (mg)	1200	1200
Magnesium (mg)	350	400
Iron (mg)	18	18
Zinc (mg)	15	15
Iodine (μg)	150	150
Copper (mg)	2.0–3.0	2.0–3.0
Manganese (mg)	2.5–5.0	2.5–5.0
Fluoride (mg)	1.5–2.5	1.5–2.5
Chromium (mg)	0.05–0.2	0.05–0.2
Selenium (mg)	0.05–0.2	0.05–0.2
Molybdenum (mg)	0.15–0.5	0.15–0.5
Sodium (mg)	900–2700	900–2700
Potassium (mg)	1525–4575	1525–4575
Chloride (mg)	1400–4200	1400–4200
Females		
Calcium (mg)	1200	1200
Phosphorus (mg)	1200	1200
Magnesium (mg)	300	300
Iron (mg)	18	18
Zinc (mg)	15	15
Iodine (μg)	150	150
Copper (mg)	2.0–3.0	2.0–3.0
Manganese (mg)	2.5–5.0	2.5–5.0
Fluoride (mg)	1.5–2.5	1.5–2.5
Chromium (mg)	0.05–0.2	0.05–0.2
Selenium (mg)	0.05–0.2	0.05–0.2
Molybdenum (mg)	0.15–0.5	0.15–0.5
Sodium (mg)	900–2700	900–2700
Potassium (mg)	1525–4575	1525–4575
Chloride (mg)	1400–4200	1400–4200

* From Whitehead RG: Nutritional requirements of healthy adolescents and their significance during the management of PKU. Eur J Pediatr 146:A25–A31, 1987.

TABLE 8–20. Vitamin RDA Values for Healthy
American Adolescents Aged 11–18 Years[*]

NUTRIENT	11–14 YEARS	15–18 YEARS
Males		
Vitamin A (μg RE)	1000	1000
Vitamin D (μg)	10	10
Vitamin E (mg αTE)	8	10
Vitamin C (mg)	50	60
Thiamin (mg)	1.4	1.4
Riboflavin (mg)	1.6	1.7
Niacin (mg NE)	18	18
Vitamin B_6 (mg)	1.8	2.0
Folacin (μg)	400	400
Vitamin B_{12} (μg)	3.0	3.0
Vitamin K (μg)	50–100	50–100
Biotin (μg)	100–200	100–200
Pantothenic acid (mg)	4–7	4–7
Females		
Vitamin A (μg RE)	800	800
Vitamin D (μg)	10	10
Vitamin E (mg αTE)	8	8
Vitamin C (mg)	50	60
Thiamin (mg)	1.1	1.1
Riboflavin (mg)	1.3	1.3
Niacin (mg NE)	15	14
Vitamin B_6 (mg)	1.8	2.0
Folacin (μg)	400	400
Vitamin B_{12} (μg)	3.0	3.0
Vitamin K (μg)	50–100	50–100
Biotin (μg)	100–200	100–200
Pantothenic acid (mg)	4–7	4–7

[*] From Whitehead RG: Nutritional requirements of healthy adolescents and their significance during the management of PKU. Eur J Pediatr 146:A25–A31, 1987.

PREVENTION

Smoking

Because the initiation of smoking typically beins at the age of 11 years and its incidence rises steeply at the age of 14 years, early adolescence is the optimal time for introduction of strategies designed to prevent smoking.

Giving young adolescents factual information about the long-term adverse sequelae of smoking (cancer and heart disease) is probably not the best utilization of the physician's time, as most teenagers have heard

TABLE 8–21. 1973 Recommendations, 1985 Average Calculated Expenditures, and Mean Literature Energy Intakes (kcal/day) for Adolescents Aged 10–18 Years*

AGE (YEARS)	EXPENDITURE		1973 RECOMMEN- DATIONS	MEAN MEASURED INTAKES
	× BMR†	Total		
Boys				
10–11	1.76	2140	2500	2110
11–12	1.73	2240	2600	2170
12–13	1.69	2310	2700	2200
13–14	1.67	2440	2800	2280
14–15	1.65	2590	2900	2340
15–16	1.62	2700	3000	2390
16–17	1.60	2800	3050	2440
17–18	1.60	2870	3100	2490
Girls				
10–11	1.65	1910	2300	1850
11–12	1.63	1980	2350	1890
12–13	1.60	2050	2400	1930
13–14	1.58	2120	2450	1970
14–15	1.57	2160	2500	2010
15–16	1.54	2140	2500	2050
16–17	1.53	2130	2420	2080
17–18	1.52	2140	2340	2120

* From Whitehead RG: Nutritional requirements of healthy adolescents and their significance during the management of PKU. Eur J Pediatr 146:A25–A31, 1987.
† *BMR*, basal metabolic rate.

these facts and have discounted their personal relevance. The only successful antismoking programs have been directed at youngsters in the seventh grade of school and have utilized peer counselors to teach skills necessary to resist peer pressure to smoke (McAlister et al., 1979). On the other hand, the facts that smoking can impair pulmonary function and predispose to respiratory infections during adolescence may not be well known to the adolescent and should be mentioned. Furthermore, with the recent increase in use of chewing tobacco by teenagers, its potential for carcinogenesis should be discussed. It should be remembered, however, that tactics designed to frighten have never substantially discouraged the use of cigarettes or other abused substances. Programs aimed at developing peer counterpressure may be the most effective in this regard.

Cycle Safety

The high toll of accidents involving riders of bicycles or mopeds should be addressed during the routine evaluation of the early adolescent. Engaging the youngster in a conversation about the reasons that teenagers do not use helmets, for example, may be an appropriate stimulus for his or her reassessment of safety practices without having been put on the spot.

Automotive Passenger Safety

Along similar lines, discussion about prevention of morbidity and mortality from automobile accidents is appropriate as teenagers enter the age category of highest risk for their occurrence. The two issues that may most profitably be examined are the use of seat belts and anticipation of strategies for coping with the situation in which the driver has become intoxicated. These should be addressed in a problem-solving rather than a lecture format. Some physicians have taken leading roles in organizing "safe ride" programs in their communities, in which parents arrange to provide an anonymous pick-up service, with "no questions asked," for any teenager or driver who reports that he or she has become functionally impaired.

Sports Safety

Epidemiologic data suggests that there are more sports-related injuries during adolescence than earlier or later periods of life. A number of factors contribute to these injuries, including:

1. The nature of the sport
2. Conditions of the environment
3. Adequacy of protective gear
4. The physical status of the athlete
5. Supervision

The Nature of the Sport

The type of sport in which the adolescent is involved will influence the number and severity of injuries. Contact and collision sports are associated with more injuries and more serious injuries than noncontact sports, but there are differences within these categories as well. For example, among the noncontact sports, softball is responsible for the most and badminton for the least number of injuries. Garrick and Requa's study (1978) of girls' high school athletic injuries further showed that the sport associated with the longest period of disability following an injury was track and field.

In softball most injuries occurred during the competitive event, whereas in gymnastics and track and field most injuries occurred during practice. In those sports with the highest rates of injury, more than two thirds of injuries occur during practice sessions.

Most athletic injuries involve soft tissue (contusions, sprains, and strains) and more than half affect the lower extremities. The type of sport affects the nature of the injury. Most football injuries of the lower extremity are to the knee or involve the ligaments of the ankle. Ice hockey and equestrian activities are associated with a high incidence of head injury, and vaginal lacerations and/or rupture may result from the impact of a fall of a waterskier. The most serious of injuries (quadriplegia resulting from cervical spine injury) occur in football, diving, and amateur ice hockey.

Conditions of the Environment

The types of playing field is related to the frequency of accidents. Bramwell et al. (1972) found the rate and severity of injuries to be significantly higher when high school football games were played on a synthetic field than on a grass field. The wetness of either natural or artificial turf may also contribute to the likelihood of injury.

Adequacy of Protective Gear

As in the case of automotive injuries, those injuries that occur in athletics are markedly reduced in number and severity by wearing appropriate protective equipment. An appropriately fitted helmet is vital in football and equestrian events. Devices for the football player that involve "bird cage" face protection combined with shells and suspension systems are ideal for prevention of serious head injury unless the helmet is used as a battering ram during tackling, a practice that is condemned. Padding of knees and elbows reduces injury in contact sports. Basketball ankle injuries can be reduced by wearing high-top shoes or taping the ankle. Eye protection afforded by wearing closed safety goggles is vital in sports such as racketball, in which it has been demonstrated that the ball can reach a speed of 127 mph. The development of face masks for use in ice hockey has similarly decreased the incidence of eye injury. Contact lenses, and soft lenses in particular, can improve comfort and visability and reduce the incidence of injuries associated with wearing corrective glasses.

The Physical Status of the Athlete

A number of factors contribute to the physical status of the adolescent athlete, including gender, stage of pubertal development, nutritional and health status, and conditioning.

With increasing participation of females in athletics, there is a growing literature on the differences between their experiences and those of their male counterparts. In order to evaluate this literature on possible experiential differences, it is important to include consideration as well of the sex differences in pubertal development, which have implications for physical activity.

In males, puberty increases particularly muscle strength and bulk, with increases in cardiac output, hemoglobin, and vital capacity of the lungs. All of these contribute to a higher total oxygen-carrying capacity, to higher maximum aerobic capacity, and hence to better exercise tolerance and performance in male adolescents than in females.

Puberty in females is responsible for increases in adipose tissue (which enhance buoyancy in swimming), a decrease in hemoglobin concentration (which lowers the total oxygen-carrying capacity), and increases in the angle that the femur makes at the knee and in the laxity of ligaments (disposing female athletes to greater risk than in males of ligamentous injuries of the lower extremity). Breast and genital injuries are rare.

Males have generally grown up involved in some athletic activity, whereas many females come to a sport in high school without such a background. Garrick and Requa (1978) note that in many cases of female high-school athletes "the sport experience had to transform the non-athlete to athlete as well as create a volleyball player, swimmer, or gymnast."

The physical status of the adolescent athlete includes his or her stage of pubertal development. It has been well documented that injuries in contact and collision sports are markedly decreased when players are matched on the basis of size, as a manifestation of pubertal development, rather than according to chronologic age. Moreover, according to a policy statement of the American Academy of Pediatrics (1983), children and teenagers should not be permitted prior to attainment of SMR 5 to participate in long-distance competitive running events such as a full marathon.

Weight training has been shown to increase muscle mass and strength in the limbs of adolescent males after attainment of SMR 2. The risk of epiphyseal injuries from weight lifting will be a continuing concern for adolescents whose pubertal development is not yet completed.

When a teenager has a single functional member of a pair of vital organs, the threat of injury to that organ should preclude participation in contact or collision sports. The presence of sustained hypertension is a contraindication for sports that involve isotonic exercise such as weightlifting. Whenever a teenager is prohibited from playing a contact sport for medical reasons, every effort should be made to substitute a noncontact alternative. Exercise-induced bronchospasm is an indication for prescription of an inhaler to be used prior to sports participation, rather than as a reason for exclusion from involvement. (Table 8–22 indicates the recommendations of the American Academy of Pediatrics for exclusions from sports participation.)

The amount of physical training and conditioning of the adolescent athlete bears on the rate and severity of injuries. For example, it has been shown that weight training to strengthen neck muscles can decrease the risk of cervical spine injuries in football.

Supervision

Safe sports require good communication between physician, trainer, coach, and the teenager. Working together they can prevent injuries, recognize them promptly when they occur, treat them, and allow for adequate healing after their occurrence.

Immunizations (see Table 8–23)

Early adolescence is a good time to update immunizations, as 10 years typically have elapsed since the last dT booster. Immunization against rubella and rubeola is now routinely provided at 15 months of age, but that

TABLE 8-22. Classification of Sports and Recommendations for Participation[8]

CLASSIFICATION OF SPORTS

Contact/ Collision	Limited Contact/Impact	Non-Contact		
		Strenuous	*Moderately Strenuous*	*Non-Strenuous*
Boxing	Baseball	Aerobic dancing	Badminton	Archery
Field hockey	Basketball	Crew	Curling	Golf
Football	Bicycling	Fencing	Table tennis	Riflery
Ice hockey	Diving	Field:		
Lacrosse	Field:	discus		
Martial arts	high jump	javelin		
Rodeo	pole vault	shot put		
Soccer	Gymnastics	Running		
Wrestling	Horseback riding	Swimming		
	Skating:	Tennis		
	ice, roller	Track		
	Skiing:	Weight lifting		
	cross-country			
	downhill			
	water			
	Softball			
	Squash, handball			
	Volleyball			

RECOMMENDATIONS FOR PARTICIPATION IN COMPETITIVE SPORTS

	Contact/ Collision	Limited Contact/Impact	Non-Contact		
			Strenuous	Moderately Strenuous	Non-Strenuous
Atlanto-axial instability * Swimming: no butterfly, breast stroke, or diving starts	No	No	Yes*	Yes	Yes
Acute illnesses * Needs individual assessment, eg, contagiousness to others, risk of worsening illness	*	*	*	*	*
Cardiovascular Carditis	No	No	No	No	No
Hypertension mild	Yes *	Yes *	Yes *	Yes *	Yes *
moderate	*	*	*	*	*
severe	†	†	†	†	†
Congenital heart disease † Needs individual assessment * Patients with mild forms can be allowed a full range of physical activities; patients with moderate or severe forms, or who are postoperative, should be evaluated by a cardiologist before athletic participation					
Eyes Absence or loss of function of one eye	*	*	*	*	*
Detached retina * Availability of American Society for Testing and Materials (ASTM) approved eye guards may allow competitor to participate in most sports, but this must be judged on an individual basis † Consult ophthalmologist	†	†	†	†	†
Hernia, inguinal	Yes	Yes	Yes	Yes	Yes
Kidney, absence of one	No	Yes	Yes	Yes	Yes

Liver, enlarged	No	No	Yes	Yes	Yes
Musculoskeletal disorders *Needs individual assessment	*	*	*	*	*
Neurologic					
History of serious head or spine trauma, repeated concussions, or craniotomy	*	*	Yes	Yes	Yes
Convulsive disorder well controlled	Yes	Yes	Yes	Yes	Yes
Convulsive disorder poorly controlled	No	No	Yes†	Yes	Yes‡
†Needs individual assessment					
†No swimming or weight lifting					
‡No archery or riflery					
Ovary, absence of one	Yes	Yes	Yes	Yes	Yes
Respiratory					
Pulmonary insufficiency	*	*	*	Yes	Yes
Asthma	Yes	Yes	Yes	Yes	Yes
*May be allowed to compete if oxygenation remains satisfactory during a graded stress test					
Sickle cell trait	Yes	Yes	Yes	Yes	Yes
Skin: boils, herpes, impetigo, scabies	*	*	Yes	Yes	Yes
*No gymnastics with mats, martial arts, wrestling, or contact sports until not contagious					
Spleen, enlarged	No	No	No	Yes	Yes
Testicle, absence or undescended	Yes*	Yes*	Yes*	Yes*	Yes*
*Certain sports may require protective cup					

§ From Dement P: Ross Laboratories, 1987.

TABLE 8–23. Recommended Schedule for Active Immunization of Normal Infants and Children[*]

RECOMMENDED AGE	IMMUNIZATION(S)[†]	COMMENTS
2 months	DTP, OPV	Can be initialized as early as 2 wk of age in areas of high endemicity or during epidemics
4 months	DTP, OPV	2-mo interval desired for OPV to avoid interference from previous dose
6 months	DTP, (OPV)	OPV is optional (may be given in areas with increased risk of poliovirus exposure)
15 months	Measles, mumps, rubella (MMR)	MMR preferred to individual vaccines; tuberculin testing may be done
18 months	DTP, OPV	
4–6 yr	DTP, OPV	At or before school entry
14–16 yr	Td	Repeat every 10 yr throughout life

[*] From American Academy of Pediatrics: *Report of the Committee on Control of Infectious Diseases,* 21st ed. Elk Grove Village, Ill., American Academy of Pediatrics, 1988.

[†] *DTP,* diphtheria and tetanus toxoids plus pertussis bacterial antigens; *OPV,* oral poliomyelitis vaccine; *Td,* tetanus and diphtheria toxoids.

was not the practice when many of the current cohort of older adolescents were that age.

It has been estimated that as many as 25 per cent of adolescent females do not have measurable antibody titers to rubella. The low risk from rubella immunization has prompted a recent recommendation that all young adolescent girls be immunized or reimmunized without a need for prior determinations of rubella antibody titer. The potential hazard of rubella vaccine virus to a fetus should be explained and it should not be administered to any patient who might be pregnant. Recent studies have found that the fetus does not become infected, but a sexually active adolescent should be assisted in not becoming pregnant within 3 months of rubella immunization.

Nearly three quarters of cases of rubeola and mumps now occur among adolescents and young adults. For males, absence of a history of mumps should be an indication for mumps immunization in an attempt to prevent the occurrence of orchitis and sterility.

It has been suggested that the immunization status of all adolescent patients be assessed by serologic surveillance and that vaccination be provided to those found lacking in protective titers.

Pregnancy Prevention

The need for contraception is discussed in Chapter 9 (pp. 312–315).

Prevention of Sexually Transmitted Disease

This issue also is addressed in Chapter 9 (pp. 315–316).

ANTICIPATORY GUIDANCE

Preparation for Puberty

The onset of puberty is typically associated with a number of concerns as the self-conscious early adolescent may view him or herself as too early or too late in pubertal onset, too fat, too short, or in some way abnormal (e.g., because of acne or of asymmetric breast development in girls or any breast development at all in boys).

The physician should instruct the early adolescent as to the wide range of normal developmental patterns with the aid of pictures of stages of pubertal development and charts indicating the timing and duration of each. Showing the young adolescent female her actual present stage and using this as a marker for anticipating the likely time either of menarche or of the growth spurt is reassuring to her.

Preparation for the possibility of asymmetry of breast development and the adiposity associated with female development can be most useful in preventing anxiety, should or when these occur. The young gymnast or ballet dancer concerned about her lack of onset of pubertal development should be counseled that with discontinuation of training for a period of about 2 months, pubertal development may begin and may progress more rapidly than usual so long as there are no other problems and the timing is consistent with the family pattern.

Comparisons in the locker room often lead to anxiety among males in early adolescence as to the adequacy of development of their external genitalia or the presence of breast tissue. Accordingly, the physician should instruct males as to the wide range of timing of normal development. Indicating where the young man falls with respect to SMR is often reassuring, as it is with females, particularly if coupled with estimates of the time interval until progression to the next stage. Boys who have not yet had their height spurt may be relieved to learn that the recent growth of testes (or hands and feet) indicates that the height spurt is imminent.

It is also important in the case of boys to comment upon the frequency with which gynecomastia occurs (30 to 50 per cent), as well as to reassure the youngster of the likelihood of its resolution within 18 months of onset.

Preparation for Menarche

Because 10 per cent of girls have menarche during early adolescence (SMR 2), it is appropriate that this issue be addressed during any routine evaluation before the age of 11 years. Not only should menses be explained, but the variability of timing of the event should be stressed in order to allay anxiety if the patient should be earlier or later than her peer group. In addition, there should be discussion about menstrual cramps, their etiology, and their prevention with use either of prostaglandin inhibitors or of oral contraceptives. Discussion about the use of tampons is appropriate, both because of concern about risks for toxic shock syndrome (TSS) and to provide an opportunity for the young girl to express any reluctance she may have about touching her own genitalia. TSS is associated with use of superabsorbant tampons and still occurs in the United States at a frequency of 30 reported cases per month, 40 per cent of which currently occur in adolescents (Litt, 1983b).

Development of Independence

Because early adolescence is the time when independence from parents typically begins to be negotiated (see pp. 259–260), the physician may provide assistance in facilitating this process. By acknowledging the teenager's maturity and explaining that he or she is now capable of assuming a greater role in his or her own health care, the physician may stimulate parents to delegate responsibility in other areas. In the health care setting, this principle is made operational by taking most of the medical history from the teenager, rather than from the parent, by examination in privacy, by extending confidentiality, by discussing plans for treatment and follow-up first with the teenager, and by handing any prescription directly to him or her. The parents are then informed of the plans in the presence of the adolescent patient, after the physician has received permission from the latter to do so. In this way, as a role model in the context of the routine health examination, the physician may be in a position to assist parents in the process of granting some independence to their early adolescent offspring.

Parents' willingness to allow their sons to separate and gain independent from them is often a function of the sons' rate of pubertal development. For example, parents of sons who are late maturing, albeit within the normal range, have lower expectations of them than do parents of early-maturing boys. Parents of chronically ill adolescents should be encouraged by the physician to allow their youngster involvement in age-appropriate activities (e.g., overnights, parties) that acknowledge and/or promote development of independence.

Chapter 9

MIDDLE ADOLESCENCE

Middle adolescence comprises stages (SMRs) 3 and 4 of pubertal maturation. As seen in Tables 8–1, 8–2, 8–3, and 8–4, there is a wide range of chronologic age at each of these stages. The majority of 12 to 14-year-old white females, 12-year-old black females, and 13-year-old white and black males are at this stage of adolescence, along with 14- and 15-year-old Latino males and 13- and 14-year-old Latino females.

ENDOCRINOLOGY

The earlier pubertal pattern of pulsatile release of the gonadotropins LH and FSH continues through middle adolescence, with persistence of sex differences in plasma levels. In girls, the FSH levels have reached a plateau by this time, whereas the LH levels begin to rise. In boys, FSH levels continue to rise through middle adolescence, whereas the LH level had its steepest rise earlier during stage 2. The impact of these changes in gonadotropin levels is that plasma testosterone levels continue to increase during middle adolescence. The greatest increase occurs between bone ages 12 and 13 years in boys, whereas the increase in this hormone in girls is gradual from SMR 2 through SMR 4.

A fourfold increase in estradiol level occurs in girls upon entry into middle adolescence (SMR 3, breast), with further increases to levels of 30 ng/dL achieved by SMR 4. The advent of menarche (which occurs during middle adolescence for 80 per cent of normal females) initiates cyclic variations in estradiol levels, which range from 15 ng/dL in the follicular phase to 45 ng/dL during the luteal phase. Estrone levels reach a plateau during middle adolescence following their early adolescent rise. Estrone and estradiol levels rise in males during middle adolescence, but to significantly lower levels than in females. A sex difference in prolactin levels can be appreciated toward the end of early adolescence and the beginning of middle adolescence. Somatomedin-C levels peak during middle adolescence (SMR 4) in both sexes (537 ± 155 ng/mL in females and 530 ± 142 ng/mL in males) (see Fig. 8–5).

PHYSICAL GROWTH AND DEVELOPMENT

Physical

Height and the Skeletal System

The peak in height velocity for both sexes occurs during middle adolescence (for about 80 per cent of males and 60 per cent of females), at about 12 years for females and 14 years for males. The Harpendin Growth Study found growth velocity at the peak to average 10.3 cm/year (± 1.54) for males and 9.0 cm/year (± 1.03) for females (Tanner and Marshall, 1974). As a result, males grow 7 to 12 cm and females 6 to 11 cm during the year in which peak height velocity occurs. For the entire growth spurt, the gain for males averages 28 cm, and for females 25 cm. The earlier the age at the time of the peak of the height velocity curve, the greater is the peak velocity.

The pattern of linear growth is orderly, beginning with the foot, followed approximately 6 months later by that of the calf and then the thigh. This early acceleration of foot growth contributes to the awkward appearance of many adolescents, who may be reassured to learn that foot growth ceases before that of the rest of the body. More than half of the growth of the lower limbs occurs at the distal epiphysis of the femur (Ogden, 1982). The upper extremity begins its growth spurt later than the lower extremity, with the radius and humerus reaching their maximum growth rates at approximately the same time. The carrying angle of the arm of the male is less than that of the female as a result of differential pubertal growth of cartilage at the lateral humeral epicondyle.

The approximate ages of children and adolescents at the times of radiologic appearance of secondary ossification centers and of physical closure of the epiphyses of the long bones are given in Figures 9–1 and 9–2 (see also Table 1-6).

Growth of the trunk also accelerates after that of the lower extremity, with a greater gain in sitting height during the growth spurt than in leg length. Leg length, in relation to total body length, is greater in men than in women because of the later age of the growth spurt and the correspondingly longer period of prepubertal growth in boys.

The biacromial and biiliac measurements experience peaks in growth velocity approximately 4 months after the peak of leg length growth. The biacromial growth is of greater magnitude in males and the biiliac in females, leading to wider shoulders in boys and broader hips in girls. Ossification is seen in the crest of the ilium within 6 months of menarche in most girls. This occurs approximately 1.5 years later in males (Ogden, 1982).

Most of the bones of the face also undergo growth spurts during middle adolescence, shortly after the peak of the height velocity curve or, in the case of the mandible in girls, coincident with it. As a result of the increase in mandibular length and in height of the mandibular ramus, the jaw projects more and appears thicker than in earlier childhood, particularly

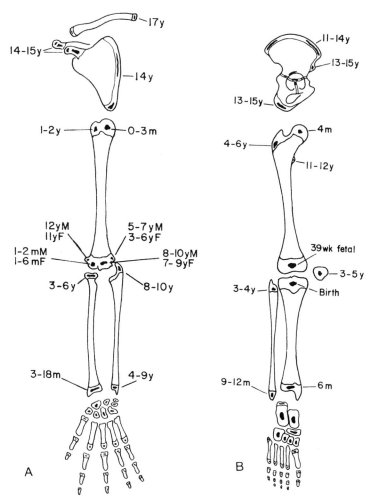

Figure 9–1. Ages of onset of secondary ossification centers. *A*, Arm. *B*, Leg. From Ogden JA: *Skeletal Injury in the Child*. Philadelphia, Lea & Febiger, 1982, pp 56–57.

in boys. Lowering of the hyoid bone as a result of growth in length of the pharynx also occurs during the pubertal growth spurt.

Weight and Growth of Soft Tissues

The peak of the weight velocity curve occurs during middle adolescence, approximately 6 months after that for height velocity. For males, the increase in weight is largely due to an approximately fourfold increase in the number of muscle cells. The peak in muscle strength is noted about 14 months after the peak of the height velocity curve and corresponds to SMR 4. For males, the relative amount of fat in the body falls from 8 to 7 per cent at the time of the pubertal growth spurt. For females, the puber-

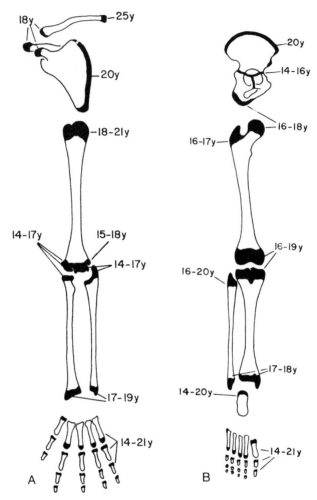

Figure 9–2. Ages of physical closure of the epiphyses. *A*, Arm. *B*, leg.
From Ogden JA: *Skeletal Injury in the Child*. Philadelphia, Lea & Febiger, 1982, pp 56–57.

tal weight spurt is predominantly due to increase in number and size of adipocytes. The fat content of the body in females increases from about 8 per cent before puberty to more than 20 per cent at the time of the peak of the weight velocity curve.

The viscera of the chest and abdomen experience growth spurts during middle adolescence; lymphoid tissue undergoes involution at this time. Accordingly, tonsils and lymph nodes become smaller. The peak increase in transverse diameter of the heart and width of the lungs parallels that of the peak of the height velocity curve, whereas that for lung length occurs approximately 6 months later. The pancreas, the nonlymphatic components of the spleen, the liver, and the kidneys also participate in the growth spurt during middle adolescence.

In males, in addition to the structural changes of the pubertal growth spurt, such as those in lung, heart, and muscle (increase in number and size of cells and strength of muscle), there occur at this time certain physiologic changes, such as slowing of pulse rate, increase in systolic blood pressure, and increase in hemoglobin concentration. These changes combine to make the middle adolescent male stronger and endow him with greater endurance than his younger male counterpart or females at any age. These changes also require that participation in contact or collision sports such as football, soccer, or hockey should be based on criteria of physical maturation rather than on chronologic age in order to prevent the late-maturing adolescent from being overpowered or injured by his or her earlier maturing peer of the same chronologic age (see also pp. 284–285).

Primary Sex Characteristics

Males

The volume of the testes during middle adolescence ranges from approximately 10 to 14 mL (see Table 8–6). There is a growth spurt in the seminal vesicles, epididymis, and prostate at this time and the first morning urine frequently contains spermatozoa by approximately 14.5 years of age, although the timing of spermarche is quite variable (see Fig. 8–16). First ejaculation may occur during this period, although more typically at SMR 2.

Females

Ovaries enlarge in the year prior to menarche, at which time their average weight becomes about 6 g each. Just prior to menarche the endometrium develops, the cervix and corpus of the uterus enlarge, and cervical glands begin to secrete a milky, nonmalodorous, mucoid material in large amounts (a "physiologic" discharge). Vaginal fluid is also secreted in larger amounts than earlier, and its pH becomes acid, owing to production of lactic acid by the bacilli that come to inhabit the vagina.

Eighty per cent of girls achieve menarche during middle adolescence (SMR 3 and 4). Most early menstrual periods are anovulatory, but there is sufficient variability in time of onset of ovulatory periods to make this unreliable as a method of contraception.

Secondary Sex Characteristics (See Figs. 8–13, 8–14, and 8–15)

Males

The average age for attainment of *SMR 3 (genital)* is 12.85 (± 1.04) years, and this stage lasts for an average of 0.8 year, with a range from 0.2 to 1.6 years. At SMR 3 the external genitalia continue to grow, the penis in length and at this stage, for the first time, in width as well, owing to growth of the corpora cavernosa. During this stage, the pubic hair becomes darker and coarser and begins to curl. It extends upward from the base of the penis and somewhat laterally. The average age for attainment of *SMR 3* (*pubic hair*) is 13.9 (±1.04) years, and this stage of pubic hair persists on the average for 0.4 year, with a range from 0.3 to 0.5 year.

At *SMR 4* (*genital*) the testes and scrotum continue to enlarge and the skin of the scrotum darkens. In addition to further growth in the length and breadth of the penis, the glans develops. The average age for reaching SMR 4 (genital) is 13.7 (±1.02) years, and it lasts for an average of 0.8 year, with a range from 0.4 to 1.9 years.

The pubic hair reaches its adult texture and spreads to cover most of the mons. *SMR 4* (*pubic hair*) in the male is reached at an average age of 14.36 (±1.08) years, and persists for an average of 0.7 year with a range from 0.2 to 1.5 years.

During middle adolescence axillary and circumanal hair appears, the voice deepens, and axillary perspiration acquires its characteristic odor.

Females

At *SMR 3* (*pubic hair*) development is identical with that for males (above). SMR 3 (pubic hair) is reached at an average age of 12.36 (±1.10) years, and lasts for an average of 0.5 year with a range from 0.2 to 0.9 year.

The breast at this stage has enlarged further and taken a continuous, rounded shape. SMR 3 (breast) is reached at an average age of 12.15 (±1.09) years and persists for an average of 0.9 year with a range from 0.1 to 2.2 years.

At *SMR 4* (*pubic hair*) is again comparable to that of males (above). This stage occurs at an average age of 12.95 (±1.06) years, and lasts an average of 1.3 years with a range from 0.6 to 2.4 years.

The areola and the papilla enlarge at this stage and form a mound on the underlying breast tissue. *SMR 4* (*breast*) is reached at an average age of 13.11 (±1.15) years and persists for an average of 1.96 years, with a range from 0.1 to 6.8 years. In contrast with other stages, which are fairly universal, some girls appear to pass directly from SMR 3 (breast) to SMR 5 (breast) without an intervening SMR 4. Alternatively, the duration of SMR 4 (breast) may have been unusually transient in them and therefore unnoticed.

Other Secondary Sex Characteristics

Axillary hair may precede the appearance of pubic hair, but the more typical pattern is for it to follow, appearing during middle adolescence (see Fig. 8–12). Circumanal hair usually appears shortly before that in the axillary region. Facial hair in males tends to appear approximately 1 year after axillary hair, usually during middle adolescence.

Deepening of the male voice begins during middle adolescence as a result of stimulation by testosterone of the growth of cells of the thyroid and cricoid cartilages, and of laryngeal muscle cells.

Apocrine sweat glands become functional at about the time of appearance of axillary hair. Acne worsens with advancing sexual maturation.

In males, as in females, the areola of the breast typically widens during puberty. In 30 to 50 per cent of middle adolescent boys there occurs, in addition, enlargement of the underlying breast tissue in one or both breasts (see p. 251). This enlargement is transient in most, persisting less than 18 months.

Dentition

The second permanent molar generally erupts (see Table 1–7) during late early adolescence or early middle adolescence (from 11 to 13 years of age). As with dentition in general, this occurs earlier in females than males. There is a close correlation between the timing of this event and menarche.

Neurodevelopment

There is no further neuromaturation during middle adolescence, so far as we know currently. During SMR 3 and 4, sleep latency time decreases, and daytime sleepiness increases (Anders et al., 1980).

Cognitive Development

In the piagetian scheme of classification, middle adolescents would be expected to have reached the stage of formal operations (see Table 8–12). It is probably more appropriate, however, to consider them to be continuing toward achievement of adult processing capabilities along the lines described by Flavell (see pp. 256–257).

Moral Development

The chronologic ages that encompass middle adolescence correspond roughly to those at which Kohlberg and Gilligan (1971) thought the individual would have attained Stage 3 of moral development. At this stage, there is mutuality in interpersonal relationships and right is defined in terms of shared feelings and of agreements that supersede individual concerns (p. 257).

Psychosocial Development

Despite the eriksonian characterization of adolescence as a time of "identity crisis," studies of this construct over the course of the adolescent years suggest that stability is the norm, rather than marked disruption. When instability is found, it tends to be among those adolescents whose *self-image* was negative at the time of first testing in early adolescence.

Problems of self-image tend to arise among middle adolescents who view their pubertal development, or lack thereof, as problematic. Among these, for example, are males who mature later than their peer group and females who view the normal pubertal increase in adiposity with disgust. Any departure from the peer group norm may give rise to anxiety, but this is a particular problem for later maturing males, who have been consistently found to have poorer self-image than do early-maturing males. On follow-up of these youngsters into adulthood, there appear to be sequelae of the feelings of insecurity and inadequacy. Gross and Duke (1980) suggest that the progressive stages of pubertal maturation in females evoke increasing feelings of being fat and the desire to become thinner. Such feelings of negative self-worth often lead to dieting and may contribute to the development of anorexia nervosa and bulima, particularly in a social environment such as ours, which values slenderness as the ideal of feminine beauty.

Functional Contexts of Middle Adolescence

The family, peer group, and school remain the primary contexts for function during middle, as in early adolescence. Family interaction tends to be calmer than during the early adolescent years, when rebelliousness was most likely to surface if it was to occur at all. Offer (1973) characterized adolescents entering high school as having become "amateur psychologists," having gained "an intuitive grasp of [their] own psychological being," and in so doing, having gained mastery over many of their impulses and feelings. Included in the latter category were sexual feelings, which most middle-class youngsters in Offer's sample controlled through such other outlets as sports, academic pursuits, and same-sex social activities.

Interpersonal Relationships

For males, who manifest strong needs for achievement and independence, peer activities tend to occur mainly in the context of a group.

For females, who at this stage appear to need to develop interpersonal skills and secure loving relationships, peer interactions are more likely to be centered in a dyadic friendship characterized by loyalty, commitment, and the intimacy of shared secrets and experiences (Douvan and Adelson, 1966).

The peak level of anxiety, insecurity about friendships, and fear of rejection tends to occur during middle adolescence for both sexes. Perhaps as a result of these insecurities, it is during middle adolescence that there is the greatest emphasis on conformity of behavior within the peer group. Interestingly, self-blame parallels the emphasis on conformity, and like the latter is highest during middle adolescence. An interesting paradox thus develops during this period of life: as youngsters proclaim their independence from their families and their individuality, they substitute confirmity to the standards of another group, of their own age rather than older.

The emphasis on conformity and tendency toward self-blame have important implications for the middle adolescent whose physical development deviates in any way from his or her peer group norm, even if it falls within the normal range as defined by larger populations. The physically impaired adolescent is at a particularly serious disadvantage at this stage of development. Accordingly, the physician caring for such youngsters must be aware of and responsive to their discomfort and inevitable feelings of inadequacy. Reassurance is indicated and should be given in concrete terms, such as predictions of when a growth spurt will occur or what the progression of development of secondary sex characteristics will be. An ongoing commentary is useful as to the normality of each organ or organ system examined during the course of the physical examination.

Same-sex groupings characterize this period of development, but it is also during middle adolescence that social groups become extended to include members of the opposite sex and paired dating may begin (Chess et al., 1976).

Heterosexual Relationships

Dating behavior undergoes a developmental progression that has been described by Schofield (1965), and typically begins with talking, to the exclusion of physical contact (Stage 1). The next stage (Stage 2) includes kissing with touching of clothed breasts. In Stage 3 there is touching of unclothed breasts or genital apposition. Intercourse with a single partner characterizes Stage 4, and in Stage 5 there are often multiple partners. Among middle adolescents who date, it is unusual that Stage 4 is reached, and among adolescents who engage in intercourse at all, it is typically with a single partner.

Sorensen's survey (1973) of teenagers' sexual attitudes and behaviors found that among 13- to 15-year-olds 22 per cent reported absence of any sexual contact other than kissing (20 per cent of males and 25 per cent of females). Petting (sexual touching or viewing of another's body for sexual pleasure) described the level of sexual involvement of another 17 per cent of this sample (14 per cent of males and 19 per cent of females). The importance of petting as a link to later adult heterosexual encounters has been recognized. It teaches adolescents about each other's bodies, emotional and sexual responses, notions of masculinity and femininity, and social rules and customs of sexual behavior and thus allows for beginning consolidation of the disparate components of sexual identity.

The determinants of the age at which dating behavior begins have been studied with conflicting results. Blyth et al. (1981) reported that biologic factors appeared dominant, whereas Dornbusch et al. (1981) found dating in females to be more closely linked to grade in school than to stage of sexual maturation. The complexity of this issue is underscored by the finding in one study that timing of pubertal maturation interacted with environmental factors in determining both the onset of dating behavior and its associations. Simmons et al. (1979) found that earlier maturing females who entered junior high school and began dating early had lower self-esteem and a lower grade point average than those who had not yet commenced dating.

Those who date late tend to be better students and to be involved in religious activities, but the cross-sectional nature of the studies that have examined these issues precludes definition of the direction of these relationships. Another study of determinants of early dating not surprisingly found that physical attractiveness in general and absence of obesity in particular were important factors.

In studies of the transition from virginity to intercourse activity during the high school years, Jessor and Jessor (1975b) conclude that those who would make this transition tended to be those who valued independence more than achievement and who were more influenced by the views of friends than parents. In this study, as well as in the study by Sorensen (1973), virgins were characterized as having greater religiosity, less tolerance for drug usage by friends, and higher levels of scholastic achievement.

The ages for initiation of sexual activity for females are given in Fig. 9–3. The average age of initiation of sexual intercourse has remained fairly constant at 16 years over the past few decades. For white females it is 16.4 years, and for black females 15.5 years. However, during the 1970s there was a significant increase (approximately two thirds) in the number of teenagers who become sexually active; the increase is largely attributable to unmarried whites. It has been found that 18 per cent of boys and 6 per cent of girls become sexually active during middle adolescence. Those males who have had intercourse by the age of 14 years appear more likely to become what Sorsensen has termed "sexual adventurers"—those who have multiple sexual partners.

Teenage Pregnancy

More than half of sexually active teenage couples use no birth control at the time of first intercourse, and young adolescents are less likely than those who are older to obtain or to continue to use effective contraceptives. Accordingly, it is not surprising that the risk of pregnancy is very high among them. One fifth of adolescent pregnancies occur within the first month and 50 per cent occur within 6 months after the onset of intercourse activity. In 1985 in the United States there were 31,000 pregnancies among adolescents under the age of 15 years.

The Alan Guttmacher Institute (1981) estimated that of every 10 girls who were then 14 years of age, about four would get pregnant while still a teenager; two would bear a live child; 1.5 would have a therapeutic abortion; and 0.6 would experience a spontaneous abortion. Among adolescents under 15 years old abortions surpassed births in the year following the 1973 Supreme Court decision legalizing abortions, and since then there have been about 1.4 abortions for each live birth among middle adolescents.

The frequency of medical complications of pregnancy during middle adolescence is significantly higher than for adult women or for older adolescents. For example, the risk of death for women under the age of 15 years was 18 per 100,000 live births, a rate 2½ times higher than that for

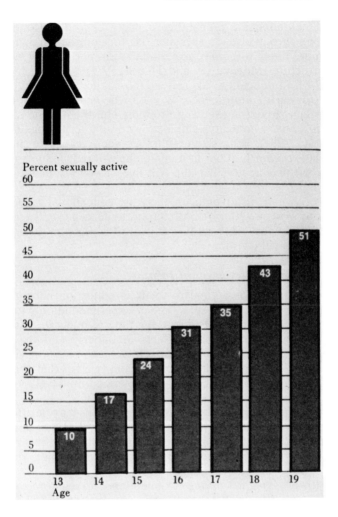

Figure 9–3. Percent of 13- to 19-year-old females that are sexually active, by single years of age, United States, 1974–1975.
From Alan Guttmacher Institute. *11 Million Teenagers.* New York, Alan Guttmacher Institute, 1976.

mothers between the ages of 20 and 24 years. Their risks of developing nonfatal complications such as toxemia and anemia are also correspondingly higher. Obstetrical complications such as prolonged labor, uterine dysfunction, contracted pelvis, and need for cesarean section for cephalopelvic disproportion are also more frequent in this age group.

For the infant born to a mother under 15 years of age there is twice the risk of being born small for gestational age and/or premature than that for infants born to adult women. The reasons for these findings are multifactorial and relate to the fact that adolescents are less likely than older women to seek adequate prenatal care, more likely to belong to a low socioeconomic group already at higher risk for poor health and malnutrition, and more likely to be physically immature, particularly with regard to pelvic structure (McAnarney and Thiede, 1983).

Nonmedical complications also attend those who become pregnant during middle (or early) adolescence. Women who give birth before the age of 16 years can expect in the future to have half the income of a female head-of-household who delays childbearing until after the age of 20 years (Moore et al., 1981). Data suggest that for each year after menarche a woman delays the birth of her first child, she will reduce by two percentage points the probability that she will live in poverty at the age of 27 years.

Besides economic disadvantages, there are educational sequelae. Only 50 per cent of women who give birth during adolescence will achieve their high school diplomas, whereas 97 per cent of those who do not become teenage parents will do so.

Progress toward Achievement of Identity

Middle adolescence is a time to focus attention on educational and vocational goals. It is, therefore, a time of experimentation with possible roles. It is, in the scheme of Erikson, the time to integrate with societal pressures the profound physical effects of puberty and the cognitive changes of adolescence, and in so doing to achieve a subjective identity. It is only after successful resolution of the identity crisis that one is free to progress to the next stage, which is characterized by developing the capacity for intimacy.

Developing educational and vocational aspirations may be affected by a variety of factors in addition to the obvious ones of school performance and of experience (whether planned or serendipitous). Parents remain the dominant force when it comes to planning for the future, despite the influence of peers in other domains.

The health professional caring for middle adolescents needs to know that something as seemingly far-removed as timing of pubertal maturation may have an effect on this process. Not only can synchrony or lack thereof with the peer group pattern have an influence on school performance and self-image, but asynchrony appears for males to have a significant impact both on the teenager and on his parents' aspirations and expectations. Gross and Duke (1980) found that later maturing males have lower educational aspirations and expectations than do those who mature early, even when both groups were within the range defined as normal for pubertal development. These lowered expectations were found to be mirrored in the expectations of parents.

Steinberg (1988) found that relationships between the middle adolescent and parents appear to be influenced by pubertal maturation. Middle adolescent males and their mothers interrupt each other more than before or after this period of development. Females in middle adolescence have more arguments with their mothers and distance themselves from their fathers. There appears to be more rigidity in patterns of interaction within the family at this time, as well.

Not only is self-image and educational identity solidified during middle adolescence, but so also is sexual identity and a sense of sexual adequacy. As indicated above, heterosexual experimentation begins, typically in the form of petting. In addition, for the individual whose sexual preference is homosexual, middle adolescence tends to be the time when this issue is confronted.

Homosexuality

It is estimated that 8 per cent of females are lesbian and 13 per cent of males gay, figures that suggest that most health professionals dealing with this age group will have contact with someone grappling with issues of homosexuality and likely in need of support, whether or not this need is overtly expressed or sought. The issues that are likely to confront the homosexual midadolescent include: 1) acceptance of one's homosexuality; 2) dealing with the family's reaction to discovery; 3) peer relations within the nonhomosexual community; 4) career planning; and 5) health sequelae.

Porowski (1987) described the process of acceptance of one's homosexuality as consisting of eight stages:

1. Realization of the desire to have same-sex relationships.
2. Guilt, shame, and fear about the feelings and behavior because of concern that they are abnormal.
3. Attempts to change to heterosexual interests, even to the extent of marriage and becoming a parent.
4. Poor self-esteem following failure to change.
5. Denial, associated with assumption of asexuality and involvement in stereotypically masculine behavior for males and feminine behavior for females.
6. Exploration of the gay/lesbian life-style. For males this typically involves frequenting places attractive to homosexuals and multiple sexual encounters. For females, involvement in lesbian support groups is more common.
7. Acceptance of homosexuality.
8. Development of a positive attitude toward one's sexual preference.

The nature of the interface of the homosexual adolescent with the health care system will depend upon the youngster's stage of progress in realization of and adjustment to his or her homosexual orientation. If the stage is early, there may be attempts to avoid physicians because of fear of "being found out" through a physical examination. For example, most male teenagers with gynecomastia have at some time or another some question as to their maleness. Fear is accentuated for the gay teenager who, if he happens to have gynecomastia, may be concerned that his breasts will signal his homosexuality to the physician. The physician should suspect that this may be the cause when a teenager refuses a physical examination; this occurrence should be met by reassurance and by provision of opportunity to discuss personal concerns.

The teenager who is at the stage of attempting to change to a heterosexual orientation may become involved in promiscuous heterosexual behavior with its attendant risks of pregnancy for the female and of sexually transmitted disease, or premature heterosexual marriage and childbearing. When the physician discovers that an adolescent is having sexual intercourse without any interest in contraception, there should be prompt exploration of the possibility that homosexual fear is the underlying cause, albeit the majority of sexually active adolescents who shun contraception do so for other reasons.

The poor self-esteem that often follows failure at attempts to change to a heterosexual life-style may precipitate profound depression. As with depression of any etiology, this may portend a suicide attempt and should therefore be a signal for the need for counseling. Depression in the homosexual youngster may be even more serious than with others, owing to the frequently associated isolation that results from the need to hide sexual orientation from peers.

Pursuit of asexuality and total immersion in stereotypically same-sex behavior may also have medical sequelae. Male homosexuals often cope with this stage by involvement in "macho" activities, with the attendant risk of injury. There is no apparent counterpart of this stage for lesbian teenagers.

The next stage, that of exploration of the gay life-style, often places the gay teenager in jeopardy as far as the risk of sexually transmitted diseases. In addition to those infections that often result from heterosexual activity, gays appear to be at heightened risk for amebiasis, hepatitis B, anal condyloma accuminata, giardiasis, salmonella, and shigella, as well as for the acquired immunodeficiency syndrome (AIDS). The extensive publicity about AIDS has understandably contributed to widespread anxiety and hypochondriasis among gay adolescents and young adults.

Once the acceptance of his or her homosexuality occurs, the next issue to be faced is the decision to inform parents. There is no simple answer to the question of whether and how parents might best be informed. The physician can play an important role in assisting the teenager to sort out the pros and cons of informing parents. If the decision is affirmative, further help is needed in deciding on timing. The best time would be when the family and teenager are not under stress and surely not at a time of anger. By being present when the family is told, the physician may assist them in raising specific concerns and then guide them through an exercise in reality testing.

Career decisions are often influenced by stereotypic thinking about homosexuals. The former classification of homosexuality as a psychiatric disorder surely served as a barrier to acceptance into professional schools. The American Psychiatric Association's *Diagnostic and Statistical Manual of Mental Disorders* (third edition, revised) (DSM III-R) (1987) no longer supports this view of homosexuality. The lack of knowledge of or access to gay and lesbian role-models is a more subtle influence on career choices for homosexual teenagers.

In order to be helpful to the homosexually oriented adolescent, the physician must first identify him or her as gay or lesbian. Occasionally, the youngster may be referred to the physician by a parent who is worried about this possibility. More often, however, he or she does not appear with such a label, but may be recognized through sensitive questioning in the context of obtaining a sexual history. For example, asking a male adolescent if he has a girlfriend and dropping the subject if he says "no" will miss an opportunity to identify a gay male. The same holds true for the adolescent female, who is typically asked only if she has a boy friend.

Chronic Illness

The task of developing a sense of sexual adequacy during middle adolescence is also difficult for the teenager with a chronic illness. If the illness is one that delays development of secondary sex characteristics, such as sickle cell anemia, cyanotic congenital heart disease, cystic fibrosis, inflammatory bowel disease, or diabetes mellitus, the youngster may be made to feel abnormal and to doubt his or her future chances for normal heterosexual relationships and procreative potential. This concern is accentuated when a proscription against pregnancy is given by the physician concerned about its potential harmful effects on the progression of the disease or about the effects of medication on the fetus.

For example, should a chronic illness affect the genitourinary tract, the teenager may erroneously assume that the anatomic proximity of urinary with genital organs reflects functional overlap and he or she may worry about reproductive implications (Cogan et al., 1975). It is rare that such concerns are expressed spontaneously. Anticipation that they exist should prompt reassurance by the physician.

Chronic illness associated with physical disability may prevent the middle adolescent from the opportunities for peer interaction so vital for acquisition of knowledge about sexuality and for experimentation. Parents of such teenagers may have even more difficulty than do those of physically healthy youngsters in recognizing their need for information about reproductive and sexual matters. This has, for example, been well documented among girls with meningomyelocele, who are at a particular disadvantage because of their early maturation and limitations of physical mobility (Hayden et al., 1979).

DEVELOPMENTAL ASSESSMENT AND DELIVERY OF HEALTH CARE

The elements of assessment of the middle adolescent are listed in Table 9-1.

Physical Examination

Females

In addition to the issues raised in the discussion of the physical examination of the early adolescent (pp. 264–270), examination of the middle adolescent female should focus on those organs or organ systems likely to manifest pathology at this stage of development. Accordingly, breast examination should be undertaken because of the frequency of development

TABLE 9–1. Package of Care for the Well Adolescent, Visit II: Mid–Late Adolescence (Tanner 3–5)*,†

	FEMALES	MALES
Screening		
Physical	Vision testing	Vision testing
	Hearing testing	Hearing testing
	Genetically transmitted diseases	Genetically transmitted diseases
If sexually active	Pap smear	—
	VDRL	VDRL
Prevention	Gonorrhea and chlamydia culture	Gonorrhea and chlamydia culture
	Automotive safety	Automotive safety
	Venereal disease prevention	Venereal disease prevention
	Prevention of pregnancy	Prevention of pregnancy
Anticipatory Guidance	Planning for marriage	Planning for marriage
	Vocational/educational planning	Vocational/educational planning
	Cults	Cults
	Becoming a health-care consumer	Becoming a health-care consumer
Physical Examination	Breast masses	Gynecomastia
	—	Testicular tumor
	Vaginal discharge	Urethral discharge
	Pregnancy	—
Treatment	Corrective surgery (after growth complete)	Corrective surgery (after growth complete)

* Adapted from Litt IF: Adolescent health care. In Green M, Haggerty RJ (eds): *Ambulatory Pediatrics III*. Philadelphia, WB Saunders Company, 1984, pp 80–103.
† Incremental with items listed for early adolescence in Table 8–13.

of cysts and fibroadenoma at this time. If the technique for self-examination of the breast has not previously been taught, it is appropriate at this time; if so, a review may be in order. The possibility of a vaginal discharge should be investigated first by history, and then by pelvic examination if the history indicates.

The pelvic examination is not generally a routine procedure for physicians who are not gynecologists, and certainly not for all patients, regardless of age. For the adolescent patient, it is even more a special procedure than for adults. The first pelvic examination is often a dreaded event, for which the young girl has been poorly or inappropriately prepared. Emotions called fourth by this event include modesty, fear of pain, and anxiety about the possibility of being found to be abnormal, or to be "found out" if she has experienced masturbation or sexual intercourse. Reassurance may come from explanation of the procedure to be followed, preferably with demonstration on a pelvic model, and from reassuring commentary as to what is being done and found during the course of the examination. In addition, ample time for questions will help alleviate some of the anxiety.

No patient should ever be forced to have a pelvic examination, and a complete pelvic examination (that is, bimanual and speculum examination) is not always indicated. For example, if the patient is not sexually active yet is experiencing a vaginal discharge, the necessary culture specimens for detecting *Candida albicans* may be obtained by the patient's insertion of a sterile swab into the vagina under supervision. Similarly, concern about the possibility of an ovarian mass may be addressed by a bimanual examination, without the added discomfort of a speculum examination. When both are needed, it has been our experience that reversal of the traditional order of the pelvic examination is better tolerated by the adolescent (see Appendix A). Accordingly, the digital and bimanual examination is performed first, using water and patience as lubricators. Following this, examination with the speculum is made and necessary visualization and collection of specimens undertaken. When the speculum examination is done first, as is usual in the traditional pelvic examination of adults, the young patient often becomes so fearful that neither element of the examination can be carried out satisfactorily.

Some clinicians advocate performance of a pelvic examination for all adolescent females, whereas others suggest waiting until the 18th birthday. It is our impression that such age-related criteria are arbitrary and that the yield from early pelvic examination is quite small. Accordingly, we suggest that the procedure be performed when the cost-benefit ratio is low, i.e., when one of the following indications exist:

When the patient is sexually active. Sexual activity is associated with risk of contracting venereal disease (see above) or pregnancy. As both of these conditions may be present in the asymptomatic individual, performance of a pelvic examination, in conjunction with collection of material for culture, is the only satisfactory way in which they may be detected. A pelvic examination is also necessary prior to prescription of most effective contraceptive methods, as well as to obtain a Pap smear.

When there is a symptom that may be gynecologic in origin. If abdominal pain, vaginal discharge, or irregular, excessive, or absent menstrual bleeding occurs, a pelvic examination is indicated.

When the patient has a history of exposure in utero to diethylstilbestrol (DES). Such patients are at risk for developing adenocarcinoma and/or adenosis of the vagina following puberty or of having anomalies of the internal genitalia, conditions that may be detected by a careful examination by a skilled gynecologist.

When the young women is curious about the normality of her anatomy. Some adolescents, as a result of unsuccessful attempts at tampon insertion, or of infections of the vagina or urinary tract, are concerned that they may have abnormal genitalia and worry that they will be unable to have intercourse or to bear children. Some have an increased interest in their own bodies that comes during adolescence. Such concerns may be stated explicitly or indirectly through a request for contraception, even if the latter is not needed. Reassurance should accompany a pelvic examination for any indication, but is especially important when the patient's concerns have motivated its performance.

Males

From 30 to 50 per cent of middle adolescent males will have transient breast development (gynecomastia) (see p. 251). The examiner should be alert to this possibility and, if it is found, should explain and reassure.

The fact that about one quarter of middle adolescent males are sexually active should prompt concern that a sexually transmitted disease may be present, even if the patient is asymptomatic. Accordingly, examination of the urethra, with collection of a specimen for culture of *Neisseria gonor-*

rhoeae and of *Chlamydia trachomatis*, as well as examination of the prostate and epididymis, should be undertaken. Examination of the scrotum for testicular masses, which at this age may suggest malignancy, or of varicocele should also be performed, and should be coupled with instruction about self-examination of these structures (see Appendix B).

Screening

Laboratory Tests

Like early adolescent females, those in middle adolescence are at increased risk for iron-deficiency anemia because of the suppressive effect of increasing estrogen levels on erythropoietin, menstrual blood loss, and often inadequate dietary intake. Consequently, it is appropriate that a hematocrit be obtained at least yearly during this period of development (see Table 8–11).

Similarly, those factors that increase the risk of asymptomatic urinary tract infection during early adolescence also pertain during middle adolescence and mandate screening urinalysis or urine culture as part of the routine assessment at this time.

If rubella immunization status has not been evaluated during early adolescence, this should be done during middle adolescence, with care to assess the possibility of pregnancy, and taking measures to ensure that pregnancy will not occur during the 3 months following vaccination.

Sexually active adolescents should be screened by examination of urine for white cells, as well as by cultures for sexually transmitted disease, and should have cervical smears examined for neoplasia at yearly intervals (see p. 267).

A yearly tuberculin test continues to be indicated during the years of active physical growth, with prophylactic administration of isoniazid for 1 year following discovery of a positive test in any middle adolescent female who has not been previously treated.

Consideration should be given at this time to the performance of screening tests for genetic diseases (see p. 268).

Physical

Hearing. Continuing exposure to highly amplified music places the adolescent at increased risk for elevation of the audiometric threshold. This possibility can be adequately evaluated through an audiogram.

Vision. The adolescent growth spurt is reflected in the optic globe, which in genetically predisposed individuals may elongate at this time to produce myopia. Vision screening should therefore be performed during this phase of adolescence.

Blood Pressure. The need of the early adolescent for careful measurement of blood pressure continues (see p. 269), and this is a vital part of the evaluation of the middle adolescent.

Scoliosis. Since most adolescents experience their growth spurt during middle adolescence, the chances of developing scoliosis are highest at this time, particularly for females. Accordingly, the spine should be examined in the upright and bent-forward positions to detect curvature (see pp. 269–270). If curvature greater than 10 degrees is discovered the youngster should be referred to an orthopedist to be followed until growth is complete.

Psychosocial Screening

Issues of self-image, depression, sexuality, school, and substance abuse continue to be major concerns during middle adolescence, and the techniques for their detection, discussed in Chapter 8, continue to be appropriate (see pp. 270–276).

HEALTH PROMOTION

Breast Self-Examination

If this procedure has not previously been taught (see p. 277), it should be at this time. If it has been taught, it is appropriate to provide a refresher course of instruction at this time, and in so doing to take advantage of the opportunity to offer reassurance as to the progress of breast development and to be available to respond to any concerns about it.

Scrotum Self-Examination

As indicated above for the breast self-examination, the middle adolescent should be instructed or reinstructed in the procedure for self-examination of the testes (Appendix B).

Nutrition Counseling

For a discussion of nutrition counseling in the middle adolescent, see pp. 277–281.

PREVENTION

Smoking

For approximately 13 per cent of adolescents, middle adolescence is the time of onset of smoking, with slightly more females than males embarking on what is predictably a lifelong health hazard. Primary prevention, through use of techniques designed to teach adolescents to resist peer pressure to smoke, is the most effective approach (see pp. 281–282).

Vehicle Safety

It is during middle adolescence that most persons begin to drive automobiles or motorcycles. The accident rate is higher among this age group than in any other, and such accidents are the leading cause of death at this time of life. Moreover, the leading cause of fatal automotive accidents is driving under the influence of alcohol. Accordingly, in the course of providing health care to this age group, educational efforts at accident prevention are of major importance (see pp. 282–285).

Immunizations

For information on immunizations in middle adolescents, see pp. 285–289 and Table 8–23.

Pregnancy Prevention

As middle adolescence is often the time when sexual intercourse is considered or actually engaged in for the first time, it is appropriate that prevention of adverse sequelae be addressed at this point.

Primary prevention of adolescent pregnancy consists of postponement of sexual intercourse until adulthood. Although this goal is shared by most adults, it is unrealistic to believe that it can be accomplished by prohibitions or lectures by parents, teachers, or health professionals. What may be effective, however, is an approach that provides the adolescent with factual information and assists him or her in the process of clarifying thinking about the matter. It may be a useful strategy to stimulate the youngster to consider whether or not engaging in intercourse is something he or she actually desires or is simply a capitulation to pressures from a date one is anxious not to lose. For the girl, for example, has she considered whether or not her relationship with her boyfriend is meeting her needs and is not exploitive on his part?

In asking such questions, the health professional must take care to avoid sounding judgmental, as this will surely terminate any chance of a dialogue on the subject. The process may be facilitated by such questions as: "Is there anything in your relationship with (name of boyfriend) that could be better, or that you would wish to change?" or, more directly, "Do you actually enjoy the sexual part of your relationship with (name)?"

Secondary prevention of adolescent pregnancy involves the use of effective and safe contraceptive methods by those already sexually active. In choosing a contraceptive method for a teenager, risks of the method must be weighed against the risk of pregnancy for this age group. The possibility that compliance with a method that requires active planning may present problems for the adolescent must also be considered. The adolescent's past experience with compliance both with contraceptive and with noncontraceptive medications will give information as to whether the prescription of a contraceptive method is likely at this time to face problems in compliance (Litt, 1984b).

The importance of peer pressure in accepting a contraceptive method cannot be underestimated. For girls, the opinions of girlfriends and, most importantly, of the sexual partner should be ascertained. Even more desirable is that the sexual partner come to the physician's office so that any concerns he may have about any proposed method may be discussed, along with a general review of the situation.

It is helpful to determine the extent of parents' knowledge of their daughter's sexual activity, as this may also influence choice of method. In our experience, approximately half of our adolescent patients indicate that their parents are aware of their sexual activity. For those adolescents who wish to keep such knowledge confidential, it is legal in all states of the United States (at the time of this writing) for a physician to do so and to provide contraception.

A proposed Federal regulation that would have had the effect of requiring parental notification when a minor received contraception through any program funded by Federal Title X funds (the so-called squeal law) was defeated, but publicity surrounding its consideration has frightened many sexually active adolescents into not seeking the protection they need, in the mistaken belief that physicians are bound by such a law to notify their parents. The physician will need to take the initiative in clarifying the legal situation and in offering confidentiality.

The method of contraception for a sexually active adolescent must be individualized to account for the frequency and circumstances of intercourse, her partner's opinions as well as her own about each method, her past compliance, and the presence of medical contraindications. As indicated above, any method risk must be weighed against the possible risk of pregnancy itself.

The fact that adolescents are at greater risk for sexually transmitted disease must also be taken into account, as this may increase their risk for infertility with use of an intrauterine device. Similarly, the fact that they are at relatively greater risk for toxic shock syndrome would affect the decision to use any device that remains in the vaginal cavity for a long period of time, such as a diaphragm, contraceptive sponge, or possibly a cervical cap. Conversely, their youth places them in a very low risk category for developing cardiovascular complications from use of estrogen-containing oral contraceptives.

Besides the special biologic issues that must be taken into account when choosing a contraceptive method for an adolescent, attention needs to be paid to psychosocial and cognitive considerations. Prior to entry into the stage of formal operational thinking it is difficult for a young person to envision realistically the consequences of his or her own sexual intercourse; the concepts of pregnancy or of sexually transmitted disease are relatively abstract, information notwithstanding. As a result, it is often difficult to motivate such patients to use birth control inasmuch as they do not feel at risk for pregnancy. Adolescents generally feel invulnerable and are often willing to take risks.

Another factor complicating making contraceptive choices is the young teenager's difficulty in accepting her change in status and in admitting to herself that she is "sexually active" even when she has had sexual intercourse. Such sexual behavior is often rationalized by her as having been unanticipated and out of her control and having been "swept off her feet"; she rationalizes that it is unlikely to recur. In such a context, use of contraception would imply intentionality and require that she confront her new status, a process that takes time.

The teenager's fear of repercussions from parental discovery of sexual activity also often precludes obtaining a contraceptive method, because of fear either that a physician will notify or send a bill to the parent, or that the parents will discover the contraceptive itself.

Adolescents are also very much influenced by the opinions and experiences of their peers. If these have included unsuccessful use of a contraceptive method or complications arising from it, it is unlikely that the patient will use that method, even if she appears to accept it from the physician.

Adolescents typically feel self-conscious and imagine that they are being observed by others. This phase of development creates a formidable barrier to the obtaining of an "over-the-counter" contraceptive method, often making it too embarrassing for them to do so, even when they are otherwise motivated.

Finally, it is important to know that adolescents have limited knowledge about reproductive physiology and are subject to myths of their subculture as to the causes of pregnancy. Because of these myths, as well as because of common fears about their own sterility, they often feel that they cannot become pregnant, even though they are sexually active. Religious beliefs often preclude the use of effective contraception by adolescents.

Once having accepted an effective contraceptive method, half of adolescent patients fail to continue to use it for more than 6 months. Compliance with contraceptive use has many of the same barriers or determinants as obtaining the method initially, but is also dependent upon the adolescent's self-image and degree of achievement of independence.

Studies have shown that teenagers with good self-image and who are acting autonomously can be expected to be compliant with their contraceptive method (DuRant and Jay, 1987). It is important, therefore, that the health care provider learn about the teenager's beliefs and stage of psychosocial development in order to provide the most effective method available. For example, the patient who eschews planning for intercourse might do well with use of a method that is chronologically unrelated to the act itself, such as daily administration of an oral contraceptive, insertion of an intrauterine device, or use of an injectable, long-acting hormonal preparation. The latter two methods are easily concealed from parents, should it be necessary to do so. Spermicidal foam is prepackaged in applicators covered in white paper that look like tampons and make detection unlikely.

When poor compliance is anticipated, a method that requires little involvement of the patient, such as an injectable hormone or intrauterine device, may be advisable. Whatever methods are chosen, however, frequent follow-up is indicated to ensure continued compliance.

Provision of contraceptive care within the context of a general medical program helps to overcome the self-consciousness of the adolescent, who may be embarrassed to be seen buying contraceptives or entering a building that is known for family planning services. School-based health clinics that provide a variety of health services to this underserved age group can be very effective in this regard, by overcoming many of the systemic and psychologic barriers to access to contraception.

Sexually Transmitted Disease

Adolescents have the highest rate of sexually transmitted disease of any age group. Factors responsible for this include sexual experimentation, which often follows initiation of intercourse activity among adolescents, as well as certain features of pubertal development as previously described (p. 252). In addition, emergence of β-lactamase–producing, penicillin-resistant strains of *Neisseria gonorrhoeae* have hampered attempts at control of transmission. Moreover, the realization that males, as well as females, may harbor asymptomatic, yet transmissable, disease has only recently been appreciated.

Adolescents' reluctance to use contraceptives, including those such as condoms and spermicidal chemicals that may protect against transmission of these organisms, further contributes to the increased susceptibility of this age group. Moreover, teenagers are typically reluctant to consider the possibility that a potential sexual partner may have a venereal disease and often lack the communication skills necessary to discuss this possibility, placing them at even greater risk for contracting one.

Accordingly, the task of prevention of sexually transmitted disease in the adolescent is a complicated one. It includes sensitizing the young, newly sexually active or soon-to-be sexually active person to the fact that he or she may be at risk for contracting such a disease, as well as providing instruction about methods of decreasing this risk. These include use of spermicidal foam or a condom or, preferably, both together. Girls should be encouraged to carry a condom, which is easily concealable. As mentioned above, some contraceptive foams are packaged in single-dose applicators wrapped in plain white paper that look like a tampon and are similarly easy to conceal. The teenaged female with multiple sexual partners should be discouraged from choosing an intrauterine device as a contraceptive method because of her increased risk for contracting salpingitis, with its risk for sterility.

The physician should also encourage sexually active teenagers to request screening cultures for *N. gonorrhoeae* and *Chlamydia* at regular intervals. Routine testing for human immunodeficiency virus is not now recommended, except when another sexually transmitted disease has been diagnosed, if the patient or her sexual partner is an intravenous drug user, or if the patient is a prostitute.

ANTICIPATORY GUIDANCE

Vocational/Educational Planning

One of the major tasks for the middle adolescent is to begin planning realistically for his or her future role in society. Physicians should consider ways in which they may assist in this process. Occasionally, realities of physical growth potential may not be as apparent to the patient as they are to the physician, for example, and such knowledge may have bearing on career choice. The aspiring jockey may benefit from learning that he is destined to be 6 feet tall and weigh in excess of 150 lb. Similarly, the young woman deciding between a career as a ballet dancer or as a physician may choose the latter upon hearing that she, too, will not have the physique to match her fantasy. The physician's knowledge of prognosis of a chronic illness may also be relevant to career choice, as in the case of the newly diagnosed but still well-functioning teenager with Freidreich's ataxia who was planning to be a teacher of physical education.

Becoming a Health Care Consumer

Middle adolescents have an interest in health and physical development, sometimes to the point of slight hypochondriasis; and their growing cognitive capacities, coupled with their quest for justice, may all be captured by the physician to stimulate interest in health consumerism. Discussions of patients' rights, choosing a physician, and the obligations both of physicians and patients in their partnership may be undertaken in this context. Issues for discussion will include, on the physician's side, availability and confidentiality, and on the patient's side, such things as compliance with medications and appointment-keeping.

Chapter 10

LATE ADOLESCENCE

Late adolescence defines the last stage of pubertal development, SMR 5, the stage just before adulthood. The chronologic age at which this stage is reached is, as with earlier stages, quite variable (Tables 8–1, through 8–4). As with earlier stages of adolescence, sex and ethnic differences are apparent in the timing of late adolescence. In sum, by the age of 17 years, 74 to 84 per cent of females and 92 to 94 per cent of males have reached the final physical stage of pubertal development. It is noteworthy that although females tend to have the peak height velocity of their growth spurt an average of 2 years earlier than males, both sexes tend to achieve full sexual maturation at approximately the same age.

ENDOCRINOLOGY

With the achievement of SMR 5 pubertal growth is complete, and the diurnal differences in patterns of secretion of LH and FSH disappear, to be supplanted by equal waking and sleep levels of these hormones.

For females, it is at SMR 5 that LH levels reach the highest point in pubertal rise (2 to 3 ng/mL), whereas FSH levels have neared a plateau in the range of 2 to 3 ng/mL.

For males, completion of pubertal development is associated with a slight rise in LH, to approximately 2.0 ng/mL, and a high point for FSH, averaging 3.0 ng/mL. Responsiveness to stimulation by luteinizing hormone–releasing hormone (LH-RH) is maximal during late puberty, with the result that gonadotropin levels are approximately twice those achieved during midpuberty (an LH rise of approximately 12 mU).

In females, the development of a positive feedback loop between estradiol and pituitary gonadotropins is not fully functional until late adolescence, after which the ovary secretes sufficient estradiol to stimulate a regular midcycle LH surge. This final condition is reached by approximately 5 years after menarche.

Estradiol and testosterone reach their highest levels in serum at SMR 5, the former exceeding 40 ng/dL in women during the follicular phase, and the latter in excess of 800 ng/dL in males. Serum testosterone levels rise in females also, but reach values of only about 85 ng/dL by late adolescence. Serum prolactin levels in females reach their adult levels of approximately 18 mIU/ml shortly after menarche, but the timing of the rise has been the subject of some controversy. Serum growth hormone levels fall in late adolescence to about 6 mIU/mL, and its secretion continues to occur in bursts during sleep. Somatomedin-C levels begin to fall following their middle adolescent peak at SMR 4 (see Fig. 8–5).

PHYSICAL DEVELOPMENT

Height and the Skeletal System

The data of Tanner and Marshall (1974) indicate that one fifth of males do not experience the peak of their height velocity curve until they achieve SMR 5. After this peak is achieved, however, there is little additional growth of the skeletal system. That which does occur during this time is generally limited to the chin, as a result of "apposition of bone at the mandibular symphysis." This is accompanied by forward growth of the maxilla and results increased prominence of the jaws.

Roentgenographic studies of the long bones show characteristic fusion of epiphyses, which progresses from the distal to the proximal bones (see Fig. 9–2) (see also Table 1-6). The last epiphysis to fuse tends to be the sternal end of the clavicle.

Weight and Growth of Soft Tissues

Muscle cell number and strength in males continue to increase after growth has leveled off or ceased in other areas. As a result, according to Tanner and Marshall, by the age of 16 to 17 years, males in late adolescence have one third more muscle than girls.

Primary Sex Characteristics

Males. By late adolescence, testes have attained their adult size of approximately 25 mL each, with a weight of 20 g. Roughly one third is composed of Sertoli cells, and the remainder of germinal epithelium. Full reproductive capability is reached by SMR 5.

Females. All normal females will have achieved menarche by the end of SMR 5. Approximately 10 per cent do so during this stage of development. Accordingly, as with males, the potential for reproduction exists for all normal women by late adolescence.

Secondary Sex Characteristics

Males. The external genitalia are fully developed (SMR [genital] 5) in both size and configuration. The pubic hair has also reached its adult form (SMR [pubic hair] 5): curly, coarse, dark, and extending to the medial aspects of the thighs. A few males experience extension of pubic hair up the linea alba to the umbilicus during the early 20s, a stage earlier designated as SMR 6.

By the time of completion of growth of the external genitalia and pubic hair, hair generally appears on the chin. Recession of the hairline (male pattern baldness) commences in approximately one third of late adolescent males, who have a genetic predisposition.

Females. Breast development proceeds to SMR (breast) 5 in most, but not all, girls. The adult rounded contour is characteristic, the secondary mound of SMR 4 having disappeared by this stage.

As with boys, SMR (pubic hair) 5 represents in girls that stage of pubic hair growth at which the adult texture and distribution is reached: curly, coarse, dark, and extending to the medial aspects of the thighs.

Dentition

The third molars ("wisdom teeth") begin to erupt during late adolescence. They may not all be fully erupted until the early years of the third decade (see Table 1–7).

NEURODEVELOPMENT

There is no further neuromaturation during late adolescence.

COGNITIVE DEVELOPMENT

According to the piagetian scheme, late adolescents should have achieved the stage of formal operational thinking. More recent understanding of cognitive development, however, suggests that it is probably more appropriate to view the late adolescent as having progressed further toward the adult level of information-processing ability (see pp. 254–257).

Moral Development

Stage 4 of moral development according to the schema of Kohlberg and Gilligan (1971) should be reached during late adolescence. During this stage of development, the individual focuses on the maintenance of the social order by doing what he or she considers to be his or her duty and by obeying the law. This has been referred to as the stage of maintenance of the social system and of conscience (see p. 257).

PSYCHOSOCIAL DEVELOPMENT

Late adolescence is characterized by its orientation to the future. Career planning follows solidification of role identity. Involvement in peer groups gives way to pairing typically with a member of the opposite sex and with progression toward establishment of the capacity for intimacy.

According to Mitchell (1976), durable intimacy does not occur until late adolescence because "it demands selfless giving and genuine sharing." Prior to that time the need for intimacy conflicts with conformity pressures and the need for security and/or independence. "Intimacy and role-playing are existential antitheses. They cannot be brought into true harmony because neither can flourish in the presence of the other.''

Friendships that develop in late adolescence, whether with a member of the opposite sex or not, tend to be more relaxed and, according to Douvan and Adelson (1966), ''less haunted by fears of being abandoned and betrayed.'' With this relaxation comes increased appreciation of individual differences among friends and a deemphasis on conformity within the peer group. Susceptibility to peer pressure gradually decreases during late adolescence. Costanzo and Shaw (1966) found such susceptibility returning to the level found in 7- to 9-year-olds by the time the age of 19 years is reached.

Relationships with parents tend to stabilize at a new, more democratic level of interaction by late adolescence.

Sexuality

As indicated in the previous section, the average age of initiation of sexual intercourse activity for white females is 16.4 years, and that for black females 15.5 years. In 1978 Zelnik and Kantner (1980) found that among 15- to 19-year-old black and white urban female teenagers, one third of 16-year-olds, one half of 17-year-olds, more than one half (58 per cent) of 18-year-olds, and two thirds of 19-year-olds were sexually active. The same study found that among males 45 per cent of 16-year-olds, 52 per cent of 17-year-olds, 67 per cent of 18-year-olds, and 79 per cent of 19-year-olds were sexually active.

In sum, more than half of late adolescents were found to be sexually active. More recent data on groups of this size from different socioeconomic strata are not available for comparison, but it has been estimated that 12 million of the 29 million adolescents over the age of 12 years in this country are sexually active.

Sexual activity among late adolescents is more likely to be associated with use of contraceptives than among younger teenagers, though the rates of use are still abysmally low. Two thirds of sexually active female adolescents do not use birth control consistently.

Zelnik and Kantner (1980) found that in 1972 medically prescribed contraceptive methods tended to be used by 18- to 19-year-old females, whereas those few younger adolescents who used any contraception at all tended to rely on less reliable male methods. This trend notwithstanding, there are many late adolescents who do not protect themselves from pregnancy. On one college campus, for example (Dorman, 1981), 36 per cent of sexually active students who had unwanted pregnancies had not used any contraceptive method and 20 per cent had used methods that are unreliable.

The Alan Guttmacher Institute reported (1981) that nearly 7 per cent of late adolescent females and just under 2 per cent of late adolescent males were married. These figures reflect a decrease in comparison with the rates of marriage a decade earlier and suggest a change in attitude toward marriage for the purpose of legitimizing a pregnancy. The growing number of Latino adolescents in this country and their tendency to marry earlier than whites or blacks may soon influence these national statistics.

There has been increase in the number of out-of-wedlock births to adolescents in the last decade. Between 1960 and 1977, out-of-wedlock births to teenagers increased by almost 200 per cent. In addition, there has been a growing trend among adolescents toward keeping their babies rather than placing them for adoption. In 1971 86 per cent of teenagers kept their babies, in 1976 this figure was 93 per cent, and by 1986 it had risen to 96 per cent.

OTHER DEVELOPMENTAL ISSUES

Cults

Some late adolescents, predominantly upper- and middle-class Caucasians, appear to be particularly vulnerable to the influence of a growing number of cults in this country. It has been estimated that there are between 2500 and 3000 of these organizations in the United States, many with international affiliations. A number of individual, family, and situational factors have been cited as predisposing youth to joining a cult.

Vulnerable teenagers appear to be those with low self-esteem; who are depressed, lonely, uncertain, and/or with dependent personalities; who have strong needs for affection; and who are searching for answers to society's problems, as well as to their own. Joining a cult is one reaction to the pressure on late adolescents to commit themselves simultaneously, in eriksonian terms, to physical intimacy, to definitive occupational choice, to energetic competition, and to psychosocial self-definition. In earlier eras these youngsters might have become Flower Children, but in the 1980s they are susceptible to the lures of the instant and unquestioning acceptance ("love-bombing") and of the well-defined and rigidly structured environment that are offered by the cults.

Changes in child-rearing practices have also been implicated in the etiology of this trend. The increased permissiveness of parents since World War II has been cited by some as a cause of confusion and impotence in relationship to their child-rearing role. Teenagers, as a result, have been given more freedom and greater decision-making responsibility than those in previous generations, for which they are often ill-prepared. The willingness to accept the strong cult leader as a substitute for the weak father has been interpreted as a reaction to this premature pressure.

Zerin (1982) has described other family factors that characterized youth who joined cults. In these families there was a tendency to reward performance rather than personal qualities ("just being"). Offspring had been placed in what Zerin called "double-binds": injunctions to think/don't think, feel/don't feel (particularly anger), grow up/don't grow up, and the like. She found also a lack of meaningful religiosity (i.e., more than just membership in a church or synagogue), a lack of training in values clarification, and lack of generational boundaries in these families.

In addition to these background factors that tend to characterize youth vulnerable to cult recruitment, there are situational factors that appear to increase vulnerability. For example, times of stress in the life of the late adolescent, such as examination time or a broken romance, or periods of transition, such as that between graduation from school and onset of a new activity or school, have been identified as problematic in this regard.

Depression

Depression occurs in a high number of late adolescents, for most of whom the condition never comes to medical diagnosis. For those who are recognized as depressed, the rate of prescription of psychopharmacologic agents rises precipitously during late adolescence, particularly for female patients. In fact, at the age of 19 years the rising curve describing the frequency of initiation of prescribed psychoactive drugs crosses that for the rate of self-administration of illicit drugs.

The reasons for the high rate of depression among late adolescents relate, in part, to the many pressures these young people are under to make decisions about careers, marriage, and childbearing, and to assume responsibilities for which many do not feel adequately prepared. Limitations on choice imposed by a high rate of unemployment within this age group, particularly for late adolescent black males, adds to the stress.

A major consequence of depression is *suicide* (or suicidal behavior: unsuccessful attempts or gestures, or suicidal ideation). Suicide represents the second leading cause of death among late adolescents and young adults (15- to 24-year-olds), with a rate of 12.5/100,000; the rate has nearly tripled since 1950. The rate of completed suicide was highest in 1980 among white males (21.4/100,000), with black males next (12.3/100,000), followed by white females (4.6/100,000) and black females, (2.3/100,000). Suicide attempts, on the other hand, are more frequent in females than in males.

It is often difficult to know at first whether an apparently unsuccessful attempt is actually a gesture intended to be a cry for help or a cry of anger without truly lethal intent, or whether what appears to have been a gesture without lethal intent was actually an act of utter hopelessness, carried out imperfectly or naively. Knowledge of the details of the circumstances and of the content of suicidal ideation may resolve the uncertainty. In any case, *every* attempt or gesture or suicidal comment of an adolescent must be taken seriously, and calls for informed investigation and skillful management. A sense of *hopelessness* on the part of the adolescent thinking about, contemplating, or attempting suicide should be regarded as a particularly ominous sign.

Drug Abuse

In a 1987 survey of high school seniors, Johnston et al (1988) found that by the time of their early adolescence (grades 6–8), 40 per cent had tried cigarettes, 13 per cent had used marijuana, and 31 per cent had tried alcohol. By middle adolescence (grades 9–11), an additional 24 per cent had tried cigarettes, 32 per cent more had tried marijuana, and 55 per cent more had used alcohol. By late adolescence (12th grade) a total of 67 per cent had used cigarettes, 50 per cent had tried marijuana, and 92 per cent had tried alcohol. Among late adolescents 38 per cent were heavy drinkers; that is, they had had 5 or more drinks in a row at least once in the two-week period prior to the survey.

Kandel and Logan (1984) found that the rate of onset of use of alcohol begins to increase at approximately 18 years of age, at which time those who have not used alcohol previously have a 0.87 probability of initiating use. Failure to do so by the age of 18 years is associated with a greatly reduced risk of initiation in later years.

The peak rate of initiation of marijuana use is also at the age of 18 years, with a sharp decrease between the ages of 19 and 20 years. The pattern for abuse of psychedelics is similar to that of marijuana, with the major period of risk ending at the age of 18 years.

Cocaine use, however, follows a very different pattern, with less than 10 per cent trying the drug prior to 18 years but 30 per cent having done so by the age of 24, according to Kandel. Cigarette use rises slowly from 11 years to approximately the age of 16 years. By the end of adolescence, 90 per cent of users of alcohol, cigarettes, marijuana, and psychedelics had initiated their use. These data should influence the timing of preventive efforts directed at teenagers.

Periods of highest use of marijuana and alcohol occur prior to the age of 20 years, with their peak ages occurring 1 year later for males than females (19 to 20 and 18 to 19 years, respectively). These findings are interpreted by Kandel and Logan to reflect a "process of psychosocial maturation [which] coincides with the assumption of the roles of adulthood . . . such as getting married, entering the labor force, or becoming a parent . . . that may be incompatible with involvement in illicit drugs and deviant lifestyles." In support of this interpretation are the results of a longitudinal study by Jessor and Jessor (1975a) that found that only one half of males who are problem drinkers during adolescence remain so by early adulthood. For females, only one in four adolescent problem drinkers can be so classified by the time they reach 25 years of age.

Over the past decade there have been changes in the types of illicit substances used by late adolescents. Longitudinal studies of high school seniors (Johnston et al., 1988) have shown that cigarette use peaked in the mid 1970s, whereas alcohol use increased in the late 1970s and has gradually declined to 66 per cent in 1987. Marijuana use increased throughout the 1970s and began to decrease in the early 1980s. By 1987, it had fallen to an annual prevalence of 36 per cent. Cocaine use, still low compared with these other substances, doubled among high-school seniors during the early 1980s and had a sharp downturn in 1987. Barbiturate use has decreased since the 1970s and use of LSD has remained steady at approximately 2 per cent over this period.

Drugs have varied in their popularity among teenagers, but the characteristics of teenagers who use them appear to have been rather stable. For example, six consecutive studies by Bachman et al. (1981) found adaptation to the school environment to be strongly correlated with drug use such that those with above-average drug use were also those with more absenteeism and poorer grades. Similarly, the Jessors' longitudinal studies (1975a) showed that substance abuse was associated with other forms of problem behavior such as premature sexual intercourse, delinquency, and aggression. Sixty-one per cent of marijuana users and 41 per cent of those who drank alcohol were sexually experienced by the end of their senior year, in contrast to only 18 per cent of non–marijuana users and 4 per cent of non–alcohol users.

The Jessors found an inverse relationship between church attendance and drug use. They also found personality and child-rearing differences between the drug-involved and noninvolved high-school seniors. The former group was characterized as placing a higher value on independence than on achievement, as more tolerant of transgression, and as more disposed toward risk-taking than the latter group. The parents of the drug users tended to be less strict, to have less influence over the teenager than friends, and to be perceived as less supportive and as more likely to be models for drug use.

DELIVERY OF HEALTH CARE

Assessment

The late adolescent, in transition to adulthood, benefits from completion of the medical agenda for adolescence, as previously described, which should include establishing a healthy life-style that will prevent morbidity in later years. The latter should be based on a review of family history for risk factors for chronic illness of adult onset, genetic counseling, review of exercise and nutritional habits, and risk factors for depression and substance abuse, as well as issues of family planning (see Table 9–1). The assessment of the late adolescent should always occur without parents being present, unless the patient requests their presence to discuss a specific issue.

Physical Examination

The items listed for special attention during examination of the early and middle adolescent continue to be appropriate for the late adolescent. In addition, since pubertal development is completed during late adolescence, consideration should be given to those body organs and systems impacted by this late growth. For example: adult height has now been nearly reached; asymmetry in breast size can no longer be expected to correct itself; and growth of facial bones has ceased. These last two are important in discussing any possible need for corrective surgery.

Late adolescence and early adulthood are the peak times for development of certain neoplasms, including carcinoma of the thyroid gland and the testes, and such solid tumors as Hodgkin and non-Hodgkin lymphoma. Careful examination should be made of the sites of their possible occurrence.

Essential hypertension often begins in late adolescence. (The technique for determination of blood pressure is reviewed on p. 269). Male pattern baldness typically has its onset during late adolescence in those genetically disposed to it, and may need counseling or reassurance.

Inasmuch as the majority of late adolescents are likely to have had experience with sexual intercourse, the possible need for a pelvic examination for females and of prostatic and urethral examinations for males should be considered. For those with same-sex partners, examination of other areas for the possibility of sexually transmitted disease is indicated.

Screening

Detection of asymptomatic disease and of risk factors for diseases of later life remains the agenda for screening in late adolescence. Because considerations of marriage become more salient at this age, screening for genetically transmissible conditions is indicated if the family history suggests this possibility and if testing has not been done previously. Should the patient prove to be a carrier, he or she may be invited to bring a potential spouse for testing in the future.

With the completion of pubertal growth, the risk for activation of latent tuberculosis becomes unlikely. It is therefore no longer necessary that tuberculin testing be performed yearly in the previously screened late adolescent who is asymptomatic.

If the patient is sexually active, cultures for sexually transmissible disease should be performed at least yearly in both sexes, and a Pap smear also for females. Cholesterol testing should be done yearly. If a rubella titer was not previously obtained or the patient has not been reimmunized during adolescence, this should definitely be done at this time. Hematocrit and urinalysis are useful, as well.

Psychosocial Screening and Anticipatory Guidance

As in the case of middle adolescents, the issues of self-image, depression, substance use, sexuality, family relationships, and school performance should be explored with the late adolescent. The most salient issue for the late adolescent will be the transition from the family home to college, to the work place, and/or into a living arrangement with friend or spouse. That such decisions be reasonable will require implicitly that the late adolescent be secure in decision-making, in self-assessment, and in goal direction.

When the pressure is particularly intense to make seemingly definitive decisions such as those above, such tension may for some prove to be the precipitating factor for depression, for entering a cult, or for retreat to abuse of drugs or alcohol, as indicated earlier. Knowing that a physician with special understanding of this period of life is available and interested in providing support at this difficult time can be very reassuring to the adolescent, and argues against routine transfer of the patient from a long-standing physician/counselor to an internist at this potentially vulnerable period of life.

Assisting the adolescent to become an informed consumer of health care, including issues of choosing adequate health insurance, is appropriate at this time. The late adolescent with a chronic illness will benefit from frank and sensitive discussion about the risks, benefits, and realities of future parenthood.

Health Promotion

Helping the late adolescent prepare a health agenda for the future is a useful undertaking, given the probability that life-style will change in the direction of decreased exercise, altered eating habits, and increased stress associated with entry into college or the workplace. Family planning can, at this age, be addressed without the embarrassment and uncertainties of earlier adolescence. Review of techniques of breast or scrotum self-examination are timely, as are reminders of the importance of receiving a Td booster every 10 years. Automotive safety continues to be an important issue to discuss. It may at this age include that of responsibility for the safety of passengers.

CONCLUSION

"When does adolescence end?" This question is often asked, with various motivations and in various settings. For the adolescent who asks the question, it is often a plea for independence. The parent may, in posing such a query, be yearning for relief from the pressures of parenting a teenager at a time in our history when drug abuse, suicide, violence, unwanted pregnancy, sexually transmitted diseases, and deaths in automobile accidents pose conspicuous threats to the well-being of their offspring. The pediatrician may be asking when he or she should transfer the care of the patient to another medical care setting.

The answer to the question of when adolescence ends is not easy to find. In a society that prolongs the economic dependency of many of its young people through long periods of education, or that cannot make jobs for nearly half of the black male youngsters who are ready to enter the work force, it is difficult to define the end of adolescence and the beginning of adulthood.

Chronologic criteria might define adolescence as the "teen" years, with an end after the 18th or 20th birthday. Biologic criteria might have the end of adolescence coincide with the completion of pubertal development, as measured by the final differentiation of the secondary sex characteristics (anywhere from 14 to 18 years), by the achievement of reproductive capacity (from 12 to 18 years), or by closure of the epiphyses and the completion of skeletal growth (14 to 18 years). The mature stage of cognitive development (formal operations) may be achieved in middle adolescence by some, yet never reached by others. Erikson has suggested that adult psychosocial development is reached with the stage of *intimacy*, with resolution of the conflict between identity and role diffusion.

There may, then, be no good answer. Perhaps the simplest may be that the adolescent becomes an adult in our society when he or she leaves the parental home and becomes self-supporting. Not all who accomplish this will have resolved all the problems of adolescent development.

Appendix A

Technique of Pelvic Examination in an Adolescent

1. Have the patient placed in lithotomy position after general examination is completed.

2. *Inspection*: of the pubis for Tanner staging, or for pediculosis; of the external genitalia for malformations, lesions, lacerations, bleeding, or discharge; and of the vaginal mucosa for evidence of excoriation.

A foul odor would suggest a foreign body, gonorrhea or trichomonas, whereas an acrid odor would suggest candidosis.

The hymen is next viewed to determine if it is intact or imperforate. The vagina is examined for bleeding and the urethra inspected for inflammation, caruncle, or prolapse.

3. *Digital examination*: A gloved, non-lubricated finger is inserted. The mucosa normally feels rugose. Are there any polyps or masses? Does the cervix point forward or backward? Does it feel soft or firm (like the tip of a nose)? Is there any irregularity, nodularity, or tenderness on palpation of the tip of the cervix? Do you feel strings or plastic at the os (when IUD has been placed)?

4. *Bimanual examination*: Place the other hand on the abdomen and gently push down in the midline until you feel downward pressure on cervix. This will allow you to judge the height of the uterine fundus, which normally is below the pelvic brim.

Next palpate the adnexae. The ovaries should be about the size of walnuts. Don't be alarmed if you cannot feel the ovaries. If there is marked asymmetry in ovarian size, or if you feel a discrete mass or marked tenderness upon palpation, consultation with a gynecologist is advisable.

Finally, gently rock the cervix and note the patient's reaction. If there is marked abdominal tenderness on cervical motion in either or both directions this would suggest inflammation or a mass in the tube or ligaments of the uterus.

5. *Speculum examination*: This is done in order to visualize the vaginal vault and cervix, and to facilitate obtaining specimens for a Pap smear and cultures.

A disposable plastic speculum is preferable, since it allows visualization of the entire vaginal vault, is more comfortable for the patient and can be connected to its own fiberoptic light source. The speculum may be lubricated, unless cultures and Pap smears are to be taken, in which case lubricant should be avoided.

Introduce the closed speculum with its narrowest diameter perpendicular to the labia (the handle pointing to the thigh) while the index finger of the opposite hand applies pressure posteriorly at the fourchette. Once the speculum is inserted as far posteriorly as it goes with ease, the handle is turned medially, so that it points toward the anus and the speculum is opened. The cervix is inspected for lacerations, lesions, cyanosis, or discharge from the os.

A sterile swab is inserted into the os and then discarded, after which subsequent swabs may be inserted into the os for cultures.

Pap smears are obtained as follows: the wider end of the spatula is inserted into the cervical os and rotated in order to obtain a sample of endocervical cells. The thinner end is inserted and rotated in such a way as to obtain a specimen from the vaginal fornix.

The specimens are spread on separate slides and *immediately* sprayed with a fixative.

Many physicians perform the speculum examination before the digital and bimanual evaluations. We prefer to do the speculum examination last, since it is the part most feared by adolescents. When the more comfortable maneuver is done first, the patient may relax and become more receptive to later insertion of a speculum.

If a pelvic examination is refused and cultures are necessary, an attempt should be made to insert a swab far into the vagina for culture, or (less satisfactorily) to have the patient do this herself under the physician's guidance.

How to do Testicular Self-Examination

Men can increase their chances of finding a tumor promptly by routinely performing a simple procedure called testicular self-examination (TSE).

TSE should be performed once a month—after a warm bath or shower. The heat causes the scrotal skin to relax, making it easier to find anything unusual. The procedure itself is simple and only takes a few minutes:

Stand naked in front of a mirror. Look for any swelling on the skin of the scrotum

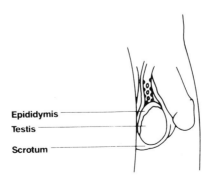

Examine each testicle gently with both hands. The index and middle fingers should be placed underneath the testicle while the thumbs are placed on the top. Roll the testicle gently between the thumbs and fingers. One testicle may be larger than the other.

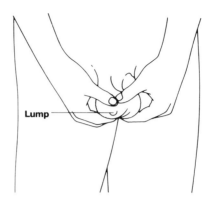

Lump

Find the epididymis (a cord-like structure on the top and back of the testicle that store and transports the sperm). Do not confuse the epididymis with an abnormal lump.

Feel for a small lump—about the size of a pea—on the front or the side of the testicle. These lumps are usually painless.

If you do find a lump, you should contact your doctor right away. The lump may be due to an infection, and a doctor can determine the proper treatment. If the lump is not an infection, it is likely to be cancer. Remember that testicular cancer is highly curable, especially when treated promptly. Testicular cancer almost always occurs in only one testicle, and the other testicle is all that is needed for full sexual function. Testicular self-examination performed regularly is an important health habit, but it cannot substitute for a physician's examination. Your doctor should examine your testicles when you have a physical exam. You also can ask your doctor to check the way you do TSE.

Reference

Testicular Self-Examination. A pamphlet of the National Cancer Institute, National Institutes of Health Publication No. 87-2636. Washington DC, U.S. Government Printing Office, 1987 (1987-193-770).

BIBLIOGRAPHY

Alan Guttmacher Institute: *11 Million Teenagers*. New York, Alan Guttmacher Institute, 1976.

Alan Guttmacher Institute: *Teenage Pregnancy: The Problem That Hasn't Gone Away*. New York, Alan Guttmacher Institute, 1981.

AMA White Paper on Adolescent Health. Chicago, American Medical Association, 1986.

American Academy of Pediatrics. Report of the Committee on Control of Infectious Diseases. 21st ed. Elk Grove Village, IL. American Academy of Pediatrics, 1988.

American Academy of Pediatrics Committee on Early Childhood, Adoption and Dependent Care: *Health in Day Care: A Manual for Health Professionals*. Elk Grove Village, IL, American Academy of Pediatrics, 1987.

American Academy of Pediatrics Task Force on Children and Television: *Children, Adolescents, and Television*. Elk Grove Village, IL, American Academy of Pediatrics, 1984.

American Academy of Pediatrics Committee on Sports Medicine: *Sports Medicine: Health Care for the Young Athlete*. Evanstons, IL, American Academy of Pediatrics, 1983.

Amundsen SW, Diers CJ: The age of menarche in Medieval Europe. Human Biol 45:363–369, 1973.

Anders TF: Night-waking in infants during the first year of life. Pediatrics 63:860–864, 1979.

Anders TF, Carskadon MA, Dement WC: Sleep and sleepiness in children and adolescents. Pediatr Clin North Am 27:29–43, 1980.

Andrews S, Blumenthal J, Bache W, Wiener G: Parents as early childhood educators: the New Orleans model. Paper presented at the Society for Research in Child Development, Denver, April 1975. Cited by Slaughter (1983), p. 7.

Anthony S: *The Child's Discovery of Death*. New York, Harcourt, Brace, World, 1940.

Armstrong GD, Martinsorol M: Death, dying and terminal care: dying at home. In Kellerman J (ed): *Psychological Aspects of Childhood Cancer*. Springfield, IL, Charles C Thomas, 1980.

Bachman JG, Johnston LD, O'Malley PM: Smoking, drinking, and drug use among American high school students: correlates and trends, 1975–1979. Am J Pub Health 71:59–69, 1981.

Bachrach LK, Guido D, Katzman D, et al: Decreased bone density in adolescent girls with anorexia nervosa. Presented at meeting of Western Society for Pediatric Research. Carmel, California, February, 1989.

Bandura A: *Social Learning Theory*. Englewood Cliffs, NJ, Prentice-Hall, 1977.

Baumrind D: Effects of authoritative parental control on child behavior. Child Dev 37:887–907, 1966.

Baumrind D: Authoritarian *vs* authoritative parental control. Adolescence 3:255–272, 1968.

Baumrind D: A developmental perspective on adolescent risk taking in contemporary America. In Irwin CE (ed): *Adolescent Social Behavior and Health*. San Francisco, Jossey-Bass Inc, 1988.

Bayley N: *Bayley Scales of Infant Development*. New York, The Psychological Corporation, 1969.

Beach RV: Routine breast exams: a chance to reassure, guide and protect. Contemp Pediatr Oct:70–100, 1987.

Beck RW, Morris JB, Beck AT: Cross-validation of the Suicidal Intent Scale. Psychol Rep 34:445–446, 1974.

Bell SM, Ainsworth MDS: Infant crying and maternal responsiveness. Child Devel 43:1171–1190, 1972.

Bernstein AC: How children learn about sex and birth. Psychol Today 9(8):6–11, 1976.

Bernstein AC, Cowan PA: Childrens' concepts of how people get babies. Child Dev 46:77–92, 1975.

Blurton Jones NG: An ethological study of some aspects of social behavior of children in nursery school. In Morris D (ed): *Primate Ethology*. Chicago, Aldine Publishing Co, 1967.

Blurton Jones N: Categories of child-child interactivities. In Blurton Jones N (ed): *Ethological Studies of Child Behavior*. Cambridge, England, Cambridge University Press, 1972.

Blyth DA, Simmons RG, Bulcroft R, et al: The effects of physical development on self-image and satisfaction with body-image for early adolescent males. In Simmons RG (ed): *Research in Community and Mental Health*, Vol 2. Greenwich CT, JAI Press, 1981, pp 43–73.

Bower TGR: *Development in Infancy*. San Francisco, WH Freeman, 1974.

Bower TGR: *A Primer of Infant Development*. San Francisco, WH Freeman, 1977. (a)

Bower TGR: *The Perceptual World of the Child*. San Francisco, WH Freeman, 1977. (b)

Bower TGR: *Human Development*. San Francisco, WH Freeman, 1979, p 156.

Bower T, Turnbull JD, Wishart JG: The effects of infant research toward understanding families. In Brazelton TB, Vaughan VC III (eds): *The Family—Setting Priorities*. New York, Science and Medicine Publishing Co, 1979.

Bowlby J: Pathological mourning and childhood mourning. J Am Psychoanal Assoc 11:500–541, 1963.

Bowlby J: *Attachment and Loss: Volume I—Attachment; Volume II—Separation; Volume III—Loss*. New York, Basic Books, 1969 (Vol I), 1973 (Vol II), 1980 (Vol III).

Boyar RM, Finkelstein JW, Roffwarg H, et al: Synchronization of augmented luteinizing hormone secretion with sleep during puberty. N Engl J Med 287:582–586, 1972.

Bramwell ST, Requa RK, Garrick JG: High school football injuries: a pilot comparison of playing surfaces. Med Sci Sports 4:166–169, 1972.

Brazelton TB: *Neonatal Behavior Assessment Scale*. Clinics in Developmental Medicine Series No 50. London, William Heinemann, 1973.

Brazelton TB: Stress for families today. Infant Mental Health J. 9:65–71, 1988.

Brittain CV: An exploration of the bases of peer-compliance and parent-compliance in adolescence. Adolescence 2:445–458, 1967.

Brittain CV: A comparison of rural and urban adolescents with respect to peer vs parent compliance. Adolescence 4:59–68, 1969.

Bronson FH, Desjardins C: Aggression in adult mice: modification by neonatal injections of gonadal hormones. Science 161:705–706, 1968.

Brown JM, O'Keeffe J, Sanders SH, Baker B: Developmental changes in children's cognition to stressful and painful situations. J Pediatr Psychol 11:343–357, 1986.

Burns RB: *The Self Concept. Theory, Measurement, Development and Behavior*. London, Longman, 1984.

Campos JJ: as quoted by Goleman D: Shame steps out of hiding and into sharper focus. New York Times, September 15, 1987, pp 23 *et seq*.

Capute AJ, Accardo PJ: Linguistic and auditory milestones during the first two years of life. Clin Pediatr 17:847, 1978.

Capute AJ, Shapiro BK, Palmer FB: Marking the milestones of language development. Contemp Pediatr 4:24–41, 1987.

Carey S, Diamond R, Woods B: Development of face recognition—maturational component? Dev Psychol 16:257–269, 1980.

Carey WB: Night waking and temperament in infancy. Pediatrics 84:756–758, 1974.

Carey WB, McDevitt SC: Revision of the Infant Temperament Questionnaire. Pediatrics 61:735, 1978.

Cattell P: *The Measurement of Intelligence in Young Infants*. New York, The Psychological Corporation, 1960.

Chess S, Thomas A: *Temperament in Clinical Practice*. New York, Guilford Press, 1986.

Chess S, Thomas A, Cameron M: Sexual attitudes and behavior patterns in a middle-class adolescent population. Am J Orthopsychiatry 46:689–701, 1976.

Chilman CS: *Adolescent Sexuality in a Changing American Society: Social and Psychological Perspectives*. DHEW Publication #(NIH) 79-1426. Washington, DC, 1982. US Department of Health Education and Welfare, 1979.

Chivian E, Snow R: *There's a Nuclear War Going on Inside Me*. 1983. (Videotape recording comments of children and adolescents on the nuclear scene.) Available through Educators for Social Responsibility, 23 Garden Street, Cambridge, MA 02138.

Cogan SF, Becker RD, Hofmann, AD: Adolescent males with urogenital anomalies: their body image and psychosexual development. J Youth Adolesc 4:359–373, 1975.

Coles R: *The Moral Life of Children*. Boston, Atlantic Monthly Press, 1986.

Condon WS, Sander L: Neonatal movement is synchronized with adult speech: interactional participation and language acquisition. Science 183:99, 1974.

Copeland K, Brookman RR, Rauh JL: *Assessment of Pubertal Development*. Columbus, Ross Laboratories, 1986.

Coplan J: *The Early Language Milestone Scale*. Tulsa, OK, Modern Education Corp, 1987.

Costanzo PR, Shaw ME: Conformity as a function of age level. Child Dev 37:967–975, 1966.

Davis JR, Hindman WH, Paplanus SH, et al: Value of duplicate smears in cervical cytology. Acta Cytol 25:533–538, 1981.

DeCasper AJ, Spence MJ: Prenatal maternal speech influences newborns' perception of speech sounds. Infant Behav Dev 9:133–150, 1986.

DeLoache J: Rapid change in the symbolic functioning of very young children. Science 238:1556–1557, 1987.

Denart PG: Ross Laboratories, Columbus, Ohio, 1987.

DeVos G: As quoted by Goleman D: An emerging theory on Blacks' I.Q. scores. The New York Times, Section 12, April 10, 1988, pp 22 *et seq.*

Diagnostic and Statistical Manual of Mental Disorders, 3rd ed, revised. Washington, DC, American Psychiatric Association, 1987.

Dorland's Illustrated Medical Dictionary, 26th ed. Philadelphia, WB Saunders Company, 1981.

Dorman JM: Positive pregnancy tests at Stanford: a follow up study, 1978–1980. J Am Coll Health Assoc 29:286–288, 1981.

Dornbusch SH, Carlsmith JM, Gross RT, et al: Sexual development, age and dating: a comparison of biological and social influences upon one set of behaviors. Child Dev 52:179–185, 1981.

Dorner S: Sexual interest and activity in adolescents with spina bifida. J Child Psychol Psychiatry 18:229–237, 1977.

Douvan E, Adelson J: *The Adolescent Experience*. New York, Wiley, 1966.

Dubowitz L, Dubowitz V: *Gestational Age of the Newborn*. Reading, MA, Addison-Wesley, 1977.

Duke PM: Adolescent sexuality. Pediatr Rev 4:44–52, 1982.

Dunn J: Understanding human development: limitations and possibilities in an ethological approach. In von Cranach M, Foppa K, Lepenies W, Ploog D (eds): *Human Ethology: Claims and Limits of a New Discipline*. Cambridge, England, Cambridge University Press, 1979.

Dunn LM: *Expanded Manual for the Peabody Picture Vocabulary Test*. Circle Pines MN, American Guidance Service, 1965.

DuRant RH, Jay MS: A social psychologic model of female adolescents' compliance with contraceptives. Semin Adolesc Med 3:135–144, 1987.

Ehrhardt AA, Money J: Progestin-induced hermaphroditism: IQ and psychosexual identity in a study of ten girls. J Sex Res 3:83–100, 1967.

Ehrhardt AA, Epstein R, Money J: Fetal androgens and female gender identity in the early treated adrenogenital syndrome. John Hopkins Med. J. 122:160–167, 1968.

Ehrhardt AA, Meyer-Bahlburg MFL: Effects of prenatal sex hormones on gender-related behavior. Science 211:1312–1318, 1981.

Elder GH Jr: *Adolescent Socialization and Personality Development*. Chicago, Rand McNally, 1968.

Elkind D: *Miseducation: Preschoolers at Risk*. New York, Alfred A Knopf, 1987.

Epstein JT: Phrenoblysis: special brain and mind growth periods. I Human brain and skull development. Dev Psychobiol 7:207–216, 1974.

Erikson EH: *Identity: Youth and Crisis*. New York, WW Norton, 1968.

Erikson EH: *Childhood and Society* (35th Anniversary Edition). New York, WW Norton, 1985.

Escalona S: Children and the threat of nuclear war. In Schwebel M (ed): *Behavioral Science and Human Survival*. Palo Alto, Science and Behavior Books, 1965.

Fenson L: The developmental progression of exploration and play. In Brown CC, Gottfried AW (eds): *Play Interactions: The Role of Toys and Parental Involvement in Children's Development*. Skillman, NJ, Johnson & Johnson, 1985.

Ferber R: Sleeplessness, night awakening, and night crying in the infant and toddler. Pediatr Rev 9:1–14, 1987.

Fernald A, Mazzie C: *Pitch-marking of New and Old Information in Mother's Speech.* Paper presented at the meeting of the Society for Research in Child Development, Detroit, MI, 1983.

Fernald A: Four-month-old infants prefer to listen to motherese. Infant Behav Dev 8:181–195, 1985.

Fernald A, Kuhl P: Acoustic determinants of infant preference for motherese speech. Infant Behav Dev 10:279–293, 1987.

Fernald A: Intonation and communicative intent in mother's speech to infants: is the melody the message? Child Dev, 1989, in press.

Fernald A, Taeschner T, Dunn J, Papousek M, de Boysson-Bardies B, Fukui I: A cross-language study of prosodic modifications in mothers' and fathers' speech to preverbal infants. J Child Language, 1989, in press.

Field J: *The Development of the Concept of Death in Children.* M.A. thesis, University of New South Wales, 1979.

Field TM, Greenberg R: Temperament ratings by parents and teachers of infants, toddlers, and preschool children. Child Dev 53:160–163, 1982.

Fifer WP: Neonatal preference for mother's voice. In Krasnegor NH, Blass EM, Hofer MA, Smotherman WP (eds): *Perinatal Behavioral Development: A Psychobiological Perspective.* Orlando, FL, Academic Press, 1987.

Flavell JH: *The Developmental Psychology of Jean Piaget.* Princeton, NJ, Van Nostrand, 1963.

Flavell JH: *Cognitive Development,* 2nd ed. Englewood Cliffs, NJ, Prentice-Hall, 1985.

Forman MA, Kerschbaum WE, Hetznecker WH, Dunn JM: Assessment and interviewing. In Behrman RE, Vaughan VC III (eds): *Nelson Textbook of Pediatrics,* 13th ed. Philadelphia, WB Saunders Company, 1987. (a)

Forman MA, Kerschbaum WE, Hetznecker WH, Dunn JM: Socialization, discipline, and punishment. In Behrman RE, Vaughan VC III (eds): *Nelson Textbook of Pediatrics,* 13th ed. Philadelphia, WB Saunders Company, 1987. (b)

Frankenburg WK, Goldstein AD, Camp BW: The revised Denver Developmental Screening Test: its accuracy as a screening instrument. J Pediatr 79:988, 1971.

Frankenburg WK, Thornton SM, Cohrs ME: Pediatric Developmental Diagnosis. New York, Thieme-Stratton Inc., 1981.

Friedman IM, Litt IF, King DR, et al: Compliance with anticonvulsant therapy in epileptic youth: relationships to psychosocial aspects of adolescent development. J Adolesc Health Care 7:12–17, 1986.

Frisancho AR: New norms of upper limb fat and muscle areas for assessment of nutritional status. Am J Clin Nutr 34:2540–2545, 1981.

Frisch RE: Fatness of girls from menarche to age 18 years with a nomogram. Human Biol 48:353–359, 1976.

Frisch RE: Fatness and fertility. Scientific American, March 1988, pp. 88–95.

Furman E: *A Child's Parent Dies.* New Haven, Yale University Press, 1974.

Furstenberg FF, Brooks-Gunn J, Morgan SP: *Adolescent Mothers in Later Life.* Cambridge, England, Cambridge University Press, 1987.

Gaffney A, Dunne EA: Developmental aspects of children's definition of pain. Pain 26:105–117, 1986.

Gaffney A, Dunne EA: Children's understanding of the causality of pain. Pain 29:91–104, 1987.

Gardner H: *Frames of Mind: The Theories of Multiple Intelligences.* New York, Basic Books, Inc., 1983.

Garner DM, Olmsted MP: *The Eating Disorders Inventory Manual.* Odessa, TX, Psychological Assessment Resources, 1984.

Garrick JG, Requa RK: Girls' sports injuries in high school athletics. JAMA 239:2245–2248, 1978.

Garvey C: *Play.* Cambridge MA, Harvard University Press, 1977.

Gerard HB: Aspects of socialization among minority children. In Vaughan VC III (ed): *Issues in Human Development.* Washington, DC, US Government Printing Office, 1971.

Gerbner G: About the anxiousness of heavy viewers. Fernsehen Bildung 12:48–58, 1978.

Gerbner G: Health, medicine, and violence on TV. Trans Studies Coll Physicians Phila (Ser 5) 6:33–40, 1984.

Gerbner G, Gross L: Living with television: the violence profile. J Communication 26:172–199, 1976.

Gerbner G, Gross L, Morgan M, Signorielli N: Charting the mainstream: television's contributions to political orientations. J Communication 32:100–127, 1982.

Gerbner G, Gross L, Morgan M, Signorielli N: Political correlates of television viewing. Public Opinion Q 283–300, 1984.

Gesell A, Amatruda CS: *Developmental Diagnosis.* New York, Paul B. Hoeber, Inc., 1941.

Gilligan C: *In a Different Voice.* Cambridge, MA, Harvard University Press, 1982.

Gilsanz V, Gibbons DT, Roe TF, et al: Vertebral bone density in children: effect of puberty. Radiology. 166:847–850, 1988.

Ginsburg H, Opper S: *Piaget's Theory of Intellectual Development.* Englewood Cliffs, NJ, Prentice-Hall, Inc, 1979.

Glasser M: Homosexuality in adolescence. Br J Med Psychol 50:217–225, 1977.

Goldman J, Stein Cl'E, Guerry S: *Psychological Methods of Child Assessment.* New York, Brunner/Mazel, 1983.

Goldstein G, Hersen M: *Handbook of Psychological Assessment.* New York, Pergamon Press, 1984.

Goodnow JJ: Childrens' household work; its nature and functions. Psychol Bull 103:5–26, 1988.

Goren C, Sarty M, Wu P: Visual following and pattern discrimination of face-like stimuli by newborn infants. Pediatrics 56:544–549, 1975.

Gottfried AW: The relationship of play materials and parental involvement to young childrens' development. In Brown CC, Gottfried AW (eds): *Play Interactions: The Role of Toys and Parental Involvement in Children's Development.* Skillman NJ, Johnson & Johnson, 1985, pp 181–185.

Gould MS, Shaffer D: The impact of suicide in television movies: Evidence of imitation. N Engl J Med 315:690–694, 1986.

Green M: Helping children and parents deal with grief. Contemp Pediatr 3:84–98, Oct 1986.

Green R: Childhood cross-gender behavior and subsequent sexual preference. Am J Psychiatry 136:106–108, 1979.

Greenberger E, Steinberg L (eds): *When Teenagers Work: The Psychological and Social Costs of Adolescent Employment.* New York, Basic Books, 1986.

Greenspan SI: *Psychopathology and Adaptation in Infancy and Early Childhood: Principles of Clinical Diagnosis and Preventive Intervention.* New York, International Universities Press, 1981.

Greulich WW, Dorfman RI, Catchpole HR, et al: Somatic and endocrine studies of puberal and adolescent boys. Monogr Soc Res Child Dev VII, 1942.

Greulich WW, Pyle SI: *Radiographic Atlas of Skeletal Development of the Hand and Wrist,* 2nd ed. Stanford, CA, Stanford University Press, 1959.

Grøn A-M: Prediction of tooth emergence. J Dental Res 41:573–585, 1962.

Gross RT, Duke PM: The effect of early versus late physical maturation on adolescent behavior. Pediatr Clin North Am 27:71–77, 1980.

Grumbach M: The neuroendocrinology of puberty. In Krieger DT, Hughes JC (eds): *Neuroendocrinology.* Sunderland, MA, Sinauer Assoc, 1980, pp 249–258.

Hamill PVV, Drizd TA, Johnson CL, Reed RB, Roche AF, Moore WM: Physical growth: National Center for Health Statistics percentiles. Am J Clin Nutr 32:607–629, 1979.

Hammond J: Hearing and response in the newborn. Dev Med Child Neurol 12:3–5, 1970.

Harlan WR, Grillo GP, Cornoni-Huntlay J, et al: Secondary sex characteristics of boys 12 to 17 years of age: the U.S. Health Examination Survey. J Pediatr 95:293–297, 1979.

Harlan WR, Harlan EA, Grillo GP: Secondary sex characteristics of girls 12 to 17 years of age: the U.S. Health Examination Survey. J Pediatr 96:1074–1078, 1980.

Harlow HF, Harlow MK: The affectional systems. In Schrier AM, Harlow HF, Stollnitz F (eds): *Behavior of Non-human Primates,* Vol 2. New York, Academic Press, 1965.

Harris DB: *Children's Drawings as Measures of Intellectual Maturity; a Revision and Extension of the Goodenough Draw-a-Man Test.* New York, Harcourt, Brace and World, 1963.

Harris DE, Clark KE, Rose AM, Valasek F: The relationship of children's home duties to an attitude of responsibility. Child Dev 25:29–33, 1963.

Harter S: The perceived competence scale for children. Child Dev 53:87–97, 1982.

Harter S: Developmental perspectives on the self-system. In Mussen PH (ed): *Handbook of Child Psychology*, 4th ed, vol IV. New York, John Wiley & Sons, 1983, pp 275–385.

Hass H: *The Human Animal*. New York, Putnam, 1970.

Hatcher RA, Guest F, Stewart F, et al (eds): *Conceptive Technology 1988–89*, 14th ed. New York, Irvington Publ, 1988.

Havighurst RJ, Robinson HZ, Dorr M: The development of the ideal self in childhood and adolescence. J Educ Res 40:241–257, 1946.

Hayden PW, Davenport SLH, Campbell MM: Adolescents with myelodysplasia: impact of physical disability on emotional maturation. Pediatrics 64:53–59, 1979.

Healthy People: The Surgeon General's Report on Health Promotion and Disease Prevention. Washington, DC, US Government Printing Office, 1979.

Hein K, Dell R, Pesce M, et al: Effects of adolescent development on theophylline half-life. Pediatr Res 19(Suppl):173A, 1985.

Hetherington EM, Parke RD: *Child Psychology: A Contemporary Viewpoint*. New York, McGraw-Hill, 1975, pp 279–306.

Hill JP: *Understanding Early Adolescence: A Framework*. Carrboro, NC, Center for Early Adolescence, 1980.

Hill JP, Holmbeck GN: Attachment and autonomy during adolescence. Ann Child Dev 3:145–189, 1986.

Hogan GR, Milligan JE: The plantar reflex in the newborn. N Engl J Med 285:502–503, 1971.

Holder AR: Minors' rights to consent to medical care. JAMA 257:3400–3402, 1987.

Holmes KK, Mardh PA, Sparling PF, et al (eds): *Sexually Transmitted Diseases*. New York, McGraw-Hill, 1984.

Horne A: Quoted by Kutner L: Parent and Child. In dealing with bullies, solutions can start at home. New York Times National Edition, May 5, 1988.

Hughes J: Quoted by Kutner L: Parent and Child. In dealing with bullies, solutions can start at home. New York Times National Edition, May 5, 1988.

Jacklin CN, Maccoby EE, Dick AE: Barrier behavior and toy preference: sex differences (and their absence) in the year old child. Child Dev 44:196–200, 1973.

Jacklin CN, Maccoby EE: Issues of gender differentiation. In Levine MD, Carey WB, Crocker A, et al. (eds): *Developmental-Behavioral Pediatrics*. Philadelphia, WB Saunders Company, 1983, pp. 175–183.

Jackson RL, Kelly HG: Growth charts for use in pediatric practice. J Pediatr 27:215–229, 1945.

James W: *Principles of Psychology*. New York, Holt, 1890.

Jeffries-Fox S, Gerbner G: Television and the family. Fernsehen Bildung 11:222–234, 1977.

Jensen AR: *Bias in Mental Testing*. New York, Free Press, 1980.

Jersild AT, Holmes FB: *Children's Fears*. New York, Columbia University Teachers College, 1935.

Jessor R: Adolescent development and behavioral health. In Matarazzo JD, Weiss SM, Herd JA, et al (eds): *Behavioral Health: A Handbook of Health Enhancement and Disease Prevention*. New York, John Wiley & Sons, 1984.

Jessor R, Jessor SL: Adolescent development and the onset of drinking: a longitudinal study. J Studies Alcohol 36:27–51, 1975. (a)

Jessor SL, Jessor R: Transition from virginity to nonvirginity among youth: a socio-psychological study over time. Dev Psychol 11:473–484, 1975. (b)

Johnston LD, O'Malley PM, Bachman JG, Illicit drug use, smoking, and drinking by America's high school sudents, college students and young adults, 1975–1987. NIDA, USDHAS, PHS, Alcohol, Drug Abuse, and Mental Health Administration, 1988.

Kagan J: *The Second Year: The Emergence of Self-Awareness*. Cambridge, MA, Harvard University Press, 1981.

Kagan J: Early influences and social class. In Vaughan VC III (ed): *Issues in Human Development*. Washington, U.S. Government Printing Office, 1971.

Kagan J, Reznick JS, Snidman N: Biological bases of childhood shyness. Science 240:167–171, 1988.

Kandel DB, Logan JA: Patterns of drug use from adolescence to young adulthood: 1. Periods of risk for initiation, continued use, and discontinuation. Am J Public Health 74:660–666, 1984.

Kandel DB, Lesser GS: *Youth in Two Worlds*. San Francisco, Jossey-Bass, 1972.

Kassowitz KE: Psychodynamic reactions of children to the use of hypodermic needles. Am J Dis Child 95:253–257, 1958.

Kastenbaum R: Time and death in adolescence. In Feitel H (ed): *The Meaning of Death*. New York, McGraw-Hill, 1965.

Kaufman AS, Kaufman NL: *K-ABC: Kaufman Assessment Battery for Children*. Circle Pines MN, American Guidance Service, 1983.

Kaye K: *The Mental and Social Life of Babies: How Parents Create Persons*. Chicago, University of Chicago Press, 1982.

Kellogg R: *Analyzing Children's Art*. Palo Alto, National Press Books, 1970.

Kessen W: "Stage" and "structure" in the study of children. In *Cognitive Development in Children: Five Monographs of the Society for Research in Child Development*. Chicago, University of Chicago Press, 1970.

Kessler RC, Downey G, Milavsky JR, Stipp H: Clustering of teenage suicides after television news stories about suicides: A reconsideration. Am J Psychiat 145:1379–1383, 1988.

Kinsey AC, Pomeroy WB, Martin CL: *Sexual Behavior in the Human Male*. Philadelphia, WB Saunders Company, 1948.

Kinsey AC, Pomeroy WB, Martin CL: *Sexual Behavior in the Human Female*. Philadelphia, WB Saunders Company, 1953.

Kirchner P, Vondraek S: Perceived sources of esteem in early childhood. J Genet Psychol 126:169–176, 1975.

Klaus MH, Kennell JH: *Parent-Infant Bonding*, 2nd ed. St Louis, CV Mosby, 1982.

Knobloch H, Pasamanick B: *Gesell and Amatruda's Developmental Diagnosis*, 3rd ed. New York, Harper & Row, 1974.

Knobloch H, Stevens F, Malone AF: *Manual of Developmental Diagnosis*. New York, Harper & Row, 1980.

Kohlberg L: Development of moral character and moral ideology. In Hoffman ML, Hoffman LW: *Review of Child Development Research*. New York, Russell Sage Foundation, 1964.

Kohlberg L, Gilligan C: The adolescent as a philosopher: the discovery of the self in a post-conventional world. Daedalus 100:1051–1086, 1971.

Koocher GP, O'Malley JE: *The Damocles Syndrome: Psychosocial Consequences of Surviving Childhood Cancer*. New York, McGraw-Hill, 1981.

Korner AF, Thoman EG: Relative efficiency of contact and vestibular stimulation on soothing neonates. Child Dev 43:443–453, 1972.

Krietler H, Krietler S: Children's concepts of sexuality and birth. Child Dev 37:363–378, 1966.

Kübler-Ross E: *On Death and Dying*. New York, Macmillan, 1969.

Levine MD: Developmental dysfunction. In Levine MD, Carey WB, Crocker AC, et al (eds): *Developmental-Behavioral Pediatrics*. Philadelphia, WB Saunders Company, 1983.

Levine MD: Developmental dysfunction in the school-aged child. In Behrman RE, Vaughan VC III (eds): *Nelson Textbook of Pediatrics*, 13th ed. Philadelphia, WB Saunders Company, 1987.

Lewis M, Brooks J: Self, other and fear: infants' reaching to people. In Lewis M, Rosenblum LA (eds): *The Origins of Fear*. New York, John Wiley & Sons, 1974.

Litt IF: Menstrual problems during adolescence. Pediatr Rev 4:203–212, 1983. (a)

Litt IF: Toxic shock syndrome—an adolescent disease. J Adolesc Health Care 4:270–274, 1983. (b)

Litt IF: Adolescent health care. In Green M, Haggerty RJ (eds): *Ambulatory Pediatrics III*. Philadelphia, WB Saunders Company, 1984, pp 80–103. (a)

Litt IF: Know thyself: adolescents' self-assessment of compliance. Pediatrics 75:693–696, 1984. (b)

Litt IF: Adolescent development. In Behrman RE, Vaughan VC III (eds): *Nelson Textbook of Pediatrics*, 13th ed. Philadelphia, WB Saunders Company, 1987.

Litt IF, Cohen MI: Age of menarche: a changing pattern and its relationship to ethnic origin and delinquency. J Pediatr 82:288–289, 1973.

Litt IF, Martin JA: Development of sexuality and its problems. In Levine MD, Carey WB, Crocker AC, et al (eds): *Developmental-Behavioral Pediatrics*. Philadelphia, WB Saunders Company, 1983.

Lohman TG, Roche AF, Martorell R (eds): *Anthropometric Standardization Reference Manual.* Champaign, IL, Human Kinetics Books, 1988.

Londe W, Johanson H, Kronemer NS, et al: Blood pressure and puberty. J Pediatr 87:896–900, 1975.

Lorenz KZ: *On Aggression.* New York, Harcourt, Brace and World, 1963.

Lorenz KZ: *The Foundations of Ethology.* New York, Springer-Verlag, 1981.

Lowenfeld V: *Your Child and His Art.* New York, Macmillan, 1954.

Lozoff B, Zuckerman B: Sleep problems in children. Pediatr Rev 10:17–24, 1988.

Luna AM, Wilson DM, Wibbelsman CJ, et al: Somatomedins in adolescence: a cross-sectional study of the effect of puberty on plasma insulin-like growth factor I and II levels. J Clin Endocrinol Metab 57:268–271, 1983.

Lynch MD: Self-concept development in childhood. In Lynch MD, Noren-Hebeisen AA, Gorgen K (eds): *Self-Concept: Advances in Theory and Research.* Cambridge, MA, Ballinger, 1981.

Maccoby E: *Social Development.* New York, John Wiley & Sons, 1980.

Mack JE: The perceptions of U.S.-Soviet intentions and other psychological dimensions of the nuclear arms race. Am J Orthopsychiatry 52:590–599, 1982.

Mahler MS, Pine F, Bergman A: *The Psychological Birth of the Human Infant: Symbiosis and Individuation.* New York, Basic Books, 1975.

Malina RM, Boucher C: Subcutaneous fat distribution during growth. Curr Top Nutr Dis 17:63–84, 1988.

Malina RM: Menarche in athletes: a synthesis and hypothesis. Ann Hum Biol 10:1–24, 1983.

Marino DD, King JC: Nutritional concerns during adolescence. Pediatr Clin North Am 27:125–139, 1980.

Marks A: Health assessment and screening during adolescence. Pediatrics 80(Suppl), July, 1987.

Marshall WA, Tanner JM: Puberty. In Davis TA, Dobbing J (eds): *Scientific Foundations of Paediatrics,* 2nd ed. Baltimore, University Park Press, 1974, pp 176–209.

Martorell R, Mendoza F, Mueller WH, Pawson IG: Which side to measure: right or left? In Lohman TG, Roche AF, Martorell R (eds): *Anthropometric Standardization Reference Manual.* Champaign, IL, Human Kinetic Books, 1988, pp 87–91.

McAlister AL, Perry C, Maccoby N: Adolescent smoking: onset and prevention. Pediatrics 63:650–658, 1979.

McAnarney ER, Thiede HA: Adolescent pregnancy and childbearing: what we have learned in the 1970's and what remains to be learned. In McAnerney ER (ed): *Premature Adolescent Pregnancy and Parenthood.* New York, Grune & Stratton, 1983.

McCarthy D: *Manual for the McCarthy Scale of Children's Abilities.* New York, The Psychological Corporation, 1972.

McDermott JF: As quoted by Kutner L: Parent and child: teasing and being teased are ways children practice some of the social skills needed as adults. New York Times, April 18, 1988.

McGrath PJ, Unruh AM: *Pain in Children and Adolescents.* Amsterdam, Elsevier, 1987.

McGrew WC: Aspects of social development in nursery school children with emphasis on introduction to the group. In Blurton Jones N (ed): *Ethological Studies of Child Behaviour.* Cambridge, England, Cambridge University Press, 1972.

Mechanic D: Adolescent health and illness behavior; review of the literature and a new hypothesis for the study of stress. J Human Stress 9:4–13, 1983.

Mitchell JJ: Adolescent intimacy. Adolescence 11:275–280, 1976.

Montemayor R: Parents and adolescents in conflict: all families some of the time and some families all of the time. J Early Adolesc 3:83–103, 1983.

Moore K, Hofferth S, Wertheimer R, et al: Teenage childbearing: consequences for women, families, and government welfare expenditures. In Scott K, Field T, Robertson E (eds): *Teenage Parents and Their Offspring.* New York, Grune & Stratton, 1981.

Morris R, Kralochwill T: *Treating Children's Fears and Phobias: A Behavioral Approach.* New York, Pergamon Press, 1983.

Murphy G, Murphy LB, Newcomb TM: *Experimental Social Psychology.* New York, Columbia University Press, 1937.

Mussen PH, Conger JJ, Kagan J: *Child Development and Personality,* 3rd ed. New York, Harper and Row, 1969.

Nagy M: The child's theories concerning death. J Genetic Psychol 73:3–27, 1948.

National Caries Program, National Institute of Dental Research: *The Prevalence of Dental Caries in United States Children—1979–1980.* NIH Publication #82-2245. Washington, DC, US Government Printing Office, Dec. 1981, pp 5–8.

Newcombe N, Dubas JS: Individual differences in cognitive ability: are they related to timing of puberty? In Lerner RM, Foch TT (eds): *Biological-Psychosocial Interactions in Early Adolescence.* Hillsdale, NJ, Lawrence Erlbaum Assoc, 1987.

Newson J, Newson E: *Seven Years Old in the Home Environment.* London, Allen & Unwin, 1976.

Nielsen CT, SkakkebAek NE, Richardson DW, et al: Onset of the release of spermatozoa (spermarche) in boys in relation to age, testicular growth, pubic hair, and height. J Clin Endocrinol 62:532–535, 1986.

Noam GG, O'Connell Higgins R, Goethals GW: Psychoanalytic approaches to developmental psychology. In Wolman BB (ed): *Handbook of Development Psychology.* Englewood Cliffs, NJ, Prentice-Hall, 1982.

Nottelman ED, Susman EI, Inoff-Germain G, et al: Developmental processes in early adolescence: relationships between adolescent adjustment problems and chronologic age, pubertal stage and puberty-related serum hormone levels. J Pediatr 110:473–480, 1987.

Nydick M, Bustos J, Dale JH, et al: Gynecomastia in adolescent boys. JAMA 178:449–454, 1961.

Offer D: *The Psychological World of the Teenager.* New York, Basic Books, 1973.

Ogden JA: *Skeletal Injury in the Child.* Philadelphia, Lea & Febiger, 1982, pp 56–57.

Olness K, Gardner GG: *Hypnosis and Hypnotherapy with Children.* Philadelphia, Grune & Stratton, 1988.

Olweus D, Mattsson A, Shalling D, et al: Testosterone, aggression, physical and personality dimensions in normal adolescent males. Psychosomat Med 42:153–269, 1980.

Overby KJ, Lo B, Litt IF: Knowledge and concerns about AIDS and their relationship to behavior among adolescents with hemophilia. Pediatrics 83:204–210, 1989.

Palla B, Litt IF: Medical complications of anorexia nervosa in adolescents. Pediatrics 81:613–623, 1988.

Palumbo FM: *Television: Effects on the Development of Children.* Columbus, OH, Ross Laboratories, 1985.

Papousek H: Individual variability in learned responses in human infants. In Robinson RJ (ed): *Brain and Early Behavior.* London, Academic Press, 1969, cited by Bower (1977), p. 43.

Papousek H: Cited in Bower TGR: *A Primer of Infant Development.* San Francisco, WH Freeman, 1977, p 43.

Parmelee A: The ontogeny of sleep patterns and associated periodicities in infants. In Falkner F, Kretchmer N, and Rossi E: (Eds): *Pre- and Post-natal Development of the Brain.* Basel, S. Karger, 1974, pp. 298–311.

Patterson GR: Quoted by Kutner L: Parent and Child. In dealing with bullies, solutions can start at home. New York Times, National Edition, May 5, 1988.

Petersen AC: Pubertal change and cognition. In Brooks-Gunn J, Petersen AC (eds): *Girls at Puberty.* New York, Plenum Press, 1983.

Phillips D, McCartney K, Scarr S: Childcare quality and childrens' social development. Develop Psychol 23:537–543, 1987.

Phillips DP, Carstensen LL: Clustering of teenage suicides after television news stories about suicide. N Engl J Med 315:685–689, 1986.

Phillips DP, Paight DJ: The impact of televised movies about suicide: A replicative study. N Engl J Med 317:809–811, 1987.

Piers EV, Harris D: Age and other correlates of self concept in children. Educ Psychol 55:91–95, 1964.

Pillsbury DM, Shelley WB, Kligman AM: *A Manual of Cutaneous Medicine.* Philadelphia, WB Saunders Company, 1961.

Porowski PA Jr: Health care delivery and the concerns of gay and lesbian adolescents. Adolesc Health Care 8:188–192, 1987.

Prader A: Testicular size: assessment and clinical importance. Triangle 7:240–243, 1966.

Prechtl H, Beintema D: *The Neurological Examination of the Full Term Newborn Infant.* Clinics in Developmental Medicine Series No 12. Philadelphia, JB Lippincott, 1975.

Provence S: Remarks on receiving the C. Anderson Aldrich Award. Pediatrics 59:388–389, 1977.

Provence S, Lipton R: *Infants in Institutions*. New York, International Universities Press, 1962.

Puig-Antich J, Rabinovich H: Major child and adolescent psychiatric disorders. In Levine MD, Carey WB, Crocker AC, et al (eds): *Developmental-Behavioral Pediatrics*. Philadelphia, WB Saunders Company, 1983.

Raphael B: *The Anatomy of Bereavement*. New York, Basic Books, 1982.

Raven JC: *The Coloured Progressive Matrices Test*. New York, The Psychological Corporation, 1960.

Red Book 1988: Report of the Committee on Infectious Diseases, 21st ed. Elk Grove Village, IL, American Academy of Pediatrics, 1988.

Reiter EO: Neuroendocrine control processes: pubertal onset and progression. In the syllabus prepared for the course: *Health Futures of Adolescents*, held at Daytona Beach FL, April 2–5, 1986.

Richardson SA, Hastorf AH, Dornbusch SM: The effect of physical disability on a child's description of himself. Child Dev 35:893–907, 1964.

Roche AF, Himes JH: Incremental growth charts. Am J Clin Nutr 33:2041–2052, 1980.

Roche AF, Wainer H, Thissen D: The RWT method for the prediction of adult stature. Pediatrics 56:1026–1033, 1975.

Rochlin G: How younger children view death and themselves. In Grollman EA (ed): *Explaining Death To Children*. Boston, Beacon Press, 1967.

Rogers CR: *Client-Centered Therapy*. Boston, Houghton Mifflin, 1951.

Rosen H: *Piagetian Dimensions of Clinical Relevance*. New York, Columbia University Press, 1985.

Rosenberg M: *Society and the Adolescent Self-Image*. Princeton, Princeton University Press, 1965.

Rosenberg M, Simmons RG: *Black and White Self-Esteem: The Urban School Child*. Washington, DC, The American Sociological Association, 1972.

Rosenblith JF, Sims-Knight JE: *In the Beginning: Development in the First Two Years*. Monterey, Brooks/Cole, 1985.

Rosenthal R, Jacobson L: *Pygmalion in the Classroom*. New York, Holt, Rinehart, and Winston, 1968.

Rothbart M: Measurement of temperament in infancy. Child Dev 52:569–578, 1981.

Rothbart M: The concept of difficult temperament: a critical analysis of Thomas, Chess, and Korn. Merrill-Palmer Q 28:35–40, 1982.

Rowland TW, Deisroth MB, Green GM, et al: The effect of iron therapy on the exercise capacity of nonanemic iron-deficient adolescent runners. Am J Dis Child 142:165–169, 1988.

Rubin Z: *Children's Friendships*. Cambridge MA, Harvard University Press, 1980.

Ruggiero M: Work as an impetus to delinquency: an examination of theoretical and empirical connections. In Greenberger E, Steinberg L (eds): *When Teenagers Work: The Psychological and Social Costs of Adolescent Employment*. New York, Basic Books, 1986.

Rutter M, Tizard J, Yule W, Graham P, Whitmore K: Isle of Wight Studies, 1964–1974. Psychol Med 6:313–332, 1976.

Salapatek P: Comment. In Vaughan VC III (Ed): *Issues in Human Development*. Washington, DC, US Government Printing Office, pp. 39–42, 1971.

Sander EK: When are speech sounds learned? J Speech Hearing Dis 37:55, 1972.

Savin-Williams RC: Social interactions of adolescent females in natural groups. In Foot HC, Chapman AJ, Smith JR (eds): *Friendship and Social Relations in Children*. New York, John Wiley & Sons, 1980, pp 343–363.

Scheff TJ: as quoted by Goleman D: Shame steps out of hiding and into sharper focus. New York Times, September 15, 1987, pp 23 *et seq.*

Schofield CBS: *The Sexual Behavior of Young People*. Boston, Little, Brown & Co, 1965.

Schowalter JE: Children and funerals. Pediatr Rev 1:337, 1980.

Schwebel M: Studies of children's reactions to the atomic threat. Am J Orthopsychiatry 33:202–203, 1963.

Schwebel M: Nuclear cold war: student opinions and professional responsibility. In Schwebel M (ed): *Behavioral Science and Human Survival*. Palo Alto, Science and Behavioral Books, 1965.

Schwebel M, Schwebel B: Children's reactions to the threat of nuclear plant accidents. Am J Orthopsychiatry 51:260–270, 1981.

Schweiger U, Laessle R, Pfister H, et al: Diet-induced menstrual irregularities: effects of age and weight loss. Fertil Steril 48:746–751, 1987.

Seligman MEP: *Helplessness*. San Francisco, WH Freeman, 1975.

Shangold MM: Causes, evaluation and management of athletic oligo/amenorrhea. Med Clin North Am 69:83–95, 1985.

Shapiro T: as quoted by Collins G: The fears of children: is the world scarier? New York Times, May 19, 1988.

Siegel-Gorelick B: *The Working Parents' Guide to Child Care*. Boston, Little, Brown & Co, 1983.

Simmons RG, Blyth DA, Van Cleave EF, et al: Entry into early adolescence: the impact of school structure, puberty and early dating on self-esteem. Am Sociol Rev 44:948–967, 1979.

Simmons RG, Rosenberg F, Rosenberg M: Disturbance in the self image at adolescence. Am Sociol Rev 38:553–568, 1973.

Singer DG, Singer JL: Getting control of children's television. In *When Children Need Help. A Special Report from the Editors of the Brown University Child Behavior and Development Letter*. Providence, RI, Manisses Communications Group, Inc, 1987.

Singer DG: Children, adolescents, and television—1989: I. Television violence: A critique. Pediatrics 83:445–446, 1989.

Skinner BF: Behaviorism at fifty. Science 140:951–958, 1963.

Slaughter DT: Early intervention and its effects on maternal and child development. Monogr Soc Res Child Dev 48, Serial no. 202, 1983.

Smith N, Ogilvie B, Haskell W, et al: *Handbook for the Young Athlete*. Palo Alto, CA, Bull Publ Co, 1978, p 22.

Sorensen RC: *Adolescent Sexuality in Contemporary America*. New York, World Publ Co, 1973.

Speroff L, Glass RH, Kase NG: *Clinical Gynecologic Endocrinology and Infertility*, 3rd ed. Baltimore, Williams & Wilkins, 1983.

Spitz RA: *The First Year of Life*. New York, International Universities Press, 1965. (See also: Emde RN: *René A. Spitz: Dialogues from Infancy*. New York, International Universities Press, 1983.)

Stanford-Binet, 4th Ed. (In preparation)

Steinberg L: Reciprocal relation between patient-child distance and pubertal maturation. Dev Psychol 24:1–7, 1988.

Stuart HC, Meredith HV: Use of body measurements in the school health program. Am J Public Health 36:1365–1386, 1946.

Strasburger VC: Children, adolescents, and television—1989: II. The role of pediatricians. Pediatrics 83:446–448, 1989.

Sullivan HS: *The Interpersonal Theory of Psychiatry*. New York, Norton, 1953.

Tanner JM: *Fetus into Man: Physical Growth from Conception to Maturity*. Cambridge, MA, Harvard University Press, 1978.

Tanner JM, Whitehouse RH: Revised standards for triceps and subscapular skinfolds in British children. Arch. Dis. Childh. 50:142–145, 1975.

Tanner JM, Whitehouse RH: Standards for triceps and subscapular skinfolds from birth to nineteen years: British children, 1970. Growth and Development Chart—Ref. SKB 45 (boys) and 46 (girls). Castlemead, Hertford, Castlemead Publications, 1976.

Tanner JM, Davies PSW: Clinical longitudinal standards for height and height velocity for North American children. J Pediatr 107:317–329, 1985.

Tanner JM, Goldstein H, Whitehouse RH: Standards for children's height at 2–9 years allowing for height of parents. Arch Dis Child 45:755–762, 1970.

Tanner JM, Whitehouse RH, Takaishi M: Standards from birth to maturity for height, weight, height velocity, weight velocity: British children. Arch Dis Child 41:454–635, 1965.

Taubman B: Clinical trial of the treatment of colic by modification of parent-infant interaction. Pediatrics 74:998–1003, 1984.

Terr LC: Psychic trauma in children: observations following the Chowchilla school-bus kidnapping. Am J Psychiatry 138:14–18, 1981.

Thomas A, Chess S: *Temperament and Development.* New York, Brunner/Mazel, 1977.

Tinbergen N: *The Animal in its World.* Cambridge MA, Harvard University Press, 1972–3.

Trussell J: Statistical flaws in evidence for the Frisch hypothesis that fatness triggers menarche. Hum Biol 52:711, 1980.

Užgiris IČ, Hunt JMcV: *Assessment in Infancy: Ordinal Scales of Psychological Development.* Urbana, University of Illinois Press, 1975.

Vandell D, Minnett A, Santrock J: Age differences in sibling relationships during middle childhood. J Appl Dev Psychol 8:247–257, 1987.

Villarreal S, Martorell R, Mendoza F: Sexual maturation in Mexican-American adolescents. Am J Hum Biol 1:87–95, 1989.

Walker LJ: Sex differences in the development of moral reasoning: a critical review. Child Dev 55:677–691, 1984.

Wechsler D: *Manual for the Wechsler Intelligence Scale for Children—Revised.* New York, The Psychological Corporation, 1974.

Wechsler D: *Wechsler Preschool and Primary Scale of Intelligence Manual.* New York, The Psychological Corporation, 1976.

Weinberg S: Suicidal intent in adolescence: a hypothesis about the role of physical illness. J Pediatr 77:579–586, 1970.

Wender EH: Management of learning disabled children. A paper delivered at the 23rd Annual Pediatric Course, Miami Children's Hospital. 26 January 1988.

Wertheimer M: Psychomotor coordination of auditory and visual space at birth. Science 134:1692–1693, 1961.

Wetzel NC: Physical fitness in terms of physique, development and basal metabolism—with a guide to individual progress from infancy to maturity: a new method for evaluation. JAMA 116:1187, 1941.

White LK, Brinkerhoff DB: The sexual division of labor: evidence from childhood. Social Forces 60:170–181, 1981.

Whitehead RG: Nutritional requirements of healthy adolescents and their significance during the management of PKU. Eur J Pediatr 146(Suppl):A25–A31, 1987.

Whiting BB, Whiting JWM: *Children of Six Cultures: A Psychocultural Analysis.* Cambridge MA, Harvard University Press, 1975.

Wingerd J, Solomon IL, Schoen EJ: Parent-specific height standards for preadolescent children of three racial groups, with method for rapid determination. Pediatrics 52:555–560, 1973.

Wittmer D, Crouthamel CS: Overcoming the common fears of childhood. Contemp Pediatr 3:76–90, 1986.

Yamaguchi K, Kandel DB: Patterns of drug use from adolescence to young adulthood: II Sequences of progression. Am J Public Health 74:668–672, 1984.

Young CM, Sipin SS, Roe DA: Body composition of pre-adolescent and adolescent girls. I. Density and skinfold measurements. J Am Dietet Assoc 53:25–31, 1968.

Zelizer V: *Pricing the Priceless Child.* New York, Basic Books, 1985.

Zelnik M, Kantner JF: Sexual activity, contraceptive use, and pregnancy among metropolitan-area teenagers: 1971–1979. Fam Planning Perspectives 12:230–237, 1980.

Zerin M: The Pied Piper phenomenon: family systems and vulnerability to cults. The Script 12:1–2, 1982.

Zung WWK: Factors influencing the self-rating depression scale. Arch Gen Psychiatry 16:543, 1967.

INDEX

Page numbers in *italics* indicate figures.
Page numbers followed by t indicate tables.

A

Abandonment, fear of, 116
Abdominal circumference, measurement of, 39
Accommodation, in Piagetian learning theory, 65
Achievement tests
  most frequently used, 76
  to evaluate cognitive function, 71
Acne
  classification of, 266t
  in middle adolescence, 298
Acquired immunodeficiency syndrome (AIDS), among adolescent homosexuals, 306
Activity level, in assessment of temperament, 86
Adaptability, in assessment of temperament, 86
Adaptation, in Piagetian learning theory, 65
Adaptive behavior, in child's first year, 167, *167*, 173, 175–176
Addiction, fetal, to opiates, cocaine, phenobarbital, and alcohol, 57
Adolescence. See also *Child*; *Puberty*.
  acne in, 266t
  anxiety in, 300–301
  autonomy in, 259–260, 291
  blood pressure in, 268–269, 269t, 310
  body image in, 94, 301
  breast development in, 230, *248–249*, 252, 298, 319
  breast self-examination in, 277, *278*, 311
  cholesterol testing in, 325
  chronic illness in, 307
  cognitive development in, 254–258, 299, 319, 326–327
  concrete and formal operations in, 256
  conformity in, 300–301
  cult membership in, characteristics of youths who join, 321–322
  dental development in, 253–254, 299, 319
  depression in, 270–272, 322
  developmental assessment in, 264, 307–311, 324–326
  domain-specific knowledge in, 256
  early, 229–291
    definition of, 229
    growth and development in, 238–254
  end of, 326–327
  endocrinology in, 293
  fears in, 118–120
  friendships in, 108–109. See also *Peers*.
  functional contexts of, 300–307
  genetic disease screening in, 268
  genital growth during, 297–298, 318
  gynecologic screening in, 267
  gynecomastia in, 101, 251, 251t, 305, 309
  health care delivery in, 264–276, 307–311, 324–326
  health promotion in, 311, 326
  hearing screening in, 268, 310
  height in, 238, *244*, 252–253, 294–295, *295–296*, 318
  hematocrit in, 267, 310
  heterosexual relationships in, 301–302
  homosexuality in, 305–307
  hospitalization in, 121
  human immunodeficiency virus screening in, 267
  hypertension in, 268
  identity, progress toward achievement of, during, 299–300, 304–305

Adolescence (cont'd)
immunoglobulin levels in, 54, 55t, 56–57
immunizations in, 285, 289, 289t, 325
impact on family interaction, 261–263
infection, heightened reactivity to, 56
information-processing capacity in, 256
interpersonal relationships in, 273t, 300–301
interview in, 270–276
late, 317–327
metacognition in, 256
middle, 293–316
mineral RDA values in, 280t
moral thought development in, 257–258, 299, 319
mutual masturbation in, 275
neurodevelopment in, 254, 299, 319
neuroendocrinologic changes in, 231–238
nutritional counseling in, 277–280, 281t
orthodontic therapy in, 253–254
peers, role in, 263–264
pelvic examination in, 308–309, 329–330
physical growth and development during, 238–254, 294, 295–296, 296–297, 307–310, 318–319
play in, 107–108
pregnancy in, 302–304, 321
preparation for puberty in, 290–291
primary sex characteristics in, 242–245, 297, 318
psychosocial development in, 258–264, 299–300, 319–321
psychosocial screening in, 270–276, 311, 325–326
quantitative thinking in, 256
reactions to death and dying in, 128–129
routine laboratory tests and procedures in, 267–279, 310–311
rubella titer and immunization in, 267, 310
school performance in, 275
scoliosis in, 269–270, 311
screening tests in, 266–270, 310–311
scrotum self-examination in, 277, 311, 331–332
secondary sex characteristics in, 246–247, 247–250, 251–252, 251t–253t, 297–299, 318–319
self-blame in, 300–301
self-concept development in, 93–94
self-image in, 270
sexual activity in, 320–321
age for initiation of, 302, 303t
parental knowledge of, 313
sexual development in, 241–254
biologic factors of, 99–100
problems of, 101, 272–275
sexually transmitted disease in, 308–310, 313, 315–316, 325
skeletal development in, 46t, 294–295, 295–296, 318, 326
skinfold thickness in, 240, 240t, 241, 264
sleep patterns in, 254, 299
smoking in, 281–282, 312
soft tissue growth in, 295–297
sports safety in, 283–285, 286t–288t
substance abuse in, 275–276, 322–324
suicide in, 224, 270–271
terminally ill, 129–130
toxic shock syndrome in, 313
tuberculosis testing in, 267–268, 310
urinalysis in, 267, 310
vehicle safety in, 282–283, 312
vision screening in, 268, 310
vitamin RDA values in, 281t
weight in, 239–240, 241, 244, 252–253, 295–297, 300, 318
work role in, 109–112
Adrenarche, 98, 238
Age, mental, 72
Aggressive disposition, development of, 112–114
Alcohol
fetal addiction to, 57
use, portrayal on television, 223. See also Substance abuse.
Allergy to food, in infancy, 165–166
Amatruda, Catherine, theory of behavior, 58
Amenorrhea, causes of, 246t
Anal stage, of psychosexual development, 79, 183
Analogy, between behaviors of humans and animals, 83–84
Anxiety
castration, 96
definition of, 116

Anxiety (*cont'd*)
  in middle adolescence, 300–301
  separation, 174
Apgar rating, 156, 160, *160*
Appetite, reduced, in child's second
    year, 190
Arousal, in neonate, 153
Artwork
  of preschool child, 194–195, 202
  of school-aged child, 216
Assimilation, in piagetian learning
    theory, 65
Athlete, physical status of, 284–285
Athletic injuries, 283–285, 286t–288t
Athletic training, menarche delays
    due to, 245
Attachment, in structuralist develop-
    mental scheme, 81, 82t
Attention span, in assessment of
    temperament, 86
Authoritarian style of discipline, 205
Authoritarian-restrictive family, de-
    velopment of adolescent auton-
    omy in, 26l
Authoritative family, development of
    adolescent autonomy in, 261
Authoritative style of discipline, 205
Autonomy
  in adolescence, 259–261, 291
  in second year, 186
Average, definition of, 4

B
Babinski response, 151
Bandura, A., learning theory of, 70–
    71
Bayley Scales of Infant Development,
    58, 75, 188
BCG (Calmette-Guérin bacillus),
    immunization against, 56
Behavior
  adaptive, in child's first year, 167,
    173, 175–176
  analogies of human and animal, 3
  modification techniques, 70
  patterns of
    from 1 to 5 years, 62t, 63t
    in first year of life, 60t, 61t
Behavioral organization, initiative,
    and internalization stage in
    structuralist development
    scheme, 81, 82t
Behaviorism, learning theory in, 69

Birth weight, 132, 142
Blood pressure
  in adolescent, 268–269, 269t, 310
  in neonate, 146, *147*
  in seated males, ages 2 to 18, 51t
Body composition, measurement of,
    38–39
Body image. See also *Self-image.*
  development of, 88–89
  in adolescence, 94, 301
  self-esteem and, 91–92, 94
Body Mass Index (BMI), formula for
    calculating, 38
Body movement, translation of sound
    into, in neonate, 157
Body proportions, variability in, 40–
    42, *40–41*
Bonding, 83, 140, 157
Bones. See *Skeletal system.*
Brain. See also *Neurologic growth
    and development.*
  growth of, in second year, 179
  size of, in school-aged child, 213
Brazelton scale, 155–156
Breast development, stages of, 230t,
    248–249, 252, 298, 319
Breast self-examination, in adoles-
    cence, 277, *278*, 311

C
Calmette-Guérin bacillus (BCG),
    immunization against, 56
Caloric needs
  of neonate, 148
  relationship to area of body sur-
    face, 49–50, *52*
Calories
  daily expenditure of, in relation to
    age and weight, 52t
  definition of, 49
Cancer, testicular, 331–332
Cardiac adjustment, in neonate, 146–
    147
Cardiovascular system, growth and
    development of, 49, *50–51*
Career decisions, among adolescent
    homosexuals, 306
Career guidance, in adolescence, 316
Caste, development of sense of, in
    preschool years, 197
  relationship to IQ, 73–74
Castration anxiety, 96
Cattell Infant Scale, 58

Cephalocaudad progression, 40
Chest circumference, measurement
   of, 39
Child. See also *Adolescence*; *Growth
      and development*; *Infant*.
   adaptive behavior in first year, 167,
      173, 175–176
   artwork of
      preschool, 194–195, 202
      school-aged, 216
   assessment of development of
      in first year, 171–172, 174, 178,
         189–190
      in preschool years, 200–203
      in school-age years, 217–219, 220t
      in second year, 188–190
   behavior patterns of
      in first year, 60t, 61t
      in preschool years, 62t, 63t
   cognitive development of, 2, 64–77,
      92–93
      in preschool years, 194–195, 202
      in school-age years, 215, 218t–
         220t, 218–219
      in second year, 180–181
   communication in, development of
      in first year, 169–170, 173–174
      in second year, 181, 182t, 183,
         184t–185t
   day care of, in preschool years,
      208–212
   death and dying and, perception of,
      in school-age years, 125t, 127–
      129
   discipline of, 187, 203–208
   entry into school, 219, 221
   ethologic studies of, 199
   fears of
      in preschool years, 116–118, 203
      in school-age years, 118
      of health care and hospitalization,
         119–120
   friendships in, 108–109
   gastrointestinal development of,
      147–148, 164
   grief and mourning in, 124, 125t,
      126
   head circumference of, in first 3
      years, 8t–9t, *28, 30, 36*
   immunological development of,
      164–166
   in first 3 months, 164–172
   in first year, 8t–9t, *28, 30, 36*, 60t–
      61t, 163–178

   adaptive behavior in, 173, 175–
      176
   assessing development in, 171–
      172, 174, 178, 189–190
   behavior patterns in, 60t, 61t
   communication development in,
      169–170, 173–174
   fears in, 116–118
   gastrointestinal development in,
      164
   grief and mourning in, 124, 125t,
      126
   head circumference in, 8t–9t, *28,
      30, 36*
   head control in, 166
   immunologic development in,
      164–166
   language development in, 174,
      176–177
   motor development in, 175
   neurodevelopment in, 172–173
   physical growth in, 163–164
   physiology of, 164–166, 172
   psychosocial development in,
      174, 177
   sleep patterns in, 177
   visual fixation in, 166–167
   weight in, 8t–9t, *15, 17, 28, 30,
      34–35*
   in second year, 179–191
   assessing development in, 188–
      190
   cognitive development in, 180–
      181
   communication development in,
      180–181, 182t, 183, 184t–185t
   disciplining, 187
   fears in, 116–118
   head circumference in, 8t–9t, *28,
      30, 36*
   language development in, 181,
      182t, 183, 184t–185t, 189
   length of, 8t–9t, *14, 16, 28, 30,
      32–33*
   neurodevelopment in, 180, 188–
      189
   physical growth in, 179
   play in, 105–106
   psychosocial development in,
      183, 186–187, 189–190
   self-awareness in, 181, 183, 186–
      187
   smiling in, 186–187
   weight in, *15, 17, 28, 30, 34–35*

Child (cont'd)
  Landau response in, 166
  language development of
    in first year, 174, 176–177
    in preschool years, 189t, 196
    in second year, 181, 182t, 183,
      184t–185t, 189
  learning disabilities in, 225–227
  length of
    in first and second years, 8t–9t
      14, 16, 28, 30, 32–33
    in preschool years, 24t–25t
  motor development of, in first year,
    166, 175
  neurodevelopment of
    from 3 to 6 months, 172–173
    in first 3 months, 166–167
    in preschool years, 193–195, 202
    in school-age years, 214–215
    in second year, 180, 188–189
  peer activities in school-age years,
    217
  physical growth of
    in first year, 163–164
    in preschool years, 193
    in school-age years, 213–214, 218
    in second year, 179
  physiology of, in first year, 164–
    166, 172
  play in, 104–107
  prepubescent, 26t–27t, 29, 31
    development of self-esteem in, 92
    reactions to death and dying in,
      128–129
  preschool, 193–212
    artwork of, 194–195
    assessment of development in,
      200–203
    behavior patterns in, 62t–63t
    cognitive development in, 194–
      195, 202
    day care for, 208–212
    disciplining, 203–208
    ethologic studies of, 199
    fears in, 116–118, 203
    language development in, 189t,
      196
    length of, 24t–25t
    neurodevelopment of, 193–195,
      202
    physical growth of, 193
    play in, 106–107
    psychosocial development in,
      196–197

  sexual development in, 197–198
  sibling relationships in, 197–199
  television impact on, 208
  weight of, 24t–25t
  psychosocial development of,
    in first 3 months, 170–171
    in first year, 174, 177, 189–190
    in preschool years, 196–197
    in school-age years, 216–217
    in second year, 183, 186–187,
      189–190
  pulse rates of, 50t
  respiratory rates of, 49
  school-aged, 213–227
    artwork of, 216
    assessing development in, 217–
      219, 220t
    cognitive development in, 215,
      218t–220t, 219
    fears in, 118
    learning disabilities in, 225–227
    neurodevelopment in, 214–215
    peer activities in, 217
    perception of death and dying in,
      128–128
    physical growth in, 213–214, 218
    psychosocial development in,
      216–217
    sibling relationships in, 217
    television impact on, 221–225
  sexual behavior in, 98–99
  sexual development of, in preschool
    years, 197–198
  sibling relationships in, 197–199,
    217
  skeletal system of, development of,
    44t–45t
  sleep patterns of, in first year, 168–
    169, 177
  stature in, 10t–13t, 18–20, 26t–27t,
    29–33
  television impact on, 208, 221–225
  temperament in, 167–168
  terminally ill, 127–128
  vulnerable, syndrome of, 144
  weight of, 10t–13t, 15, 17, 19, 21,
    24t–27t, 28–31, 34, 35
  work, role of, 109–112
Childbirth, as social event, 159–161
Cholesterol testing, in late adolescence, 325
Chromosomal analysis, of amniotic
  fluid cells, 141
Circulatory system, fetal, 136–138

Cocaine, fetal addiction to, 57
Cognitive development, 2, 64–77
  evaluation of, 74–76
  in early adolescence, 254–258, 299, 319, 326–327
  in neonate, 153–156
  in preschool child, 194–195, 202
  in school-aged child, 215, 218t–220t, 219
  in second year, 180–181
  preoperational period of, 195
  self-concept and, 92–93
  sexual development and, 98
Coles, or moral development, 68
Colic, 168
Communication, development of
  in child's first year, 169–170, 173–174
  in child's second year, 181, 182t, 183, 184t–185t
Concrete operations period, of cognitive development, 65, 67, 215, 255t, 256
Conditioned reflex, 69–70
Conditioning, operant, 69
Conformity, emphasis on, in middle adolescence, 300–301
Consequence, behavior learned by, 69–70
Contraception, in adolescence, 312–315, 320
Contraceptives, oral, interactions with other drugs, 274t
Conventional level, of moral judgment development, 68
Countdown, as control device, for preschool child, 206
Criterion tests, to evaluate cognitive function, 71
Crying, excessive, of infant, 168
Cults, youths who join, characteristics of, 321–322
Cultural growth and development, 3
Curve, statistical, 5, 5t

D

Danger, fear of, in children and adolescents, 121–122
Dating behavior, beginning of, 301–302
Day care, for preschool child, 208–212
Death, perception of, development of, 123–130

Defense mechanism, in freudian theory, 78
Denial
  as coping mechanism in dealing with death, 127
  in freudian theory, 78
Dental development. See also *Teeth.*
  evaluation of, 47, 48t
  in adolescence, 253, 299, 319
Denver Developmental Screening Test (DDST), 75, 188
Depression, in adolescence, 130, 270–272, 322
Development. See also *Growth, and development.*
  assessment of
    in fetus, 141–142
    in first year, 171–172, 174, 178, 189–190
    in early adolescence, 264
    in late adolescence, 324–326
    in middle adolescence, 307–311
    in preschool child, 200–203
    in school-age child, 217–219, 220t
    in second year, 188–190
  definition of, 1
  models of, 1–3
  themes in, 85–130
Developmental quotient (DQ), as predictor of intelligence quotient, 73
Developmental structuralist scheme, of psychosocial development, 81, 82t
Developmental task, mastery of, 3
Diet, in adolescence. See *Nutritional counseling.*
Differentiation, in developmental structuralist scheme, 81, 82t
Discipline
  of infant, 170
  of preschool child, 203–208
  of 12- to 24-month-old child, 187
Distractibility, in assessment of temperament, 86
Distress to model, 181
Distribution curve, normal, 5t
Doll's eye reflex, 151
Domain-specific knowledge, in adolescence, 256
Draw-a-Person Test, 194, 214
Drug abuse. See *Substance abuse.*
Drug metabolism, developmental aspects of, 57–58

Dubowitz examination, for assessing gestational age, 134t–135t
Dying, perception of, development of, 123–130

E
Eating Disorders Inventory, 277
Ectomorph, 40
Educational planning, in adolescence, 316
Educational ramifications, of teenage pregnancy, 304
Ego, in freudian theory, 78
Egocentric period, of cognitive development, 195
Electroencephalogram (EEG), of fetus, 140
Embryonic period of intrauterine life. See also *Fetus*.
    definition of, 131
    problems and mortality during, 140–141
Endocrine system
    of adolescent, 317–318
    of neonate, 149
Endomorph, 40
Energy requirement, basal, 50
Environment
    effect on intelligence quotient, 73–74
    effect on moral judgment development, 68
Enzymatic deficiencies, in neonate, 148–149
Erikson, Erik
    identity crisis theory of, 299
    psychosocial model of development, 80, 170, 186, 196, 216
    self-concept development in adolescence, theory of, 93–94
    sexuality theory of, 97
Estrogen, in puberty, 234
Ethnic differences
    in body proportions, 41
    in menarche, 245
    in psychosocial development, of preschool children, 197
    in pubertal development, 229, 230t–231t
    in sexual behavior, in late adolescence, 320–321
    in sexual maturity, 293
Ethologic growth and development, 2, 83–85, 199

F
Failure, first experience with, 217
Family
    effects of puberty on, 103–104
    factors predisposing youth to join cult, 321–322
    interaction of, impact of adolescence on, 261–263
Fears
    age specificity of, in normal child, 115t, 115–123
    basic and primitive, 116
    in infancy, 116
    in preschool child, 116–118, 203
    of health care and hospitalization, 118–121
    of nuclear catastrophe, 122–123
    of pain, 119–120
    of world as dangerous, 121–122
Feedback, role in development of self-esteem, 92
Fetus, 131–144
    assessment of development status in, 141–142
    circulatory system of, 136–138
    electroencephalogram of, 140
    factors affecting birth weight of, 132
    gastrointestinal development of, 139
    habituation in, 140
    memory in, 140
    mortality of, 141
    neurodevelopment of, 139–140
    physical growth of, 131, 133–134, *135*, 136t, 136
    placental function and, 139
    previable, 131
    psychosocial aspects of life, 140
    respiratory system of, 138
    sexuality, development of, 94
    size of, factors affecting, 132
Flavell, on cognition, 256
Follicle-stimulating hormone (FSH). See *Puberty, gonadotropins in.*
Formal operations period, of cognitive development, 65, 67–68, 255t
Friendships
    changes in, from childhood through adolescence, 108
    in late adolescence, 320
    sex differences in structure and function of, 108–109

Freud, Sigmund
psychic structure theory of, 77–78
psychoanalytic theory of, 78–79
sexual development theory of, 96–97, 170
Funeral, child attending, preparation of, 129

G
Gastrointestinal system development
in fetus, 139
in first 3 months, 164
in neonate, 147–148
Gaussian curve, 5
Gender identity, 91, 95–97
Generativity, development of, in eriksonian theory, 81t
Genetic differences, in intelligence quotient, 73–75
Genetic disease, screening for, in early adolescence, 268
Genitalia, development of, stages of, 23, 213t, 250, 297–298, 318
Gesell, Arnold, theory of behavior, 58
Gesell Developmental and Neurologic Examination, Revised, 74, 188
Gestation, period of, 131
Gestational age, determination of, 132–133, 134t–135t, 136, 142
Gilligan, on moral development, 68, 257–258
Gonadotropins, in puberty, 232–233, 233, 235
Goodenough-Harris Draw-a-Person Test, 194, 214
Greenspan, S. I., developmental-structuralist scheme of psychosocial development, 81, 82t
Grief, in infancy, 124, 125t, 126
Growth, and development. See also *Development, assessment of; Height; Length; Weight.*
aspects of classification of, 1
behavioral, 76–81
caloric needs in relation to, 49–50,52
cardiovascular, 49, 50–51, 146–147, 147
circulatory, fetal, 136–138
cognitive, 2, 64–77
in early adolescence, 254–258
in late adolescence, 319
in middle adolescence, 299
in neonate, 153–156

in preschool child, 194–195, 202
in school-aged child, 215, 218–219, 218t–220t
in second year, 180–181
self-concept and, 92–93
cultural, 3
dental, 47, 48t, 253, 299, 319
disturbances in, measured by percentile changes, 7
endocrinologic
in late adolescence, 317–381
in neonate, 149
ethologic, 3, 83–85, 199
fetal, 131–140
gastrointestinal
in fetus, 139
in first 3 months, 164
in neonate, 147–148
hematologic, in neonate, 149
immunologic, 53–54, 55t, 56–57
in first 3 months, 164–166
in neonate, 149–150
in early adolescence, 229–291
in first year, 163–178
in late adolescence, 317–327
in middle adolescence, 293–316
in neonate, 145–162
in premature infant, 141–144
in preschool child, 193–212
in school-age child, 213–227
in second year, 179–191
interrelations between parameters of, 22–23, 24t–27t, 28–36, 37
metabolic, 148–149
metabolism and, 49–50, 52–53
models of, 1–3
motor
in first 3 months, 166
in first year, 175
self-concept and, 89
muscular, 43
neurologic, 2, 58–64
in early adolescence, 254
in first year, 166–167, 172–173
in late adolescence, 319
in middle adolescence, 299
in neonate, 150–153, 160–161
in preschool child, 193–195, 202
in school-age child, 214–215
in second year, 180, 188–189
nutrition and, 49–50, 52–53, 147–148
of adaptive behavior, in first 3 months, 167, 173, 175–176

Growth, and development (cont'd)
of communication skills
in first year, 169–170, 173–174
in second year, 181, 182t, 183,
184t–185t
of drug metabolism, 57–58
of fears, specificity by age, 115–123
of head, 40
of head control, in first 3 months,
166
of Landau response, 166
of language, 189
in first year, 174, 176–177
in preschool child, 196
in second year, 181, 182t, 183,
184t–185t, 189
self-concept and, 89, 91
of lymphoid tissue, 42
of moral judgment, 68–69, 257–258,
299, 319
of perception of death and dying,
123–130
of self-esteem, 91–93, 300, 306
of sleep patterns
in adolescence, 254, 299
in first year, 168–169, 177
of temperament, 167–168
physical and physiological, 2, 4–58
in early adolescence, 238–254,
264, 265t, 266, 294, 295–296,
296–297
in first year, 163–164, 172
in late adolescence, 318–319,
324–325
in middle adolescence, 307–312
in neonate, 156, 160
in preschool child, 193, 200–201
in school-age child, 213–214, 218
in second year, 179
political, 3
process of, 1
psychosocial, 3, 76–81
in early adolescence, 258–264,
270–276
in first year, 170–171, 174, 177
in late adolescence, 319–321
in middle adolescence, 299–300
in neonate, 156–159, 161
in preschool child, 196–197, 202,
216–217
in second year, 183, 186–187,
189–190
renal, in neonate, 149
respiratory, 49, 49

in fetus, 138
in neonate, 146
sexual. See also Puberty.
in early adolescence, 241–254
in late adolescence, 318–321
in middle adolescence, 297–299
in preschool years, 197–198
sibling relationships in, 197–199,
217
skeletal, 43, 44t–46t, 47, 318–326
task mastery as aspect of, 3
themes of, 4, 85–130
variability in, 4–7, 40, 40–42
velocity, determination of, 23
visual, 166–167
water requirement, daily, in relation
to, 52–53, 52t–53t
work, role in, 109–112
Growth hormone, in puberty, 236,
237, 238
Gynecologic screening, in early adolescence, 267
gynecomastia, 101, 251, 251t, 305,
309

H
Habituation
in fetus, 140
in neonate, 155
Hair. See also Pubic hair.
axillary and facial, progression of
development of, 246, 247t, 298
circumanal, 293
Hairline, recession of, 246, 325
Hands, development of functions of,
in first year, 176
Head circumference
in first 3 years, 8t–9t, 28t, 30t, 36t
in first year, 164
in second year, 179
measurement of, 39
of neonate, 145–146
of school-aged child, 213
Head control, development of, in first
3 months, 166
Head Start, 221
Health care
becoming consumer of, in middle
adolescence, 316
delivery of, in adolescence, 264–
276, 307–311, 324–326
fears of, among children, 118–121
Health promotion, in adolescence,
277–281, 311, 326

Hearing, testing of, in adolescence, 268, 310
Height
  in early adolescence, 238, *244*, 252–253
  in late adolescence, 318
  in middle adolescence, 294–295, *295–296*
  in second year, 179
  standing, measurement of, 37–39
  of preschool child, 193
  of school-aged child, 213
Height velocity chart, during adolescence, 38
Hematocrit, in adolescence, 267, 310
Hematologic system, of neonate, 149
Heterosexual precocity, 98
Heterosexual relationships
  development of, 102–103
  in middle adolescence, 301–302
Homeostasis, as stage in developmental structuralist scheme, 81, 82t
Homology of animal and human behavior, 3, 83–84
Homosexuality in middle adolescence, 305–307
Hospitalization, fear of, in children, 118–121
Human immunodeficiency virus (HIV), screening for, in early adolescence, 267
Hyperkinesis, paradoxic drug reactions in, 57
Hypertension, in adolescence, 268, 325
Hypnosis, with children, to cope with pain, 119

I

Id, in freudian theory, 77
Identity
  crisis, in middle adolescence, 299–300
  gender, 91, 95–97
  development of, in eriksonian theory, 80, 80t
  progress toward achievement of, in middle adolescence, 304–305
  sexual, development of, in middle adolescence, 304–305
IGF-I. See *Somatomedin C.*
Illness, chronic
  amenorrhea and menarche delays due to, 245, 246t

in adolescence, 307
Image. See *Body image*; *Self-image.*
Imitative behavior
  in first year, 176
  in neonate, 152, 158
  in second year, 180, 186
Immunities, maternal, transfer of to fetus, 53–54, 139
Immunization
  in adolescence, 285, 289, 289t, 310
  mechanism of, 56
  recommended schedule of, for normal infants and children, 57, 289t
Immunologic development, 53–54, 55t, 56–57
  in first 3 months, 164–166
Immunologic system, of neonate, 149–150
Imprinting. See *Bonding.*
Infant. See also *Child*; *Neonate.*
  disciplining, in first 3 months, 170
  fears in, 116
  food allergies in, 165–166
  gender identity in, 91
  ossification in, 44t–45t
  perception of death and dying in, 124
  play in, l05
  pleasure for, 104
  premature, 131–144
    age of mother as cause of, 303–304
    developmental features of, 142–144
    metabolic problems of, 143
    neurodevelopment of, 142–143
    neurologic problems of, 143–144
    physiologic problems of, 143
    psychosocial problems of, 144
    respiratory problems of, 143
  pulse rate in, 50t
  respiratory rate in, *49*
  self-development, stages of, 90t
  sexuality of, 78–79, 97–98
  visual recognition of self, 89, 90t
Information-processing capacity, in adolescence, 256
Initiative period, in eriksonian theory, 196
Integrity, development of, in eriksonian theory, 80t
Intelligence
  definitions of, 2–3

Intelligence (cont'd)
  problem-solving skills as measure
    of, 3
  sensorimotor, 65–66, 255t
Intelligence quotient (IQ), 3, 72t, 72–
  74
Interactive processes, of neonate, 156
Intersensory coordination, in neonate,
  152
Interview of adolescent, 270–276
Intimacy, development of, in erikso-
  nian theory, 80t
Isosexual precocity, 98

K
Kaufman Assessment Battery for
  Children, 75–76
Kilocalories, 49
Kohlberg, L., theory of moral judg-
  ment development in children,
  68–69
Kübler-Ross, E., theory on stages of
  dealing with death, 129–130
Kurtosis, 5

L
Laboratory tests/procedures, routine,
  in adolescence, 267–270, 310–
  311
Landau response, 166
Language
  biologically determined characteris-
    tics of, 169–170
  development of
    in first year, 169–170, 174, 176–
      177
    in preschool child, 189t, 196
    in second year, 182t, 183, 184t–
      185t, 189
    self-concept and, 89, 91
Latency period, of psychosexual
  development, 79–80, 80t, 216
Laughter, in second year, 186
Learning, one-trial, 71
Learning ability, in utero, 152, 154–
  155
Learning disabilities, in school-aged
  children, 225–227
Learning theories
  behaviorist, 69–70
  of Bandura, 70–71
  of Gilligan, 68

of Kohlberg, 68
of Piaget, 65–68
of Skinner, 69–70
social, 70–71
Length
  by age percentiles, 8t-9t, 14, 16
  by weight percentiles, 24t–25t, 28t,
    30t
  of neonate, 145
  recumbent, 32t–33t, 37
Libido, 77
Limits, setting of, for preschool children, 205–206
Locomotor-genital stage of development, in eriksonian theory, 80,
  80t
Love, fear of losing, 116
Luteinizing hormone (LH). See Puberty, gonadotropins in.
Lymphoid tissue, growth and development of, 42

M
Magical thinking, about death and
  dying, 126, 128
Marfan syndrome, body proportion
  variations in, 41
Malnutrition, intrauterine, effects on
  cerebral structure and function,
  141
Mastery tests, to evaluate cognitive
  function, 71
Masturbation
  in childhood, 98–99
  in infancy, 97–98
  mutual
    in early adolescence, 275
    same sex, 102
Maturation, behavior as expression
  of, 58
McCarthy Scales of Children's Abilities (MSCA), 75
Mean, statistical, 4
Measles, deferring immunization
  against, 56
Median value, statistical, 5
Memory
  in fetus, 140
  in neonate, 155
Menarche, 244–245, 246t
  average age at, 100
  preparing early adolescent for, 290–
    291

Menstruation, 297. See also Menarche.
Mental age, 72
Mesomorph, 40
Metabolism
  changing needs with age, 49–50
  in neonate, 148
  of drugs, 57–58
  problems of, in premature infant, 143
Metacognition, in adolescence, 256
Mid-arm circumference (MCA), measurement of, 38
Mid-arm muscle circumference (MAMC), measurement of, 38
Mineral RDA values, for adolescent, 280t
Modal value, statistical, 5
Models, developmental, 1–3
  role of, in learning, 70–71
Mood, quality of, in assessing temperament, 86
Moral thought development
  in adolescence, 257–258, 299, 319
  in children, stages of, 68–69
Moro response, of neonate, 150
Mortality, fetal, 141
Mother
  effective, behaviors of, 187
  immunities of, transferred to fetus, 139
  interaction of, with infant, 171
Motherese, 169
Motivation, as contributing factor to development of moral judgment, 68
Motor development
  in first year, 166, 175
  in neonate, 156
  self-concept and, 89
Mourning, in infant, 124, 125t, 126
Muscle, growth and development of, 43
Muscular-anal stage of development, in eriksonian theory, 80, 80t
Mutilation of body, fear of, in childhood, 116
Myopia, in adolescence, 101

N
Neck-righting reflex, 150
Neonatal Behavioral Assessment Scale, 155–156
Neonatal period, 145

Neonate, 145–162. See also Infant.
  assessment of development of, 160–161
  blood pressure in, 146, 147
  caloric needs of, 148
  cardiac adjustments in, 146, 146–147
  cognitive development of, 153–156
  daily water requirements of, 148
  endocrine system of, 149
  enzymatic deficiencies in, 148–149
  external characteristics of, on Dubowitz examination, 134t
  gastrointestinal system and nutritional needs in, 147–148
  head circumference of, 145–146
  hematologic system of, 149
  imitative behavior in, 158
  immunologic system of, 149
  interaction with environment, 153
  lengths of, 145
  memory in, 155
  metabolism of, 148
  neurodevelopment of, 135t, 150–153, 160–161
  orienting response of, 155
  physical features of, 145–146
  physiology of, 146–150, 160
  postural reflexes of, 150–151
  posture of, 146
  problem-solving ability of, 155
  psychosocial development of, 156–159, 161
  renal function of, 149
  respiration rates of, 146
  sexuality, development of, 94–95
  state of arousal of, 153
  susceptibility to bacterial infections of, 54, 55t, 56
  visual apparatus of, 151
  visual stimuli preferences of, 151–152
  weights of, 145
Neurodevelopmental. See Neurologic growth and development.
Neuroendocrinology, of puberty, 231–238
Neurologic growth and development, 2, 58–64
  in early adolescence, 254
  in fetus, 139–140
  in first year, 166–167, 172–173
  in late adolescence, 319
  in middle adolescence, 299

Neurologic growth and development (cont'd)
in neonate, 150–153, 160–161
in premature infant, 142–144
in preschool child, 193–195, 202
in school-aged child, 214–215
in second year, 180, 188–190
problems in, of premature infant, 143–144
testing of
arrangements and materials needed for, 58–59, 59
conducting, 135t–136t
Newborn infant. See Neonate.
Night terrors and nightmares, in children, 117–118
Nightwaking, from 6 to 12 months, 177
Normal values, statistical, 5
Nuclear catastrophe, fear of, in children, 122–123
Null hypothesis, 6
Nutrition, changing needs with age, 49–50
Nutritional counseling, in early adolescence, 277, 280, 281t
Nutritional disturbances. See also Malnutrition, intrauterine.
acute and chronic, 53
effects on dental development, 47
Nutritional needs, of neonate, 147–148

O
Object permanence
earliest sense of, 176
in preschool child, 195
Oedipal complex, 79
Oedipal period, 196
Operation, in piagetian learning theory, 66–67
Opiates, fetal addiction to, 57
Oral contraceptives, interactions with other drugs, 274t. See also Pregnancy, prevention of.
Oral stage of psychosexual development, 79–80, 80t, 170, 183
Orgasm, 101
Orienting response, of neonate, 155
Orthodontic therapy, in early adolescence, 253–254
Ovaries, enlargement of, in middle adolescence, 297
Ovulation, 244

P
Pain, in children and adolescents, 119–120
Parenting styles, relationship to development of autonomy in adolescence, 260–261
Parents
inclusion of, in sexual history taking of adolescent, 274–275
knowledge of child's sexual activity by, 313
relationships of, with adolescents, 304, 320
Peabody Picture Vocabulary Test (PPVT), 76, 226
Pediatric Examination of Educational Readiness (PEER), 226
Peers
adolescent, importance of, 263–264
contraceptive method influenced by, 313
feedback from, in development of self-esteem, 92
school-aged children and, 217
Pelvic examination, in middle adolescence, 308–309, 329–330
indications for, 264–265
Penis envy, in classic psychoanalytic theory, 96
Percentile point
definition of, 5
use in growth and development assessment, 6–7
Permissive style of discipline, 205
Phallic stage, of psychosexual development, 79
Phenobarbital, fetal addiction to, 57
Phobia, definition of, 116
Physical measurement, techniques of, 37–39
Physician, portrayal of, on television, 223
Physical examination, of healthy adolescent, 264, 265t, 266, 308t, 329–330
Physical growth and development, 2, 4–48
in first year, 163–164, 172
in late adolescence, 318–319, 324–325
in middle adolescence, 307–312
in neonate, 156
in preschool child, 193, 200–201

Physical growth and development (cont'd)
in school-aged child, 213–214, 218
in second year, 179
Physique, differences in, 40
Piaget, Jean, theories of development, 195, 215, 255–256, 256t
Placental function, and fetus, 139
Placing reflex, 151
Play
in adolescence, 107–108
in childhood, 99, 104–105, 107
Pleasure, for infant, 104
Pleasure principle, in freudian theory, 78
Political growth and development, 3
Postconventional level, of moral judgment development, 68
Postterm, definition of, 131
Postural reflexes, of neonate, 150–151
Posture
of neonate, 146
symmetrotonic, 173
Preadolescent, 26t–27t, 29, 31
development of self-esteem in, 92
reactions of, to death and dying, 128–129
Preconventional level, of moral judgment development, 68–69
Pregnancy
complications of, during middle adolescence, 302–304
normal duration of, 131
prevention of, in middle adolescence, 312–315
teenage, 302–304, 321
Premature infant. See Infant, premature.
Preoperational period of cognitive development, 65–67, 195
Preschool child. See Child, preschool.
Preschool Readiness Experimental Screening Scale (PRESS), 226
Prescreening Developmental Questionnaire (PDQ), 75
Preterm, World Health Organization definition of, 131
Pride, emergence of, in second year, 186
Probability, statistical, 6
Problem-solving skills
as measure of intelligence, 3
of neonates, 154
Projection, in freudian theory, 78

Prolactin, in puberty, 236
Psychic birth, of infant, 183
Psychic structure, freudian theory of, 77–78
Psychoanalysis, freudian theory of, 78–79
Psychoanalytic theory, of sexual development, 96, 183, 196, 216
Psychosocial aspects
of childhood sexuality, 99
of gender identity development, 96–97
of sexual development, 98, 103–104
Psychosocial development, 3
eriksonian theory of, 80–81, 80t
ethnic differences in, 197
freudian theory of, 78–80
Greenspan's developmental structuralist theory of, 81, 82t
in early adolescence, 258–264
in fetus, 140
in first year, 170–171, 174, 177
in late adolescence, 311, 319–321, 325–326
in middle adolescence, 299–300
in neonate, 156–159, 161
in preschool child, 196–197, 202–203
in school-aged child, 216–217
in second year, 183, 186–187, 189–190
Psychosocial problems, of premature infant, 144
Puberty. See also Sex characteristics.
effects of, on family, 103–104
estrogen in, 234
ethnic differences in, 229, 230t–231t
gonadotropins in, 231, 232–233, 233–234, 235, 293, 317
growth hormone in, 236, 237, 238
neuroendocrinology of, 231–238
physical manifestations of, 100
preparing early adolescent for, 290
prolactin in, 236
sex hormone binding globulin (SHBG) in, 235
testosterone in, 234
variations in timing of, 103
Pubic hair
in late adolescence, 318–319
in middle adolescence, 297–298
stages of growth of, 230t–231t, 242t, 243, 248, 250

Pulse rate in infants and children, 50t. See also *Cardiovascular system, growth and development of.*
Punishment, of preschool child, 206–207
Punitive family, development of adolescent autonomy in, 261

Q
Quartile point, definition of, 5
Quetelet index, 38

R
Raven Progressive Matrices Test, 76
Reaction, intensity of, in assessment of temperament, 86
Reaction formation, in freudian theory, 78
Recognition of self, visual, 89, 90t
Reflex, conditioned, pavlovian, 69–70
Reflex grasp, development of, in first 3 months, 167
Reinforcement of behavior, in skinnerian learning theroy, 70
Relationships, interpersonal, in middle adolescence, 300–301. See also *Heterosexual relationships; Homosexuality.*
Renal function, of neonate, 149
Repression, in freudian theory, 78
Reproductive capability, beginning of, 101. See also *Puberty.*
Reproductive development, in early adolescence, 241–254
Respiration rates, of neonate, 146
Respiratory problems, in premature infant, 143
Respiratory system
  fetal, 138
  growth of, 49, *49*
Responsiveness, threshold of, in assessment of temperament, 86
Retarded persons, intelligence quotient of, 72–72
Revised Developmental Screening Inventory (RDSI), 74
Revised Parent Developmental Questionnaire (RPDQ), 74
Rhythmicity, regularity of, in assessment of temperament, 86
Rooting reflex, 147, 151

Rubella immunization, in adolescence, 267, 310, 325

S
Safety
  cycle, 282
  passenger, 283
  sports, 283–285
Schemes, in piagetian learning theory, 65
School, entry into, 219, 221
School performance, in early adolescence, 275
School refusal, in young child, 118
School-aged child. See *Child, school-aged.*
Scoliosis, in adolescence, 269–270, 311
Screening tests
  in early adolescence, 266–270
  in middle adolescence, 310–311
  to evaluate congitive function, 71
Scrotum self-examimination, in adolescence, 277, 311, 331–332
Self, visual recognition of, 89, 90t
Self-awareness, in second year, 181, 183, 186–187
Self-blame, in middle adolescence, 300–301
Self-concept. See also *Self-esteem; Self-image.*
  cognitive development and, 92–93
  content of, 93
  definition of, 88
  development of, 88–94, 258–259
  language development and, 89
  motor development and, 89
Self-esteem
  antecedents of, 93
  definition of, 91
  development of, 91–93
  physical attributes and, 91–92, 94
  poor, of adolescent homosexual, 306
  problems in, in middle adolescence, 300
Self-image. See also *Body image.*
  in early adolescence, 270
Sensorimotor intelligence, 65–66, 255t
Sensory deprivation, premature infant vulnerability to, 144
Sensory reflexes, 151
Separation anxiety, 174

Sex
  biologic, in fetus and neonate, 94–95
  curiosity about, in preschool years, 197–198
Sex characteristics
  primary
    development of, 242–245
    in late adolescence, 318
    in middle adolescence, 297
  secondary
    development of, 246–247, *247–250*, 251–252, 251t–253t
    in late adolescence, 318–319
    in middle adolescence, 297–299
Sex hormone binding globulin (SHBG), in puberty, 235
Sex play, in childhood, 99
Sexual activity
  adolescent, parental knowledge of, 274–275, 313
  age for initiation of, 302, 303t
  in childhood, 98–99
  in infancy, 97–98
  in late adolescence, 320–321
  interpersonal, development of, 102–103
Sexual developmemt, 94–104. See also *Puberty.*
  cognition and, 98
  Erikson's theory of, 97
  in preschool years, 197–198
  of fetus, 94
  psychoanalytic (freudian) theory of, 96, 216
  psychosocial aspects of, 98, 103–104
Sexual history, of early adolescent, taking of, 272, 273t, 274
Sexual identity, development of, in middle adolescence, 304–305
Sexual Maturity Rating (SMR), 39, 229, 233–234, 236, 238, 240, 242–244, 246–247, 251–254, 264, 268, 285, 293, 295, 297–298, 317–319
Sexual relationships, development of, 102–103
Sexuality
  in adolescence, 99–101
  in childhood, 99
  in infancy, 78–78, 97–98
  portrayal of, on television, 223
  problems of, in early adolescence, 272–275

Sexually transmitted disease, in adolescence, 308–310, 313, 315–316, 325
Shame, emergence of, in second year, 186
Sibling relationships
  in preschool children, 197–199
  in school-aged child, 217
Skeletal system
  development of
    in adolescence, 46t, 294–295, *295–296*, 318, 356
    in infancy and childhood, 44t–45t
  evaluation of, 44t–45t, 47
Skinfold thickness (SFT)
  in early adolescence, 240, 240t, *241*, 264
  measurement of, 38–39
  related to age and sex, *42*
Skinner, B. F., learning theory of, 69–70
Smiling
  in first 3 months, 170
  in neonate, 158
  in second year, categories of, 186–187
Smoking. See also *Substance abuse.*
  in early adolescence, 281–282
  in late adolescence, 322–323
  maternal
    fetal reactions to, 57
    impact on birth weight of infant, 132
  prevention, in middle adolescence, 312
Sleep patterns
  in early adolescence, 254
  in first year, 168–169, 177
  in middle adolescence, 299
  in neonate, 153
Social deprivation, premature infant vulnerability to, 144
Social relationships, hierarchy of, among adolescents, 273t
Soft tissue growth, in middle adolescence, 295–297
Somatic-psychological differentiation, as stage in developmental-structuralist scheme, 81, 82t
Somatomedin-C, 236–237
Somatotype
  definition of, 40–41
  in development of self-esteem, 92
Spanking of preschool child, 207–208

Speech, problems in development of, in preschool child, 189t. See also *Communication*; *Language*.
Spermarche, 243, *243*
Sports
classification of, and recommendations for participation in, 286t–288t
safety in, 283–285
Standard deviation (SD), of mean, 4
Standards, attention to, in second year, 181
Stanford-Binet Intelligence Scale, 75
Startle response, of neonate, 150
Stature percentiles, 10t–13t, *18, 20,* 24t–27t, 32t–33t
Stepping reflex, 151
Stimulation, in behavioral growth and development, 77
Streptococcus infection, in infants and children, 56
Stress, neonatal response to, 156
Stretch reflexes, 151
Structuralist, developmental, scheme of psychosocial development, 81, 82t
Sublimation, in freudian theory, 78
Substance abuse
in early adolescence, 275–276
in late adolescence, 322–324
Suicide
in adolescence, 270–271
television effect on rates of, 224
Superego, in freudian theory, 78
Symbolic, intuitive, or prelogical thought era, of Piaget's theory, 255t
Symbolic elaboration, as stage in developmental-structuralist scheme, 81, 82t
Symbolism, preschool child's use of, 195

T
Tanner stage. See *Sex Maturity Rating (SMR)*
Teeth. See also *Dental development.*
first appearance of, 164, 179
in adolescence, 253
in preschool child, 193
in school-aged child, 213
in second year, 179

structure of, healthy, formation of, 47
Television
constructive viewing of, 224
impact on preschool child, 208
impact on school-aged child, 221–225
suicide rate and, 224
Temper tantrum, in second year, 190
Temperament
assessment of, 86–88
development of, in first 3 months, 167–168
Tertiary circular reactions, 180
Testicular self-examination, technique of, 331–332
Testicular volume, 242t, 297
Testosterone, in puberty, 234
Thelarche, premature, 98
Themes in developmental assessment, 85–130
Thinking
magical, about death and dying, 126, 128
quantitative, in adolescence, 256
Time out, as control device for preschool child, 206
Toilet training, 186, 190–191
Toxic shock syndrome, in middle adolescence, 313
Tonic neck attitude (TNA), 151
Tonic neck reflex, 150–151
Traditional family, development of adolescent autonomy in, 261
Trust, basic, stage of, in eriksonian development scheme, 80, 80t, 170
Tuberculosis testing, in adolescence, 267–268, 310

U
Ultrasonography, to assess gestational age, 133
Urinalysis, in adolescence, 267, 310

V
Variability assessment, in growth and development, 4–7
Vehicle safety, in adolescence, 282–283, 312

Violence
  exposure to, on television, 221–223
  genetic predisposition to, 114
  social aspects of, 114
Vision, testing of, in adolescence, 268, 310
Visual acuity, of neonate, 151–152
Visual fixation, in first 3 months, 166–167
Visual stimuli, preferences in, of neonate, 151–152
Vitamin RDA values, for adolescents, 281t
Vulnerable child syndrome, 144

W
Walking, beginning of, 175
Water, daily requirements of, 52–53, 52t–53t, 148
Wechsler Intelligence Scale for Children—Revised (WISC-R), 75

Wechsler Preschool and Primary Scale of Intelligence (WPPSI), 75
Weight
  by age, 8t–13t, *15, 17, 19, 21,* 28t
  by length, 24t–25t, 28t, 30t
  by stature, 24t–27t, 29t, 31t
  in adolescence, 34t–35t, 239–240, *241, 244,* 252–253
  in first year, 163
  in late adolescence, 318
  in middle adolescence, 295–297, 300
  in second year, 179
  of neonate, 132, 145
  of preschool child, 34t–35t, 193
  of school-aged child, 213
Withdrawal, in assessment of temperament, 86
Women, depiction of, on television, 222
Work, role of, in child and adolescent development, 109–112